Language Development
and Neurological Theory

PERSPECTIVES IN
NEUROLINGUISTICS and PSYCHOLINGUISTICS

Harry A. Whitaker, Series Editor
DEPARTMENT OF PSYCHOLOGY
THE UNIVERSITY OF ROCHESTER
ROCHESTER, NEW YORK

HAIGANOOSH WHITAKER and HARRY A. WHITAKER (Eds.).
Studies in Neurolinguistics, Volumes 1, 2, and 3

NORMAN J. LASS (Ed.). Contemporary Issues in Experimental Phonetics

JASON W. BROWN. Mind, Brain, and Consciousness: The Neuropsychology of Cognition

SIDNEY J. SEGALOWITZ and FREDERIC A. GRUBER (Eds.). Language Development and Neurological Theory

SUSAN CURTISS. Genie: A Psycholinguistic Study of a Modern-Day "Wild Child"

JOHN MACNAMARA (Ed.). Language Learning and Thought

I. M. SCHLESINGER and LILA NAMIR (Eds.). Sign Language of the Deaf: Psychological, Linguistic, and Sociological Perspectives

WILLIAM C. RITCHIE (Ed.). Second Language Acquisition Research: Issues and Implications

PATRICIA SIPLE (Ed.). Understanding Language through Sign Language Research

MARTIN L. ALBERT and LORAINE K. OBLER. The Bilingual Brain: Neurophysiological and Neurolinguistic Aspects of Bilingualism

HAIGANOOSH WHITAKER and HARRY A. WHITAKER (Eds.). Studies in Neurolinguistics, Volume 4

TALMY GIVON. On Understanding Grammar

CHARLES J. FILLMORE, DANIEL KEMPLER and WILLIAM S-Y. WANG (Eds.). Individual Differences in Language Ability and Language Behavior

In preparation

JEANNINE HERRON (Ed.). Left-Handedness, Brain Organization, and Learning

FRANCOIS BOLLER and MAUREEN DENNIS (Eds.). Auditory Comprehension: Clinical and Experimental Studies with the Token Test

Language Development
and Neurological Theory

EDITED BY

Sidney J. Segalowitz

Department of Psychology
Brock University
St. Catharines, Ontario
Canada

Frederic A. Gruber

Niagara Child Development Centre
Welland, Ontario
Canada

ACADEMIC PRESS   New York, San Francisco, London   1977

A Subsidiary of Harcourt Brace Jovanovich, Publishers

ACADEMIC PRESS, INC.
111 Fifth Avenue, New York, New York 10003

United Kingdom Edition published by
ACADEMIC PRESS, INC. (LONDON) LTD.
24/28 Oval Road, London NW1

Library of Congress Cataloging in Publication Data

Main entry under title:

Language development and neurological theory.

    (Perspectives in neurolinguistics and psycholinguis-
tics)
    Some of the papers were presented at a conference on
language development and neurological theory at Brock
University, St. Catharines, Ont., in May 1975.
    Includes bibliographies.
       1.   Languages—Physiological aspects—Congresses.
2.   Cerebral dominance—Congresses.   3.   Children—
Language—Congresses.   4.   Speech perception—Congresses.
I.   Segalowitz, Sidney J.   II.   Gruber, Frederic A.
[DNLM: 1.   Language development.   2.   Brain—Physiology.
WL102 S464L]
QP399.L36   612′.78   76-42979
ISBN 0—12—635650—5

PRINTED IN THE UNITED STATES OF AMERICA
79 80 81 82 83 84 9 8 7 6 5 4 3

Contents

17 Manual Specialization in Infancy: Implications for Lateralization of Brain Function

GERALD YOUNG

PART IV
SPEECH PERCEPTION

18 Invariant Features and Feature Detectors: Some Developmental Implications

RONALD A. COLE

19 The Identification of Four Vowels by Children $2\frac{1}{2}$ to 3 Years Chronological Age as an Indicator of Perceptual Processing

JOHN H. V. GILBERT

20   The Development of Speech Timing

WILLIAM E. COOPER

List of Contributors

Numbers in parentheses indicate the pages on which the authors' contributions begin.

CHARLES I. BERLIN (75), Louisiana State University Medical Center, Kresge Hearing Research Laboratory of the South, Department of Otorhinolaryngology, New Orleans, Louisiana

LINDA CHAPANIS* (107), Department of Psychiatry, The Johns Hopkins University School of Medicine, Baltimore, Maryland

RONALD A. COLE (37, 319), Department of Psychology, Carnegie-Mellon University, Pittsburgh, Pennsylvania

WILLIAM E. COOPER (357), Research Laboratory of Electronics, Massachusetts Institute of Technology, Cambridge, Massachusetts

JOHN K. CULLEN, Jr. (75), Louisiana State University Medical Center, Kresge Hearing Research Laboratory of the South, Department of Otorhinolaryngology and Biocommunication, New Orleans, Louisiana

NINA CUMMINGS (37), Department of Psychology, Carnegie-Mellon University, Pittsburgh Pennsylvania

MAUREEN DENNIS (93), Department of Psychology, The Hospital for Sick Children, Toronto, Ontario, Canada

ANNE KASMAN ENTUS (63), Department of Psychology, McGill University, Montreal, Quebec, Canada

FRED GENESEE (47), Department of Psychology, McGill University, Montreal, Quebec, Canada

JOHN H. V. GILBERT (347), The Phonetics Laboratory, Division of Audiology and Speech Sciences, The University of British Columbia, Vancouver, B. C., Canada

FREDERIC A. GRUBER† (3), Niagara Child Development Centre, Welland, Ontario, Canada

JOSIANE F. HAMERS‡ (57), Department of Psychology, McGill University, Montreal, Quebec, Canada

MERRILL HISCOCK (171), Department of Psychiatry, University Hospital, Saskatoon, Saskatchewan and Department of Psychology, University of Saskatchewan

J. JACOBS (155), Department of Pediatrics, McMaster University Medical Centre, Hamilton, Ontario, Canada

MARCEL KINSBOURNE (171), Department of Psychology, The Hospital for Sick Children, Toronto, Ontario, Canada

WALLACE E. LAMBERT (47, 57), Department of Psychology, McGill University, Montreal, Quebec, Canada

*1350 Ala Moana, #2109, Honolulu, Hawaii

†Department of Communication Studies, Torrens College of Advanced Education, Holbrooks Road, Underdale, South Australia

‡C.I.R.B., Université Laval, Quebec, Quebec, Canada

DENNIS L. MOLFESE (21), Department of Psychology, Southern Illinois University at Carbondale, Carbondale, Illinois

MORRIS MOSCOVITCH (193), Department of Psychology, Erindale College, University of Toronto, Mississauga, Ontario, Canada

C. NETLEY (133), Department of Psychology, Hospital for Sick Children, Toronto, Ontario

HELEN NEVILLE[§] (121), Department of Psychology, Cornell University, Ithaca, New York

SIDNEY J. SEGALOWITZ (3), Department of Psychology, Brock University, St. Catharines, Ontario, Canada

MICHAEL SEITZ (47), School of Human Communication Disorders, Dalhousie University, Halifax, Nova Scotia

RICHARD STARCK (47), Department of Psychology, McGill University, Montreal, Quebec, Canada

HARRY A. WHITAKER (93), Department of Psychology, University of Rochester, Rochester, New York

SANDRA F. WITELSON (213), Department of Psychiatry, Chedoke-McMaster Centre, Hamilton, Ontario, Canada

GRACE H. YENI-KOMSHIAN[||] (145), Department of Otolaryngology, School of Medicine, The Johns Hopkins University, Baltimore, Maryland

GERALD YOUNG[#] (289), Children's Hospital Medical Center, Boston, Massachusetts

[§] Department of Neurosciences, School of Medicine, University of California, San Diego, La Jolla, California

[||] Human Learning and Behavior Branch, NICHD, National Institutes of Health, Bethesda, Maryland

[#] Department of Psychology, Glendon College, York University, Toronto, Ontario, Canada

Preface

The study of language development has always interested specialists from a number of fields including, of course, psychology and linguistics. In the last decade, however, psycholinguists and experimental linguists have been increasingly concerned with and influenced by research in neurology and neuropsychological models. It has become clear that a complete understanding of the child's development of language must include the insights available from viable psychological, linguistic, and neurological models. Attempts to integrate data from the three fields are admittedly simplistic still, but these initial forays into this interdiscipline are necessary and are becoming progressively more sophisticated.

In this book, we have organized 20 papers that deal with several aspects of this synthesis. Some present new research on specific issues, others summarize the evidence for a particular theoretical position on a controversial issue, and others simply review an issue without attempting a controversial stand when it is clear such a position would be premature. As is consistent with the interdisciplinary nature of this collection, the format and length vary considerably from chapter to chapter.

The book is divided into four parts: (I) Cerebral Specialization for Language in Normals, (II) Cerebral Specialization for Language in Brain-Damaged Patients, (III) The Development of Cerebral Dominance, and (IV) Speech Perception. Much of the book is devoted to the issue of cerebral specialization, or lateralization, simply because this is one of the most highly researched questions in the field. This issue exemplifies well the growing sophistication referred to earlier: The question has changed from "When does cerebral specialization begin?" to "How does the nature of the specialization change as the child grows?" Much of the basic data contributing to this change in approach are presented here. This is a very broad issue, however, and a number of aspects are discussed. The other main intersection of neurological theory and developmental psycholinguistics concerns speech perception. In the final section of the book, several sources of data in speech perception are presented that are relevant to neuropsychological theory of language development.

The first chapter (Gruber and Segalowitz) reviews some of the methods, with their inherent limitations, used to correlate neurophysiological and behavioral functions, and also some of the issues involved in trying to unite the empirical science of neuropsychology and the rationalist science of linguistics.

Molfese's presentation (Chapter 2) of his use of evoked potentials in research on lateralization for speech sounds shown by young infants initiates the discussion of early cerebral specialization and discusses possible factors in the sound signal responsible for the differentiation. Entus (Chapter 6) finds a similar hemisphere specialization for speech sounds in young infants using a procedure that melds dichotic listening with the nonnutritive, high-amplitude sucking paradigm. Cole and Cummings (Chapter 3) present the results of a study examining asymmetries in EEG alpha in young children during continuous verbal—nonvisual and visual—nonverbal story tasks.

The effects of multilanguage elementary school program on the degree of lateralization for language are examined by Starck, Genesee, Lambert, and Seitz (Chapter 4), as is the language lateralization of bilinguals in each of their languages by Hamers and Lambert (Chapter 5).

Berlin and Cullen (Chapter 7) complete Part I of the book with a review of the dichotic listening technique with respect to the acoustic parameters involved. They indicate the fragility of the effect and the care needed for obtaining interpretable results.

Part II opens with a short introduction on the question "What is it that is lateralized?" Following this, Dennis and Whitaker (Chapter 8) report on the cognitive functioning of a group of children who had the cortex of one hemisphere removed surgically shortly after birth. They include a very interesting and useful review of equipotentiality, including the literature of the last century.

In Chapter 9, Chapanis discusses her work on intramodal and cross-modal pattern perception in stroke patients with lateralized lesions. Netly (Chapter 11) presents the results of his work with collosal agenesis and Turner's syndrome patients. He finds interesting differences on ear asymmetries in dichotic listening tasks between these groups of patients, with implications for developmental theory. Yeni-Komshian's description (Chapter 12) of the gradual recovery of language by a boy with traumatically induced brain damage is intriguing for its implications for the meaning of ear asymmetries in dichotic listening and the role of extinction in such cases. As he regained language skills, he showed a decrease in right ear advantage from the exaggerated asymmetry initially shown to the usual small but consistent difference.

Neville's chapter (Chapter 10) on visual half-field asymmetries in deaf and hearing children presents fascinating possibilities concerning the role of linguistic experience in the nature of lateralization. She finds that deaf children who do not use sign language show no asymmetry for visual recognition of household items, hearing children show a greater right hemisphere response, while deaf signers show a greater left hemisphere response.

Part II closes with a short chapter by Jacobs (Chapter 13) on some thoughts that a clinical neurologist has about research questions and problems in neuropsychology.

Part III opens with an introduction summarizing several hypotheses as to why language is lateralized to the left hemisphere rather than to the right. This section consists of four review chapters on the question "Does cerebral dominance develop?" The first is a position paper by Kinsbourne and Hiscock (Chapter 14) whose position is that the data for a developing cerebral dominance are lacking and that the assumptions of such a conceptual model are faulty. Moscovitch (Chapter 15) reviews the issue of language lateralization and its relation to cognitive and linguistic development, with an emphasis on the functions of the right hemisphere. Witelson (Chapter 16), in a massive review of the literature, summarizes the results of studies using various techniques for detecting lateralization in children. Her discussion of a theoretical stand positing both cerebral specialization at birth and continuing interhemispheric plasticity is a welcome synthesis of this complex literature. Young presents a review (Chapter 17) of studies on early manual specialization. He discusses the implications of these studies for lateralization of brain function, although, as he concludes, the relationship is yet to be well understood.

The final section of the book (Part IV) concerns speech perception and opens with a brief introduction on the differences among various models. Cole (Chapter 18) presents data supporting one such model, the feature detector approach. Such an approach has considerable implications for a neurological as well as developmental theory of language. Gilbert (Chapter 19) concurs with Cole on the need for a theory involving very early perceptual abilities, although his data come from a production task as opposed to a simple recognition task. Similarly, Cooper (Chapter 20) summarizes data on the development of timing abilities in speech production, indicating possible requirements for a neurological theory of language development.

This book, with complete rewriting, reorganization, and the inclusion of new material, was advanced from a conference on Language Development and Neurological Theory held in May, 1975 at Brock University in St. Catharines, Ontario and cosponsored by the Niagara Child Development Centre of Welland, Ontario. We would like to express our appreciation to the Canada Council for its assistance in funding the conference (grant no. S75-0010) and to Dr. Nancy Johnston who with us organized the conference. As well, thanks are due to Ms. Peggy Collins and Ms. Susan Dafoe for their assistance and patience in the preparation of the manuscripts.

Part I

Cerebral Specialization for Language in Normals

1

Some Issues and Methods in the Neuropsychology of Language

FREDERIC A. GRUBER
SIDNEY J. SEGALOWITZ

The history of the neuropsychology of language is filled with issues stemming from all three sciences, whose intersection make up this field. In this chapter, we will discuss briefly a few of the important issues and methods from the neurological, psychological, and linguistic perspectives. See Boring (1957), Luria (1966), Penfield and Roberts (1959), and Whitaker (1971) for more complete reviews from these different perspectives.

CORRELATING NEUROPHYSIOLOGICAL AND PSYCHOLOGICAL FUNCTIONS

Some Elementary Speculations

The study of brain function has had two recurring contrasting themes: (1) psychological functions are precisely localized in certain brain areas; and the opposite (2) cortical representation of psychological functions is distributed or diffuse. Since the nineteenth century, both themes have had ardent supporters (Anderson, 1974; Boring, 1957). Early in the nineteenth century, Franz Joseph Gall stressed the strict localization approach with his study of phrenology; Pierre Flourens countered with evidence of the recovery of functions in birds after brain lesions. With the discovery of Broca's speech area, the strict localizationist approach resurged. During the first half of this century, the Gestalt school countered with experiments showing that underlying perceptual processes must be global, and similarly, Lashley (1950) found it difficult to wipe out memories with disturbances of specific cortical areas. Although reconciliation between the two extreme approaches has been tried (Hebb, 1949) with some success, such "middle positions" are also open to criticism (John, 1971, 1972). Feature detector theory of vision has reopened the issue (Hubel, 1963; Weisstein, 1975), with the gradual realization that although this theory is elegant it may have little to do with how we perceive (Anderson, 1974). A modern alternative, the holistic approach defined by Pribram (1966, 1971), attempts to account for the problems raised by Lashley and the Gestalt psychologists, without relinquishing the elegance of the feature detector approach.

It is apparent, on logical as well as on experimental grounds, that some functions are localized and that patterned activity in a circumscribed cortical area corresponds to some function. The question then becomes "What is the nature of functions that are localized [Luria, 1966]?" When we ask what it is about the language function that produces its localization in one hemisphere, we can come up with a long list of possibilities, e.g., phonological competence, semantic processing, syntactic processing, rhythmic activities, communication ability, or motivation to communicate (Papçun, Krashen, Terbeek, Remington, & Harshman, 1974; see also introduction to Part II, this volume). Clearly it is erroneous to allocate the representation of complex behavior to small areas (Luria, 1970). But how should we divide up behavior in order to understand how the brain does?

Does the brain divide psychological functions in terms of language versus nonlanguage, the former being represented in most people in the left hemisphere and the latter in the right? This traditional approach is now considered much too simplistic (see introduction to Part II, this volume), but has proved to be a valuable jumping-off point from which to investigate the issue. There have been other attempts to capture distinctions that indicate which hemisphere is responsible for, or at least more adept at, some activity. These include analytic versus holistic processing (Bever, 1975), serial versus parallel processing of information (Cohen, 1973), and focal versus diffuse (Semmes, 1968). It has also been postulated that what determines which hemisphere will be more active during a particular activity has more to do with the context rather than the content of the activity (Kinsbourne, 1973); attentional factors may have been ignored while sensory input factors may have been overemphasized.

Clearly, there is more than one way to slice the behavioral pie, and neuropsychological theory is dependent not only on what brain areas are examined and how they are examined but also on how behavior is divided up.

Detecting the Correlation of Functions. If we suspect a particular area of the brain is especially involved in a specific behavior pattern, we can correlate that behavior with a given brain area by several methods: (1) by measurement of the behavioral function after excision of or interference with the brain area in question (e.g., Chapter 8); (2) by measurement of the behavioral function during electrical stimulation of the area (Penfield, 1959); (3) by correlation between change in the behavioral function with abnormal growth or death of the brain structure (Penfield & Roberts, 1959); (4) by comparison of activity at the brain site with other brain sites when the behavior is and is not being performed (e.g., with EEG recordings, as in Chapters 2 and 10; and with measurement of cortical blood flow as in Risberg & Ingvar, 1973); and (5) by measurement of the relative efficiency of the behavior with an enhanced involvement of the brain area in the functioning (e.g., with a dichotic listening task, as in Chapters 4 and 6; and with visual half field projection, as in Chapter 5).

The first three approaches, used solely in clinical situations, make use of data taken from individuals with abnormal brain functioning. Although these data are valuable and give us most of our present knowledge of functional localization, it is sometimes difficult to generalize to normal brain function.

The last two approaches are favored for work with normal subjects and split-brain patients. These methods are particularly useful for studying lateral asymmetries, as is discussed later. The application of the last technique to split-brain functioning is especially useful for examining the interhemispheric interference hypothesis (Moscovitch, 1973).

Physiological Data. The preeminence of linguistic functions in human behavior and the corresponding cerebral asymmetries naturally lead to questions of neurophysiological asymmetries. Geschwind and Levitsky (1968) found one of the areas clearly associated with the asymmetric cerebral representation of language—the planum temporale—is significantly larger in the left hemisphere than in the right. Since language is one of the most complex and yet essential of human abilities, the authors claim this is not surprising. Similar asymmetries are not found in many primates (Geschwind, 1971); although some asymmetry is reported in chimpanzees (Yeni-Komshian & Benson, 1976). The view that this asymmetry does not reflect differential experiences by the two hemispheres, but rather that the hemispheres are nonequipotential for language functions (Chapters 2, 6, and 8) is supported by Witelson and Pallie (1973), who found similar asymmetries in neonates, and by Wada, Clarke, and Hamm (1975), who found related symmetries in fetuses.

It is tempting to jump from physiological data to psychological conclusions. For example, Scheid and Eccles (1975) speculate about those individuals in Geschwind and Levitsky's sample who showed the nonusual asymmetry—the 11% who showed larger right hemisphere measurements than left. They wonder if these individuals would probably have shown especially high talents for music and if this is a manifestation of the genetic predisposition for music. Although such speculation is enticing, we have no evidence for attributing a positive correlation between the variations in size of the planum temporale of the right hemisphere and musical talents. Similarly, without measurement of linguistic abilities of the patients before death, we cannot conclude anything from a measurement of the size of portions of the left hemisphere.

Methods of Measuring Lateralized Responses

There are several main methods used in the investigations of lateralized psychological responses; each with distinct advantages and disadvantages.

Dichotic Listening Technique

The Model and Interpretation. The dichotic listening technique is one of the most popular of contemporary attempts to determine whether and to what extent one hemisphere is better than the other in the processing of certain auditory material (see Chapters 4, 6, and 11). The technique involves presenting to the subject different stimuli to each ear simultaneously and asking the subject to report or recognize the content of the signals. If reports from one ear are more forthcoming or correct than are reports from the other, then a conclusion is drawn that the hemisphere opposite the higher-scoring ear is more efficient at processing that type of signal. So, for example, researchers (e.g., Kimura, 1961a, 1961b) have claimed that there exists a consistent right-ear advantage (REA) for verbal material and a left-ear advantage (LEA) for environmental sounds (Knox & Kimura, 1970) and music (Kimura, 1973), indicating a left-hemisphere prepotency for verbal signals and a right hemisphere prepotency for nonverbal signals.

These results are generally accounted for by two claims about the structure of the auditory system: (1) that there exist a greater number of contralateral ear-to-hemisphere connections than ipsilateral connections (Hall & Goldstein, 1968; Rosensweig, 1951); and (2) that ipsilateral input from one ear is blocked by contralateral input from the other ear (Cullen, Berlin, Hughes, Thompson, & Samson, 1974). The preponderance of contralateral fibers would alone account for many of the ear advantages found, since these advantages are also found with monaural input, although they are greatly lessened (e.g., a REA for speech found by Catlin & Neville, 1976; Morais & Darwin, 1974; LEA for tones found by Doehring, 1972).

The blocking of ipsilateral by contralateral input has been well established. Work with split-brain patients indicates that although responses to monaural signals (with no dichotic competition) are received by the ipsilateral hemisphere, when dichotic signals are presented there is no ipsilateral ear-to-hemisphere connection. A physiological model for this phenomenon is presented by Cullen *et al.* (1974), who hypothesize that a

> thalamic "gate" exists which becomes effective when stimuli of similar (or identical) acoustic characters are presented to the two ears. . . . The contralateral signals occlude the ipsilateral signals. Such a gate would allow full interplay of information at a sub-geniculate level while providing separation of ear-channel information at higher cortical centers [p. 110].

They refer to Aitken and Webster (1972), who found such an occlusion mechanism in the medial geniculate body of the cat.

Although these two facets of dichotomous stimulation are well established, the interpretation of dichotic listening data is not so straightforward.

Systematic variation of the acoustic features (e.g., time of onset, intensity of signals) dichotomously presented show that the REA for speech is extremely fragile (for a review, see Chapter 7; also, Berlin & McNeil, 1976). Since the tapes used by various researchers necessarily vary with respect to these features, lack of agreement across experiments is not surprising. Also, since the degree of REA or LEA is dependent on acoustic variables, any measure of degree of laterality is automatically confounded with the particular test stimuli used (Chapter 7).

The dichotic listening test does not, however, produce consistent results even with carefully produced stimulus tapes. First of all, about 20% of right-handed subjects show a LEA for speech stimuli. This does not mean that these subjects are right lateralized for language. Estimates of the percentage of the right-handed population with language lateralized to the right vary between 0% and 8%. Therefore, the dichotic listening test cannot be considered definitive.

In an attempt to determine how reliable the technique is, Blumstein, Goodglass and Tartter (1975) tested subjects and then retested them at least one week later on three dichotic tapes consisting of consonants, vowels, and music. On the first test, the (unexpected) LEA for consonants was shown by 29% of the subjects, for vowels, by 36%, and the (unexpected) REA for music by 28% of the subjects. On the second test the figures were 22%, 36%, and 19% respectively. However, the percentages of subjects who switched ear advantages were 29%, 44%, and 24%. At least two processes may account for these unstable results.

First, it is possible that the occlusion of ipsilateral input is not complete and that there is simply an added advantage given to a contralateral signal when presentation is dichotomous. Such a conclusion is compatible with the data of Aitken and Webster (1972). It has also been reported that split-brain patients will respond verbally to left ear input during dichotomous stimulation in a situation where the message to the right ear is a list of words and a single left-ear signal coincides with one of the items on the list (Gordon, personal communication). Perhaps, then, the occlusion is not complete.

Second, just as acoustic variables are critical, so may be psychological variables. For example, Spellacy and Blumstein (1970) found a REA for vowels when embedded in a series of English words and a LEA for these same vowels when embedded in a series with melodies and sound effects. The change in expectancy of psychological set presumably changed how the subjects thought of the vowels; consonants produced a more stable REA, independent of language expectation.

Similarly, when subjects are asked to pay attention to the emotional tone of a sentence, a LEA is produced, whereas attention to linguistic or acoustic cues produces a REA (Haggard & Parkinson, 1971). A clear case for cognitive factors is also presented by Van Lancker and Fromkin (1973), who found that tone words in Thai produce a REA with Thai speakers but not with English speakers. For obvious reasons, one group considers the stimuli linguistic, the other does not.

Such studies indicate that how a subject looks at the stimulus can grossly affect the hemispheric preference (cf. Kinsbourne, 1973). This statement can be taken quite literally as well. Goldstein and Lackner (1974) show that perceived displacement of the visual field (by prisms) distorts the perceived location of the sound source and can effect ear advantage (cf. Bertelson & Tisseyre, 1975). Clearly nonacoustic variables can influence ear advantages.

Experience and Language Lateralization. Another intriguing question is whether experience can permanently effect hemispheric specialization for language. As we saw above, environmental cues and biases can influence the results of a dichotic listening task in a specific testing situation. If one group receives certain long-term experiences, will this group show a persistent ear advantage different from a group without that experience? In some cases, this is clearly so, as in Van Lancker and Fromkin's study mentioned earlier. Assuming no specific knowledge difference between the groups, perhaps such differences can still exist—possibly arising out of a "permanent" difference in psychological set (i.e., cultural differences). Thus, the later development of a REA in children from lower socioeconomic levels (Geffner & Hochberg, 1971) could be due to differences between lower- and middle-class children in how they treat the task. Similarly, Starck *et al.* (Chapter 4) find differences in monolingual children and children with multilingual experiences. Such a difference would not, of course, preclude differences due to cerebral specialization.

Visual Half Field (VHF) Asymmetries

Because of the physiological structure of the human visual system, the visual cortex of each hemisphere receives input from only the contralateral visual half field. Thus, a stimulus, projected into one VHF only, will be received first by the contralateral hemisphere. Using dichoptic presentation (simultaneous presentation of different stimuli in each VHF) of words, investigators (e.g., McKeever & Huling, 1971) found considerable right-VHF superiority, while a left-VHF superiority was found for nonverbal spatial tasks (Kimura, 1969). These results reflect the general superiority of the right hemisphere for nonverbal, spatial functions. This technique has been useful in a large number of investigations of hemispheric specialization (for reviews, see Klein, 1976; White, 1969). A drawback is that the visual stimulus must be presented to the periphery of a VHF for less than 200 msec, or the subject will be able to move his eyes to the stimulus and destroy the VHF projection.

The technique is especially useful for determining the abilities of each hemisphere in split-brain patients. In these patients, information fed to one hemisphere cannot cross to the other; thus we can be sure which hemisphere is doing the processing. Zaidel (1975) has recently devised an apparatus that allows continuous visual projection to only one hemisphere, thus allowing considerable latitude in testing the relative abilities of each hemisphere.

Dichotomous Manual Tasks

Just as hemispheric differences in the processing of linguistic versus nonlinguistic material can be inferred using visual (VHF) and auditory (dichotic listening) tasks, Witelson (1974) has compared relative hemispheric processing abilities using the tactual modality. She presents objects of various shapes dichhaptically, that is, one object to each hand at the same time for tactual exploration. She then tests the subjects using a nonverbal recognition paradigm. She finds a left-hand superiority for recognition of spatial forms in boys as young as 6 years, and no difference on verbal forms (e.g., letters). Since the finger movements made to examine the forms are controlled by the contralateral hemisphere, she concludes that these data point to an early presence of right-hemisphere superiority in a spatial task such as this.

Using results from another type of manual task—simultaneous drawing of a circle with one hand and a square with the other—Buffery and Gray (1972) conclude that females show an earlier and stronger lateralization than males for spatial skills. However, Witelson (1976) finds the opposite with her dichhaptic task.

Averaged Evoked Response (AER)

The evoked potential is a rough measure of cortical activity in a general area of the cerebral cortex. Electrodes are placed on the surface of the scalp (Jasper, 1958) and changes in electrical potential are recorded with respect to some "ground," such as the nose, forehead, or chin. Recordings, time locked to the presentation of some stimulus, are averaged. If the presentation of the stimulus has some consistent effect on the cortical activity beneath the electrode, then this effect will summate, while inconsistent responses will cancel one another out. If the responses are averaged in this way over many trials, small but consistent effects can be noted (Chapman, 1973).

The advantage of the AER over other performance tasks is that a direct cortical response is tapped, enabling investigators to attempt to determine differential localized hemispheric lobe, and even within-lobe, responses. For example, McAdam and Whitaker (1971) found a greater AER for the production of speech sounds over Broca's area in the left hemisphere, and a greater AER for tongue-produced noises over the analogous area in the right hemisphere. Similarly Callaway and Harris (1974) found greater left-hemisphere activity for read stimuli and greater right-hemisphere activity for picture stimuli.

A severe drawback of this technique is the limitation of stimuli presentable: They must have a relatively discrete onset and rise time, the response examined must be quick (e.g., within 1 sec), and must be effective over a number of presentations. Nevertheless, Neville (Chapter 10) found that interesting differences in hemispheric responses are found in hearing and deaf children for visual stimuli. Molfese (Chapter 2) uses the technique to investigate hemispheric differences in the processing of acoustic stimuli in newborns. The AER has also been used to measure responses along a variety of other dimensions (Shagass, 1972).

Relative Amount of Alpha

Synchronous EEG output of 8–13 cycles per second (alpha) indicates an interruption in organized thinking. Thus, a relative suppression of alpha implies greater organized functioning. Robbins and McAdam (1974) found a relative suppression of alpha activity in the right hemisphere when adult subjects covertly imaged shapes and colors, and in the left hemisphere when subjects covertly verbalized. Cole and Cummings (Chapter 3) found similar results with young children attending to animated or spoken stories.

Cortical Blood Flow

Since neuronal activity is a delicately balanced process, increased neuronal activity is accompanied by metabolic increases. The sensitive corticovascular system reacts to such needs, and these changes in blood flow can be measured by use of radioactive tracers. Risberg and Ingvar (1973) report increases in cortical blood flow in specific areas of the left hemisphere following memory and reasoning tasks. For example, an auditory digit-span-backward test produced augmentation mainly in anterior frontal, prerolandic, and posterior temporal regions. A visual reasoning task gave rise to increases mainly in occipital, temporo-occipital, parietal, and frontal regions. Carmon, Lavy, Gordon, and Portnoy (1975) found presentation of verbal material increased the cortical blood flow in the left hemisphere, while listening to music produced a greater right-hemisphere response.

This method has advantages over other direct measurements, such as AER and electrical stimulation of the brain (ESB) (Penfield, 1959). With the former, some measure of specific activity is taken; however, what the measure signifies is not known. All we know is that it reflects synchrony of firing and the relative amplitude of this response. The latter, ESB, reconstructs cortical activity which induces experiences that seem to the patient to be realistic; however, since the train of activity is initiated by artifical means, we cannot be sure that normal cortical functioning is mimicked. Cortical blood flow avoids these uncertainties. Since it is a direct correlate of increased metabolic rate, the increase is attributed to increased cortical activity.

We are limited in the degree of fine measurement possible with this method: The intricate vascular network in the brain does not permit, of course, as fine discriminations as the other direct-measurement methods, especially ESB. However, for determining differences in overall hemispheric or lobic activity, cortical blood flow measurement may prove to be more useful.

Temporary Hemispheric Paralysis

It is crucial to determine which hemisphere is primarily responsible for language functioning when a patient is about to undergo brain surgery. The sodium amytal injection method was devised to mimic incapacitation of one hemisphere (Wada, 1949); introduction of this drug into the carotid artery supplying blood to one hemisphere paralyzes that hemisphere for 2 or 3 min, until it is worked through the system. During that time the patient's language abilities can be tested, determining if the remaining functioning hemisphere is capable of language (Penfield & Roberts, 1959). Similar studies of capabilities of the left or right hemisphere functioning alone have been done for musical abilities (Bogen & Gordon, 1971).

Researchers who use the various tools available to measure asymmetric cerebral representation of skills are interested in the abstract abilities that underlie these tasks, especially verbal versus nonverbal and language versus spatial abilities. Clearly these tasks use different input routes to tap these skills, and therefore different results could be obtained to the extent that the input mode of the tasks differ. For example, Buffery and Gray (1972) using a bimanual drawing task report greater lateralization by females on spatial skills, while Witelson (1976) reports the opposite when testing with a dichhaptic identification task.

Similarly, it should not be too surprising to find low agreement between results from VHF and dichotic listening studies. Bryden (1965) finds a low, nonsignificant correlation ($r = .19$) between the two tests when comparing the degree of asymmetry in recognition scores (cf. Hines & Satz, 1974). As he points out, in a VHF study the major problem the subject must deal with is obtaining enough information during the brief exposure to make identification; in a dichotic listening task, the subject must try to remember all the material during recall. Therefore, one task presents an input problem, the other an output problem. It should not be surprising that sometimes these parameters should overshadow any effect due to type of cognitive processing.

Interpreting Correlated Functions

There is a persistent temptation in an interdisciplinary field to interpret correlations as explanations. However, ideas generated at one level (or discipline) cannot be simply integrated into an analysis at another (cf. Kopell, 1976). When we find a biological correlate of a psychological function (e.g., Hubel, 1963), we are tempted to say that we have in some way "explained" the psychological phenomenon. Not only does this underrate the power of psychological models (as well as misinterpret the power of biological models), it leads the investigator to erroneous conclusions. In the field of neuropsychology, for example, if one accepts the model of the brain as a sophisticated switchboard, the question becomes one of discovering the brain response to specific stimulus inputs. However, as is becoming increasingly clear in recent years (Kinsbourne, 1973; Klein, 1976), although the stimulus may be a well-specified linguistic one, the brain response may be greatly dependent on psychological functions. How the brain responds is a function of psychological set, context, motivations, and so forth—factors that are not easily specified at the neurobiological or linguistic level.

Interdisciplinary research can lead to fuller understanding of phenomena within one of the component fields as well as to an integrated theory of behavior. Theoretical and empirical discoveries in one discipline may enrich the investigation of similar topics from another viewpoint. It is therefore appropriate to discuss some of the ways linguistics and neurolinguistics have profitably influenced each other.

TYING EMPIRICAL BONDS WITH LINGUISTICS

A Statement of Orientation

"To develop a psychology of language, one must have some notions about what language is [Dember & Jenkins, 1970, p. 429]." Accordingly, linguistic input would seem crucial for neurolinguistics. But, much neurological work related to language relies on superficial linguistic analyses, and linguistic studies usually are not related to whatever neurolinguistic evidence is available. This section reviews a direct rapprochement between the two most common approaches: aphasiology in brain research and generative–transformational theory in linguistics.

A goal of neurolinguistics is to establish explicit relations between brain mechanisms and phenomenal language experience. Yet, a major stumbling block has been that neurology deals exclusively with physical entities, linguistics predominantly with mental entities—a reflection of the mind–body dilemma that has perplexed philosophers for almost 2000 years (see Feigl, 1958). The advance of neurolinguistics would seem to be dependent upon establishing forms of identity relation between the mental and the physical (Meehl, 1966).

The physical nature of brain study is reflected in the empirical method, the mental nature of language in rationalist method (see Boring, 1957; Chomsky, 1968a). Both methods of science, though emanating from incompatible assumptions, have been largely successful. However, some claim that empiricism, although responsible for establishing and advancing modern physics, has been somewhat misleading when applied to cognitive psychology and linguistics (Chomsky, 1968b; Fodor, 1968). Rationalism, the methodology that developed modern mathematics and is reflected in linguistics by the generative–transformational school, resulted in a decade of what may be unparalleled progress in understanding language.

The empirical-oriented science of neurology and the rationalist-oriented science of linguistics have found profitable interface difficult, and there has been some confusion as to how the constructs of generative linguistic theory are related to empirical fact (Cofer, 1968; Horton & Dixon, 1968; Jenkins, 1968). Certainly, there are empirical *consequences* of generative grammars, and linguistic theory *relies on* empirical fact. However, substantive structures in a grammar were not intended to reflect physical being. Linguists never claimed that the brain contains noun phrases as distinct entities (see Gunderson, 1971). Several concepts crucial to linguistic theory are, nonetheless, of potential use to empirical investigations in neuropsychology. It is reasonable, then to review here some linguistic universals, evaluation procedures, markedness—and then some examples of how neurological evidence can aid linguistic theory and how linguistic evidence can influence neurological theory.

Linguistic Universals

If, indeed, genetic endowment determines the form that human languages can assume, there ought to be language universals. But there could also be facts that are true for all human languages by chance alone, since the number of actual languages is limited, though large, while the number of languages studied in detail is small. In addition, some linguistic universals could be a consequence of limitations on such nonlinguistic mechanisms as memory, which, although interesting in their own right, would not be included as a part of linguistic theory.

In fact, linguists have proposed many language universals, for example, nesting and embedding operations, the transformational cycle, rule ordering, and so forth (Bach & Harms, 1968; Chomsky & Halle, 1968; Greenberg, 1963). The place of linguistic universals is properly in general linguistic theory, thus allowing conventions that greatly simplify the expression of the particular form of and differences between individual languages. These differences are then expressed in grammars (theories) of particular languages (Chomsky & Halle, 1968). Since universals of language are expressed in linguistic theory, and neurological facts are reflected in neurological theory, the interface of these fields begins at the level of metatheory, that is, in the structure of relationships between the general theories, not between particular brains and specific languages.

Evaluation Procedures

Suppose two or more rival theories (grammars) of a language are proposed, each of which accounts for the facts of that language. To choose between the candidate theories a criterion or some evaluation procedure is needed (Chomsky, 1957, 1965). We briefly discuss three such procedures.

Parsimony, which served empirical science well, proves insufficient for two reasons: (1) there is considerable doubt that biological fact is optimally parsimonious, as the human appendix testifies; (2) linguistic theory is multileveled, so that parsimony at one level can require proliferation at another. Which is more parsimonious, a large computer with a small program or a small computer with a large program (Postal, 1968)?

Elegance, the intuitively appealing but ill-defined alternative of the mathematician, ignores the empirical base of linguistics. Pure mathematics has no necessary empirical responsibility as does linguistics (Chomsky & Halle, 1968), and so this criterion need not be applicable.

Naturalism, the introduction of independently motivated facts of direct bearing on the theories to be evaluated, is the foremost criterion. Knowledge from language acquisition study, neurology, physiology, psychology, and so on, is introduced as metatheoretical criteria to assist in the evaluation of language theories. Such criteria guide the linguist throughout in choices between otherwise equally powerful formulations when writing a grammar; they therefore become reflected in general linguistic theory. However, the primary data base for the linguist remains the intuitions of the native speaker–hearer about his or her language.

Markedness

The application of naturalism as an evaluation metric is well developed, at least in phonology. Whether a segment is Unmarked (more normal) or Marked (less normal) represents a claim with respect to the question of innateness. We would expect, that unmarked segments, at any level, would be common to the languages of the world, would be reflected in early language acquisition, would be preferred in historical language change, and would be perceptually salient. As Postal (1968), referring to phonology, remarks:

> Ultimately, perhaps some of the strongest evidence for the assignment of Marked or Unmarked status will come from physiological and perceptual investigations. Although one must avoid overly simplistic assertions . . . it is evident that articulatory and percep-

tual factors . . . are behind the linguistic structuring of Marked and Unmarked [pp. 170–171].

Marking conventions are, of course, a part of linguistic theory and do not appear in a grammar.

Neurolinguistic Evidence in Linguistic Issues

How can evidence for linguistic theory come from neurolinguistic studies? The factual basis for construction of a grammar of a specific language is based largely on judgments of the grammaticality of language strings made by the native speaker-hearer under favourable circumstances (Chomsky, 1965). Accordingly, Schnitzer (1974) studied judgments of grammaticality made by a 21-year-old male with right hemiplegia and a medical diagnosis of motor aphasia after cerebral thrombosis. He found the subject's knowledge of English to be impoverished in ways supporting specific aspects of certain linguistic theories.

This subject produced, and judged to be grammatical, sentences that consistently deleted present-tense copulas in their full form, although contractions were found. Past-tense copulas, however, were present in the patient's speech and judgments of grammaticality with equal consistency. That is, the unmarked forms were absent. From a wide array of evidence for this patient and the assumption that this change from a normal speaker–hearer's knowledge of his or her language represented a simplification, rather than an elaboration, of the linguistic system, Schnitzer concludes that his subject did not delete copulas that were present in deep structure, as some linguistic theories would have it (e.g., Katz & Postal, 1964). Rather, he failed to create copulas when an unmarked copula would result. Contracted copulas were said to have occurred when a (probably obligatory) contraction rule was applied to the copulas he did create. This evidence, Schnitzer concludes, lends credence to the analyses suggesting that the copula is not present in deep structure (Bach, 1967; Jacobs & Rosenbaum, 1970).

The aphasic patient also left out subjects when the referent of the subject could be derived from previous discourse or when it was "I." These observations suggest that a simplification of grammatical knowledge of pronominalization carries no semantic information not carried by its referent noun, that is, if it is a sort of a place-marker (cf. Bach, 1968) not determined by a transformational rule that spans sentences, such as is consistent with Ross (1970). In general, these conclusions appear to lend credence to performative analysis in linguistics. Additional evidence for transderivational rules was noted in the subject's omission of the determiners "a" and the "the" when and only when the single semantic function was specification as to whether the NP they modified was definite.

It should be noted that, if these analyses are correct, only syntactic and no semantic errors were made in speech and grammaticality judgments by this aphasic patient. This, of course, suggests that there is some validity to the distinctions made between syntax and semantics in generative grammar. Most contemporary studies with aphasic patients, however, do not use aphasic performance in the building of linguistic theory. Usually, the evidence is related to neurological theory and the linguistic facts are incidental instruments in assessment.

While this may be a legitimate procedure, linguistic theory and associated grammars are devised to represent the necessary mental operations for the speaker—hearer of that language. Borrowing fragments of grammars may, therefore, destroy interesting linguistic facts to be gleaned from a patient. The totality of the grammar and the linguistic theory to which that grammar is related should be considered. If you wish to understand a malfunction in a computer, it may be necessary to run a program that exploits important aspects of the malfunction in question, not just to notice the error in an isolated example.

Generative Capacity: Requirements for the Brain

Somehow, the brain must accomplish the functions required by a grammar. Mathematical analyses of the minimal formal machinery required to account for (or generate) language structures have received increasing attention from linguists and psychologists (Luce, Bush, & Galanter, 1965, Vol. II; Wall, 1972). For example, sentence construction requires a mechanism considerably more powerful than associations and at least as powerful as a push-down-storage mechanism, the implication being that the brain must somehow also conduct operations of at least this power to deal with language (Bever, Fodor, & Garrett, 1968).

Therefore, neurological models of language capacity must provide for operations that have been proven formally to be required for language structures. Failure to heed these constraints on neurophysiological theory building may result in neurological theories accounting for only the most trivial of language functions.

Just as adherence to physical fact is necessary in evaluating language theories, so too are formal linguistic facts ultimately required in constructing an adequate neurological theory. As difficult as this may be for the pure theorists in each discipline, a complete neuropsychological theory of language must be sensitive to the discoveries (and also the discovered restrictions) in each of the contributing fields. Such mutual restrictions are, in the end, mutually enriching.

REFERENCES

Aitkin, L.M., & Webster, W.R. (1972) Medial geniculate body of the cat: Organization and responses to tonal stimuli of neurons in ventral division. *Journal of Neurophysiology, 35,* 365–380.

Anderson, R.M., Jr. (1974) Wholistic and particulate approaches in neuropsychology. In W.B. Weimer & D.S. Palermo (Eds.), *Cognition and the symbolic processes.* Hillsdale, New Jersey: Lawrence Erlbaum, 1974.

Bach, E. (1967) *Have* and *Be* in English syntax. *Language, 43,* 462–485.

Bach, E. (1968) Nouns and noun phrases. In E. Bach & R.J. Harms (Eds.), *Universals in linguistic theory.* New York: Holt.

Bach, E., & Harms, R.T., Eds. (1968) *Universals in linguistic theory.* New York: Holt.

Berlin, C., & McNeil, M.R. (1976) Dichotic listening. In N.J. Lass (Ed.), *Contemporary issues in experimental phonetics.* New York: Academic Press.

Bertelson, P., & Tisseyre, F. (1975) Set and lateral asymmetry in the perceived sequence of speech and nonspeech. In P.M.A. Rabbitt & S. Dornic (Eds.), *Attention and performance: V.* New York: Academic Press.

Bever, J. (1975) Cerebral asymmetries in humans are due to the differentiation of two incompatible processes: Holistic and analytic. In. D. Aaronson & R.W. Rieber (Eds.), *Developmental psycholinguistics and communication disorders.* New York: New York Academy of Sciences.

Bever, T. G., Fodor, J.A., & Garrett, M. (1968) A formal limitation of associationism. In T.R. Dixon & D.C. Horton (Eds.), *Verbal behavior and general behavior theory.* Englewood Cliffs, New Jersey: Prentice-Hall. Pp. 582–585.

Blumstein, S., Goodglass, H., & Tartter, V. (1975) The reliability of ear advantage in dichotic listening. *Brain and Language, 2,* 226–236.

Bogen, J., & Gordon, H. (1971) Musical tests for functional lateralization with intracarotid amobarbital. *Nature, 230,* 524.

Boring, E.G. (1957) *A history of experimental psychology.* New York: Appleton.

Bryden, M.P. (1965) Tachistoscopic recognition, handedness, and cerebral dominance. *Neuropsychologia, 3,* 1–8.

Buffery, A.W.H., & Gray, J. (1972) Sex differences in the development of spatial and linguistic skills In C. Ounsted & D.C. Taylor (Eds.), *Gender differences: Their ontogeny and significance.* Edinburgh: Churchill Livingstone.

Callaway, E., & Harris, P.R. (1974) Coupling between cortical potentials from different areas. *Science, 183,* 873–875.

Carmon, A., Lavy, S., Gordon, H., & Portnoy, Z. (1975) Hemispheric differences in rCBF during verbal and nonverbal tasks. *Brain Work, Alfred Benzon Symposium, IV,* Munksgaard.

Catlin, J., & Neville, H. (1976) The laterality effect in reaction time to speech stimuli. *Neuropsychologia, 14,* 141–143.

Chapman, R.M. (1973) Evoked potentials of the brain related to thinking. In F.J. McGuigan & R.A. Schoonover (Eds.), *The psychophysiology of thinking.* New York: Academic Press.

Chomsky, N. (1957) *Syntactic structures,* The Hague: Mouton.

Chomsky, N. (1965) *Aspects of the theory of syntax,* Cambridge, Massachusetts: M.I.T. Press.

Chomsky, N. (1968a) *Cartesian linguistics.* New York: Harper.

Chomsky, N. (1968b) *Language and mind.* New York: Harcourt.

Chomsky, N., & Halle, M. (1968) *The sound pattern of English.* New York: Harper & Row.

Cofer, C.N. (1968) Problems, issues, and implications. In T.R. Dixon & D.L. Horton (Eds.), *Verbal behavior and general behavior theory.* Englewood Cliffs, New Jersey: Prentice-Hall. Pp. 522–538.

Cohen, G. (1973) Hemispheric differences in serial versus parallel processing. *Journal of Experimental Psychology, 97,* 349–356.

Cullen, J.K. Jr., Berlin, C.I., Hughes, L.F., Thompson, L.L., & Samson, D.S. (1974) Speech information flow: A model. *Proceedings of a Symposium on Central Auditory Processing Disorders,* Univ. of Nebraska Medical Center, Omaha, Nebraska, 108–127.

Dember, W.J., & Jenkins, J.J. (1970) *General psychology: Modelling behavior and experience.* Englewood Cliffs, New Jersey: Prentice-Hall.

Doehring, D.G. (1972) Ear asymmetry in the discrimination of monaural tonal sequences. *Canadian Journal of Psychology, 26,* 106–110.

Feigl, H. (1958) *The mental and the physical.* Minneapolis: U.M. Press.

Fodor, J.A. (1968) *Psychological explanation: An introduction to the philosophy of psychology.* New York: Random House.

Geffner, D.S., & Hochberg, I. (1971) Ear laterality performance of children from low and middle socioeconomic levels on a verbal dichotic listening task. *Cortex, 7,* 193–203.

Geschwind, N. (1971) Some differences between human and other primate brains in cognitive processes of nonhuman primates. In L.E. Jarrard (Ed.), *Cognitive processes of nonhuman primates.* New York: Academic Press. Pp. 149–154.

Geschwind, N., & Levitsky, W. (1968) Human brain: Left-right asymmetries in temporal speech region. *Science, 161,* 186–187.

Goldstein, L., & Lackner, J.R. (1974) Sideways look at dichotic listening. *Journal of Acoustical Society of America, 55,* Supplement, S10.

Gordon, H.W. (1970) Hemispheric asymmetries in the perception of musical chords. *Cortex, 6,* 387–398.

Greenberg, J.H. Ed. (1963) *Universals of language.* Cambridge, Massachusetts: M.I.T. Press.

Gunderson, K. (1971) *Mentality and machines.* Garden City, New York: Doubleday.

Haggard, M.P., & Parkinson, A.M. (1971) Stimulus and task factors as determinants of ear advantages. *Quarterly Journal of Experimental Psychology, 23,* 168–177.

Hall, J.L. II, & Goldstein, M.H. Jr. (1968) Representation of binaural stimuli by single units in primary auditory cortex of unanesthetized cats. *The Journal of the Acoustical Society of America, 43,* 456–461.

Hebb, D.O. (1949) *The organization of behavior,* New York: Wiley.

Hines, D., & Satz, P. (1974) Cross-modal asymmetries in perception related to assymetry in cerebral function. *Neuropsychologia, 12,* 239–247.

Horton, D.L., & Dixon, T.R. (1968) Traditions, trends and innovations. In T.R. Dixon & D.L. Horton (Eds.), *Verbal behavior and general behavior theory.* Englewood Cliffs, New Jersey: Prentice-Hall. Pp. 572–582.

Hubel, D. (1963) The visual cortex of the brain. *Scientific American, 209,* 54–63.

Jacobs, R., & Rosenbaum, P. Eds. (1970) *Readings in English transformational grammar.* Waltham, Massachusetts: Ginn.

Jasper, H.H. (1958) The ten twenty electrode system of the International Federation. *Electroencephalography and Clinical Neurophysiology, 10,* 371–375.

Jenkins, J.J. (1968) The challenge to psychological theorists. In T.R. Dixon & D.L. Horton (Eds.), *Verbal behaviour and general behaviour theory.* Englewood Cliffs, New Jersey: Prentice-Hall. Pp. 538–550.

John, E.R. (1971) Brain mechanisms of memory. In McGaugh (Ed.), *Psychobiology.* New York: Academic Press.

John, E.R. (1972) Switchboard versus statistical theories of learning and memory. *Science 177,* 850–864.

Katz, J., & Postal, P.M. (1964) *An integrated theory of linguistic description.* Cambridge, Massachusetts: M.I.T. Press.

Kimura, D. (1961a) Some effects of temporal-lobe damage on auditory perception. *Canadian Journal of Psychology, 15,* 156–165.

Kimura, D. (1961b) Cerebral dominance and the perception of verbal stimuli, *Canadian Journal of Psychology, 15,* 166–175.

Kimura, D. (1969) Spatial localization in left and right visual fields. *Canadian Journal of Psychology/Review of Canadian Psychology, 23,* 445–458.

Kimura, D. (1973) The asymmetry of the human brain. *Scientific American, 228,* 70–78.

Kinsbourne, M. (1973) The control of attention by interaction between the cerebral hemispheres. In S. Kornblum (Ed.), *Attention and performance,* IV. New York: Academic Press.

Klein, C. (1976) Visual perceptual asymmetries and hemispheric specialization. Mimeo, Univ. of Toronto.

Knox, C., & Kimura, D. (1970) Cerebral processing of nonverbal sounds in boys and girls. *Neuropsychologia 8,* 227–237.

Kopell, N. (1976) Pattern formation in chemistry and biology. Paper presented at the conference, Psychology and Biology of Language and Thought, Ithaca, New York.

Lashley, K.S. (1950) In search of the engram. In Society for Experimental Biology, *Physiological mechanisms in animal behavior*. New York: Academic Press.

Luce, R.D., Bush, R.R. & Galanter, E., Eds. (1965) *Handbook of mathematical psychology*, Vol. II. New York: Wiley.

Luria, A.R. (1966) *Human brain and psychological processes*, New York: Harper.

Luria, A.R. (1970) The functional organization of the brain. *Scientific American, 222,* 66–78.

McAdam, D.W., & Whitaker, H.A. (1971) Language production: Electroencephalographic localization in the normal human brain. *Science, 172,* 499–502.

McKeever, W.F., & Huling, M.D. (1971) Lateral dominance in tachistoscopic word recognition performances obtained with simultaneous bilateral input. *Neuropsychologia, 9,* 15–20.

Meehl, P.E. (1966) The compleat autocerebioscopist: A thought experiment on Professor Feigl's mind-body identity thesis. In P. Feyerabend & G. Maxwell (Eds.), *Mind, matter and method*. Minneapolis: U.M. Press. Pp. 103–180.

Morais, J., & Darwin, C.J. (1974) Ear differences for same-different reaction times to monaurally presented speech. *Brain and Language, 1,* 383–390.

Moscovitch, M. (1973) Language and the cerebral hemispheres: Reaction-time studies and their implications for models of cerebral dominance. In P. Pliner, L. Krames, & T. Alloway (Eds.), *Communication and affect*. New York: Academic Press.

Papçun, G., Krashen, S., Terbeek, D., Remington, R., & Harshman, R. (1974) Is the left hemisphere specialized for speech, language and/or something else? *Journal of the Acoustical Society of America, 55,* 319–327.

Penfield, W. (1959) The interpretive cortex. *Science, 129,* 1719–1725.

Penfield, W. & Roberts, L. (1959) *Speech and brain mechanisms*. Princeton, New Jersey: Princeton Univ. Press.

Postal, P.M. (1968) *Aspects of phonological theory*. New York: Harper.

Pribram, K.H. (1966) Some dimensions of remembering: Steps toward a neuropsychological model of memory. In J. Gaito (Ed.), *Macromolecules and behavior*. New York: Appleton.

Pribram, K.H. (1971) *Languages of the brain*. Englewood Cliffs, New Jersey: Prentice-Hall.

Risberg, J., & Ingvar, D.H. (1973) Patterns of activation in the grey matter of the dominant hemisphere during memorizing and reasoning. *Brain, 96,* 737–756.

Robbins, K.I., & McAdam, D.W. (1974) Interhemispheric alpha asymmetry and imagery mode. *Brain and Language, 1,* 189–193.

Rosenzweig, M.R. (1951) Representation of the two ears at the auditory cortex. *American Journal of Physiology, 167,* 147–158.

Ross, J.R. (1970) On declarative sentences. In R. Jacobs & P. Rosenbaum (Eds.), *Readings in English transformational grammar*. Waltham, Massachusetts: Ginn. Pp. 222–272.

Scheid, P., & Eccles, J.C. (1975) Music and speech: Artistic functions of the human brain. *Psychology of Music, 3,* 21–35.

Schnitzer, Marc L. (1974) Aphasiological evidence for five linguistical hypotheses. *Language, 50,* 300–316.

Semmes, J. (1968) Hemispheric specialization: A possible clue to mechanism. *Neuropsychologia, 6,* 11–26.

Shagass, C. (1972) Electrical activity of the brain. In N. Greenfield & R. Sternbach (Eds.), *Handbook of psychophysiology*. New York: Holt. Pp. 304–319.

Spellacy, F., & Blumstein, S. (1970) The influence of language set on ear preference in phoneme recognition. *Cortex, 6,* 430–439.

Van Lancker, D., & Fromkin, V.A. (1973) Hemispheric specialization for pitch and "tone": Evidence from Thai. *Journal of Phonetics, 1,* 101–109.

Wada, J. (1949) A new method for the determination of the side of cerebral speech dominance. *Medical Biology, 14,* 221–222.

Wada, J.A., Clarke, R., & Hamm, A. (1975) Cerebral hemispheric asymmetry in humans. *Archives of Neurology, 32,* 239–246.

Wall, R. (1972) *Introduction to mathematical linguistics.* Englewood Cliffs, New Jersey: Prentice-Hall.

Weisstein, N. (1975) The Niagara Falls, Ontario barrel detector. Paper presented to the Lake Ontario Visual Establishment, Niagara Falls, Ontario.

Whitaker, H.A. (1971) Neurolinguistics. In W.O. Dingwall (Ed.), *A survey of linguistic science.* College Park, Maryland: Univ. of Maryland Press.

White, M.J. (1969) Laterality differences in perception: A review. *Psychological Bulletin, 72,* 387–405.

Witelson, S.F. (1974) Hemispheric specialization for linguistic and nonlinguistic tactual perception using a dichotomous stimulation technique. *Cortex, 10,* 3–17.

Witelson, S.F. (1976) Sex and the single hemisphere: Right hemisphere specialization for spatial processing, *Science, 193:* 425–427.

Witelson, S.F., & Pallie, W. (1973) Left hemisphere specialization for language in the newborn: Neuroanatomical evidence of asymmetry. *Brain, 96,* 641–646.

Yeni-Komshian, G.H., & Benson, D.A. (1976) Anatomical study of cerebral asymmetry in the temporal lobe of humans, chimpanzees, and rhesus monkeys. *Science, 192,* 387–389.

Zaidel, E. (1975) A technique for presenting lateralized visual input with prolonged exposure. *Vision Research, 15,* 283–289.

2

Infant Cerebral Asymmetry

DENNIS L. MOLFESE

Over the course of the last 100 years a large body of literature has emerged which appears to support the notion that the different hemispheres of man's brain may have quite distinct cognitive functions. Much of this work has been directed toward the study of language abilities and their relation to hemisphere functions. The result of this work has been a strong case demonstrating that the control of most language abilities is exercised by mechanisms within the left cerebral hemisphere. Supporting data have come from work with individuals who suffered brain damage as a result of missile wounds (Newcombe, 1969), corticovascular accidents (Geschwind, 1965), and epilepsy (Milner, 1958), as well as from research on hemispherectomies (Basser, 1962), and split-brain preparations (Gazzaniga, 1970). Only within the last two decades have procedures been developed that permit the study of brain–language functions in neurologically intact individuals. These methods include the use of dichotic listening procedures (Kimura, 1961) and, more recently, auditory evoked potential techniques (Cohn, 1971).

The auditory evoked potential (AEP) is the very gross response of a large population of neurons to the presentation of a stimulus. It differs from an EEG in that the AEP is time locked to the onset of some specific stimulus while the EEG characterizes ongoing, continuous neural–electrical activity relatively independent of any reference point. The AEP recording procedures have certain advantages over other techniques because they can be readily used with neurologically intact cases as well as with brain-damaged individuals. In addition, these procedures enable investigators to work with individuals who may be unable to make linguistically appropriate responses, as in the case of very young children or infants (Crowell, Jones, Kapuniai, and Nakagawa, 1973; Molfese, 1972).

Although the case for hemispheric specialization for language appears to be quite strong for adults, experimental research into the development of this lateralization has just begun. For example, in 1967 Lenneberg argued, on the basis of clinical reports dealing with hemispherectomies, that lateralization of language functions develops sometime between 2 and 3 years of age, as the child begins to acquire language. Four years later, Eimas, Siqueland, Jusczyk, and Vigorito (1971) reported that 1- and 4-month-old infants could discriminate between a number of speech sounds on the basis of their phoneme category rather than only on the basis of simple acoustic changes. Furthermore, the discriminations made by the infants appeared to parallel distinctions made by adult language users as found by Lisker and Abramson (1964). These findings show that very young infants have some language or language-like abilities. Returning to Lenneberg's argument that lateralization of language functions occurs as the child acquires language, it would seem reasonable to suspect that if infants do possess language abilities, some lateralization of function must already have occurred. That is, some areas of the infant's brain may already have developed to the point where they may differentially process different types of sounds. The first experiment (Molfese, 1972) describes our initial attempt to assess the presence of such hemispheric differences in human infants. It was hoped that a comparison of hemisphere differences in infants with those present in adults would highlight any changes in laterality that might accompany maturation and language development.

EXPERIMENT 1

Subjects: Ten infants, ranging in age from 1 week to 10 months (mean: 5.8 months), eleven children, from 4 years to 11 years (mean: 6.0 years), and ten adults, from 23 to 29 years (mean: 24 years) participated in this study.

Stimuli: Two speech syllables (/ba/ and /da/), two words (/bɔi/ and /dog/), and two nonspeech sounds (a C-major piano chord and a burst of speech noise, the latter composed of frequencies between 250 Hz and 4 kHz) were the stimuli. The syllables and words were natural speech sounds produced by an adult male speaker. All stimuli were 500 msec in duration and were recorded so that they were matched for peak loudness levels. The sounds were recorded on a continuous loop recording tape in a 6 × 6 Latin square matrix.

Procedure: Each subject was tested individually. Recording electrodes were placed on the scalp of the subject with one electrode over the left temporal area (T_3) and one over the right temporal area (T_4). Two linked electrodes were attached to the ear lobes to serve as references for the temporal leads. The stimuli were presented to the subject through a speaker positioned approximately 1 m over his head. The stimuli were presented approximately 100 times, in order to elicit a large sample of AEPs. These were later summed and averaged by a computer. The use of such averaging techniques is necessary in order to reduce the level of noise in the brain response so that the AEP will more accurately reflect the response of the brain to the stimulus rather than reflect some random artifact unrelated to the specific cortical response.

Analyses: After the AEPs had been recorded and averaged, a computer calculated the magnitude of change in the evoked potential between a maximum negative peak and a maximum positive peak, which occurred within a certain temporal range of the AEP. This temporal interval was determined by the age of the subject in question. The amplitude measure was calculated for both the left and the right hemispheres in response to each stimulus. Next, a proportion score (R) was calculated by dividing the amplitude for the left hemisphere by the sum of the amplitudes for the left and right hemispheres in response to the same stimulus.

$$R = \frac{\text{left hemisphere}}{\text{left hemisphere} + \text{right hemisphere}}$$

The resulting proportion yielded a value such that if the proportion was greater than .50, the amplitude of the left hemisphere would be greater than the amplitude of the right hemisphere. If R was less than .50, the left hemisphere amplitude would be less than the amplitude of the right hemisphere.

Results: The R for 27 of the 31 subjects in response to the speech stimuli were greater than .50 ($\bar{x}$ = 55.24), 30 of the subjects' AEPs were characterized by R of less than .50 in response to the musical chord ($\bar{x}$ = 39.68), and 29 subjects had Rs of less than .50 for the noise stimulus ($\bar{x}$ = 42.74). Indications of differential hemispheric responding were present, not only in the response of the adults but in those of the infants and children as well. In fact, an analysis of variance revealed that the degree of laterality in the infants was actually greater than that of the adults for both the speech and nonspeech stimuli ($p < .01$). A more complete review of these findings is available elsewhere (Molfese, 1972; Molfese, Freeman, and Palermo, 1975).

In Figure 1 are the averaged AEPs for one adult in response to three of the stimuli: the piano chord, a speech syllable, and the noise burst. The AEPs were recorded from the onset of the stimulus over a 500-msec interval. Note that the amplitude of the right hemisphere AEP in response to both the chord and the noise

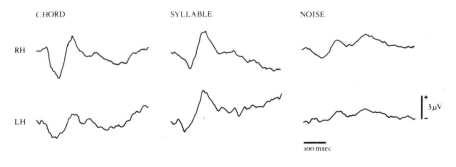

ADULT - 8

Figure 1. Averaged auditory evoked potentials recorded from the left (LH) and right hemispheres (RH) of an adult in response to 3 stimuli. The evoked potential began with stimulus onset. Duration is 500 msec. The calibration marker is 3 μV and positive is up.

is larger than the amplitude of the left hemisphere AEP. The amplitude of the left hemisphere AEP in response to the speech syllable was larger than that of the right hemisphere.

An infant's AEPs to the same three stimuli are in Figure 2; they are strikingly different in shape and involve longer latencies and higher voltage amplitudes than the adult AEPs. However, the relative hemisphere differences in amplitude of the infant AEPs as a function of the various stimuli are similar to those of the adults in Figure 1. The left hemisphere amplitude was larger than the right hemisphere in response to the speech syllable, while the right hemisphere amplitude was greater for the chord and the noise stimuli.

Discussion: It appears from the AEP data that cerebral asymmetry is present in infancy. Several recent investigations support this finding. For example, anatomical studies of premature and full-term infants indicate that some morphological differences between hemispheres are present early in development. Wada, Clark, and Hamm (1973) have reported the presence of asymmetries in the frontal operculum and the temporal planum of fetal infants as early as 29 weeks conceptual age. Witelson and Pallie (1973) and Tezner (1972) have also reported the presence of asymmetries in the temporal planum of premature and full-term infants. Furthermore, Witelson & Pallie reported that these differences were "at least as great" as those reported by Geschwind and Levitsky (1968) for adult brains.

Two recent studies employing electrophysiological recording techniques have also reported cerebral asymmetry in infants. Crowell *et al.* (1973) have found differential hemispheric responses to photic driving of the EEG, and Barnet, deSotillo and Campas (1974), employing AEP procedures, found greater amplitude responses in the left cerebral hemisphere of infants in response to hearing their names. Dichotic listening procedures have also been adapted to work with infants. Entus (1974) combined the sucking habituation technique developed by Siqueland

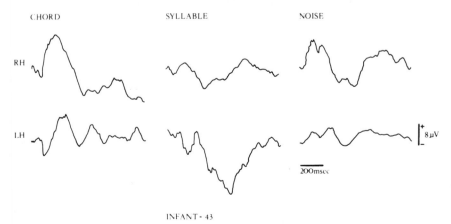

INFANT - 43

Figure 2. Auditory evoked potentials recorded from the left and right hemispheres of an infant to 3 stimuli. Duration is 1 sec. The calibration marker is 8 μV and positive is up.

and DeLucia (1969) with a dichotic listening procedure and found evidence of hemispheric specialization for speech sounds and musical notes in the left and right hemispheres, respectively.

Given these data, some degree of hemispheric specialization appears to be present in human infants long before the age of 2 years suggested by Lenneberg (1967). The two hemispheres are anatomically different from each other prior to or at least at birth, and are similar in this respect to adult brains. Furthermore, it appears that the two hemispheres of infants respond differentially to different stimuli, again similar to adults. One is struck by the number of different laboratories, employing diverse techniques, which have found evidence that appears to point to the same phenomenon—infant cerebral asymmetry. The next step, as Kimura (1967) noted, involves determining the characteristics of the stimuli that trigger these asymmetrical responses.

In adults, it appears that asymmetrical responding to auditory stimuli may be due to one of two factors: (1) linguistic meaningfulness or (2) acoustic characteristics. The effects of the first factor were investigated by Papçun, Krashen, Terbeek, Remington and Harsham (1974) who employed a dichotic listening procedure to present Morse code signals to Morse code instructors and Morse code naive college students. He found no ear differences in the college population, but the instructors reported the signals with a significantly higher degree of accuracy when the sounds were presented to the right ear. Since materials presented to the right ear are thought to be processed primarily in the left hemisphere (Kimura, 1961; Rosenzweig, 1951), it would appear that the instructors were better able to process the coded signals in their left hemispheres. Since these sounds were radically different from speech stimuli, Papçun argued that the left hemisphere may process not auditory signals per se, but rather materials that have some degree of linguistic meaningfulness.

Regarding the second factor, the acoustic characteristics, Cutting (1974) presented a strong case suggesting that the left hemisphere may also attend to specific acoustic and phonetic elements. Using a dichotic listening procedure with adults, Cutting, in the acoustic condition, presented a series of vowels and consonant–vowel syllables that were synthesized either with a narrow bandwidth (nonspeech) or with a "normal" bandwidth (speech). The nonspeech stimuli were constructed from sine waves that corresponded exactly to the central frequencies of the formants in the speech stimuli. The bandwidth of these nonspeech stimuli was "essentially zero." In contrast, the bandwidth of the formants for the speech stimuli were 60, 90, and 120 Hz for F_1, F_2, and F_3, respectively. A phonetic cue, transition, was also varied. The vowel sounds (nontransition) were steady state and did not contain an initial consonant transition; the consonant–vowel syllables (transition) did contain a rapid frquency change. Cutting found that the speech materials (normal bandwidth) produced a right-ear advantage while the nonspeech stimuli did not. The presence of transitional elements also appeared to result in a right-ear advantage, although the magnitude of this difference was not as large. In fact, the transition effect appeared to be largely due to the large right-ear advantage of the speech consonant–vowel syllable (16%). The nonspeech consonant–vowel stimuli resulted in only a 1% advantage for the right ear.

For adults, then, the acoustic and perhaps phonetic characteristics of the sounds themselves appear to play a role in determining if a sound is to be processed in the left or the right hemisphere. However, as indicated by the work of Papçun *et al.* (1974), semantic or cognitive factors would also appear to be at work. These findings present an interesting problem with respect to asymmetrical responding in infancy. Infants at birth are generally thought to have only a reflex-based cognitive system (Piaget, 1970) and little or no linguistic skills (MacNamara, 1972). There-fore, if neonates respond asymmetrically to speech stimuli, these asymmetrical responses should be based on the acoustic components of the stimuli rather than on the linguistic factors. Perhaps at a later point, when the infant acquires language skills, the left hemisphere would be responsive to either acoustic or linguistic elements. Initially, however, asymmetrical responding may be triggered only by acoustic elements. The next experiment describes an investigation of the effects of acoustic factors on asymmetry in neonates.

EXPERIMENT 2

Subjects: Fourteen neonates (seven males and seven females) were tested. Each infant was tested within 24 hr of birth.

Stimuli: Five sounds were used as stimuli: a 500-Hz sine wave, two speech stimuli (/gæ/ and /æ/), and two nonspeech stimuli, which were constructed from pure tones corresponding exactly to the central frequencies of the formants of the speech stimuli. The two speech stimuli and the two nonspeech stimuli were prepared by James Cutting on the parallel resonance synthesizer at Haskins Labora-tory. For additonal details concerning the construction of these stimuli, the reader is referred to Cutting (1974). The 500-Hz tone was generated with a Wavetek Signal Generator. All stimuli were identical in peak intensity and all were 300 msec in duration.

Forty random orderings of the five stimuli were recorded on one channel of a stereo tape recorder. The time interval between stimulus sounds was varied ran-domly between 4 and 8 sec. A 50-Hz, .5V square wave was recorded on the second channel of the tape recorder, such that the pulse preceded each stimulus by 50 msec. This pulse served as a signal to a PDP-12 computer to begin averaging.

Procedure: The procedure was similar to that described in Experiment 1.

Results: An analysis of variance indicated that there were no differences in AEP amplitude between the hemispheres for the speech stimuli and for the nonspeech stimuli ($p > .10$). However, the difference between the speech and nonspeech stimuli was significant ($p < .01$). The group Rs, on which the analyses were based, are in Figure 3.

For the neonates, the greatest amplitude change in response to the nonspeech stimuli occurred in the right hemisphere. In fact, there was no difference between

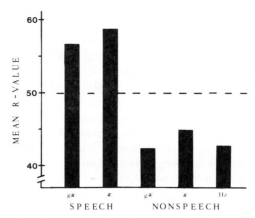

Figure 3. Mean infant *R*-value scores for the two speech and three nonspeech stimuli.

the neonates' responses to the nonspeech stimuli and the 500-Hz signal. On the other hand, the greatest amplitude change in response to the speech stimuli occurred in the left hemisphere. No differences between hemispheres were found when responses were analyzed in terms of transitional elements verses nontransitional elements ($p > .10$). The presence of a transitional element was not a critical factor in differentiating between hemispheres. Rather, the bandwidth of the stimuli was responsible for differences in hemispheric responding, as is illustrated in Figure 4.

Discussion: The results of Experiment 2 suggest that acoustic rather than phonetic cues are responsible for asymmetry in neonates. The acoustic cue, bandwidth, was responsible for a larger amplitude left-hemisphere response, providing that the bandwidth of the formants was comparable to that found in normal speech. The phonetic elements (transitions) without the acoustic cue failed to elicit a left-hemisphere response.

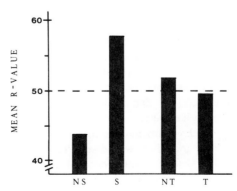

Figure 4. Mean infant *R*-value scores for the nonspeech, speech, nontransition, and transition stimuli.

The finding that vowel sounds as well as consonants triggered greater left-hemisphere responding is at variance with a large body of literature in which dichotic listening procedures have been employed to assess differential hemispheric responses (Shankweiler and Studdert-Kennedy, 1967; Studdert-Kennedy and Shankweiler, 1970). These studies have generally found that the left hemisphere is better in identifying consonant sounds, while vowel sounds produce either a slight left-hemisphere advantage or no differences between hemispheres.

A second point of discrepancy centers on the effects of transitional elements. Cutting (1974) reported that the presence of transitional elements produced a right-ear (left-hemisphere) advantage, even when the sounds contained formants that were only 1 Hz in width. When the data of the present study (Figure 4) are grouped in terms of responses to transitional versus nontransitional stimuli, there are no differences between hemispheres. If the responses are grouped according to responses to speech versus nonspeech stimuli, there is greater left-hemisphere responding to the speech stimuli and greater right-hemisphere responding to the nonspeech. As indicated earlier, Cutting's transitional effect may have been a spurious one. Nonspeech transitional stimuli produced only a 1% advantage for the left hemisphere—a difference that was not significant if viewed in isolation [personal communication].

Both discrepancies—those concerning vowel effects and those dealing with transitional effects—may be due to the differences in the techniques used to assess the hemispheric responses. Electrophysiological procedures, which involve monitoring evoked potentials in response to some stimuli, may be assessing quite different cognitive functions or physiological correlates of these functions than dichotic listening procedures. Likewise, different dichotic listening tasks that make different demands on the subjects may be assessing quite different functions (Pisoni, 1971). This could raise serious questions concerning the validity of comparing findings concerning hemispheric functions when different techniques for assessing such functions are employed.

It is also possible that the differences between Cutting's findings and our own may be due to developmental factors. Cutting employed adults as subjects in his experiments, while the AEPs reported in the present study were recorded from neonates. Developmental changes occurring between infancy and adulthood, as a result of neurophysiological and cognitive factors, might be reflected in changes in hemispheric responses. The notion that cerebral asymmtery develops into adulthood is a relatively old one (Lenneberg, 1967), and, although our data suggest that the two cerebral hemispheres of man may function somewhat differently from birth, there is no reason to believe that further changes in cerebral asymmetry do not occur. The data from Experiment 1 indicating a difference in the degree of asymmetry between infants and adults would seem to support this view.

Additional information on the development of asymmetry and on the role of acoustic and linguistic cues in hemispheric responding may be supplied by our pilot experiment on EP habituation. Research on EP habituation effects has been quite active over the last decade (Ritter, Vaughn, and Costa, 1968; Regan, 1972). In general, when a stimulus is presented repeatedly, the amplitude of the EPs elicited in response to this stimulus decrease over trials. When such a decrease occurs, the EP is said to have habituated. If a new stimulus is then presented following habituation, the amplitude of the EP will increase to its initial level (dishabituate). Dorman and Hoffman (1973) were the first to employ this procedure to assess the ability of adults to detect changes in voice onset time (VOT).[1] In general, they found that when a change in VOT crossed the phoneme boundary, the amplitude of the EP dishabituated. However, when the stimulus change did not cross this boundary, the EP amplitude remained at its habituated level.

Employing a modification of Dorman's procedures, we recorded the responses of both hemispheres in infants and adults to VOT changes.

EXPERIMENT 3

Subjects: Two groups of subjects participated in this study: eight infants (4 males and 4 females) under 24 hr of age and 6 adults (3 males and 3 females) between 18 and 23 years of age.

Stimuli: The speech syllables were constructed on the Haskins parallel resonance synthesizer and consisted of a bilabial stop consonant and vowel (/ba/). The stop consonant was produced in 20-msec steps: Ba_0, Ba_{20}, Ba_{40}, Ba_{60}. A second stop consonant and vowel (/da/), characterized by a different place of articulation, was also produced. A separate group of 10 adults identified Ba_0 and Ba_{20} as "ba," and Ba_{40} and Ba_{60} as "pa;" Da_0, the only other place stimulus used, was recognized as "da." Two stimulus tapes were then constructed with eight different series of these syllables. Each series contained 30 syllables. The series were separated from one another by silent intervals varying between 15 and 25 sec in length. The sounds within each series were separated by 3-sec intervals. The first 15 sounds of a series (preshift) were repetitions of one syllable, while the second 15 stimuli (postshift) were repetitions of a different syllable. The change from the first to the second set of 15 stimuli involved either a change in voicing which did not cross the phoneme boundary (i.e., $Ba_{40}-Ba_{60}$ and Ba_0-Ba_{20}), a change across the boundary (i.e., $Ba_{20}-Ba_{40}$), or a change in place of articulation with voicing held constant (i.e., Ba_0-Da_0). These four pairs of stimuli, and the reverse of these pairs (i.e., $Ba_{60}-Ba_{40}$), were used.

Procedure: The testing procedures employed were similar to those of Experiment 1.

[1] Voice onset time characterizes the temporal relation between laryngeal pulsing and articulatory release of the speech sound (Lisker & Abramson, 1964). Generally, adults characterize a stop consonant speech sound with a VOT of +20 msec as a voiced consonant (e.g., /b/) while the same acoustic elements if combined with a VOT of +40 msec would be identified as an unvoiced consonant (e.g., /p/).

Results: The AEPs elicited in response to the last seven sounds of the preshift condition were averaged together, as were the AEPs recorded in response to the first seven presentations of the postshift condition. Each series of stimuli was analyzed separately.

For adults, a place change elicited differential hemispheric responding. For five of the six subjects, the AEPs recorded from the right hemisphere continued to decrease in amplitude during the postshift condition, but the left-hemisphere response showed a noticeable increase in amplitude. An example of this is in Figure 5. Here, the right-hemisphere (RH) response is at the top of the figure while the left-hemisphere response (LH) is immediately below it. The left-hemisphere AEP for the postshift condition is larger than the average for the preshift condition. However, the right-hemisphere AEP for the postshift condition is smaller than that for the preshift condition. Similar differences between the preshift and postshift conditions occurred in response to a voicing change which crossed the phoneme boundary. However, when the voicing change did not cross the phoneme boundary, the AEPs for both hemispheres showed further habituation in the postshift condition.

Different findings emerged when these procedures were repeated with neonates. The place change elicited no differential hemispheric activity in any of the neo-

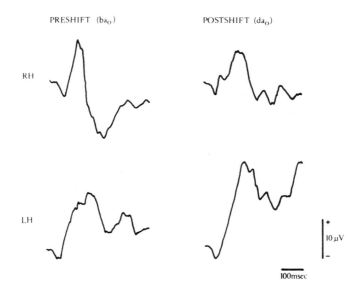

PRESHIFT (ba$_0$)   POSTSHIFT (da$_0$)

RH

LH

+
10 μV
-

100msec

ADULT-6

Figure 5. Averaged auditory evoked potentials recorded from the left and right hemispheres of an adult first to the syllable /ba/ (ba$_0$) and then to the syllable /da/ (da$_0$). Both syllables had voice onset times of 0. The evoked potential began with stimulus onset. Duration is 450 msec. The calibration marker is 10 μV with positive up.

nates. Both hemispheres responded in the same manner. For voicing changes which crossed the phoneme boundary, the AEPs of six of the eight infants showed dishabituation in both hemispheres during the postshift condition. An example of this is in Figure 6. Note the increased amplitudes for both hemispheres in the postshift condition. Unlike the adults, both hemispheres of the infants responded to the voicing change. When a voicing change occurred which did not cross the phoneme boundary, neither hemisphere of the infants responded to the change.

Discussion: Finding that adults respond asymmetrically to place and voicing changes appears to support the notion that the hemispheres have different roles in the processing of phonetic elements. Only the left hemisphere was particularly sensitive to such linguistically relevant cues as place of articulation and voicing

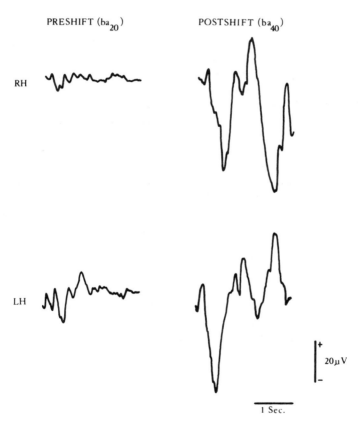

INFANT-2

Figure 6. Averaged auditory evoked potentials recorded from the left and right hemispheres of a newborn infant first to the syllable /ba/ with a voice onset time of +20 msec and then to the syllable /pa/ with a voice onset time of 40 msec. Duration was 2.6 sec. The calibration marker is 20 μV with positive up.

changes which cross phoneme boundaries. Both hemispheres, however, responded the same to within-boundary voicing changes. Neonates, on the other hand, did not respond like adults to place or voicing changes. Rather, both hemispheres dishabituated when a voicing change occurred which crossed a phoneme boundary, and both hemispheres failed to dishabituate when a place change or a within-boundary voicing change occurred. Differences between the neonates and the adults may indicate developmental differences in hemispheric functioning.

The neonates' responses present some interesting developmental data. For example, the neonates did respond differently to voicing changes which crossed the phoneme boundaries as compared to within-boundary voicing changes. These results are similar to those found with the adult subjects and similar to the findings reported by Eimas *et al.* (1971), who used older infants. Although the adults and Eimas's infants may also have used linguistic cues to differentiate changes in voicing boundaries, the neonates most likely are responding to acoustic rather than linguistic cues, since the presence of an innate lingusitic system is doubtful, as Butterfield and Cairns (1974) have argued. There may be nonlinguistic mechanisms present in the auditory system that enable neonates to detect certain acoustic changes while ignoring others.

A paper by Kuhl and Miller (1975) appears to support the notion that sensitivity to voicing boundaries may be due to acoustic factors. They trained chinchillas on a go—no go avoidance task with exemplars from each end of the voicing continuum for "ba—pa" as the discriminative stimuli. When "ba" was presented repeatedly through a speaker overhead, the animals could drink a sugar solution without fear of being shocked. However, if "pa" was presented, the animals were allowed only three seconds to escape to an adjoining chamber to avoid the shock. The animals were then tested with other stimuli differing in VOT values from the original training stimuli. Kuhl and Miller reported that the chinchillas differentiated between VOT values of the bilabial stop consonants much like humans. Voice onset time values of 0 and +20 were responded to as instances of "ba," while values of +40 and +60 were treated as "pa."

The detection of voicing boundaries, then, could well be an acoustic phenomenon. Interestingly, it is one that humans have incorporated into their linguistic systems to differentiate between various speech sounds. Voicing cues carry linguistic significance in most of the language families of the world, and, generally, there is little variability in voicing distinctions between languages. The majority of the language families utilize either two classes (e.g., English) or three classes (e.g., Thai) of voicing. This is not true for place of articulation. Place differences vary widely across languages (Greenberg, 1963) and seem to be based primarily on the types of linguistic distinctions needed in particular language families. Place discrimination, then, may be a linguistic cue that must be learned.

Support for this hypothesis is provided by the results of Experiment 3, which showed that the neonates failed to dishabituate to a place change; this may indicate that they failed to detect such a change. The adult subjects, on the other hand, showed dishabituation and asymmetrical responding to place changes. Since Eimas (1974) has reported behavioral data showing that 2- to 4-month-old infants can discriminate place changes, it is possible that some amount of linguistic experience is necessary for the detection of place changes. Interestingly, some recent work by Kuhl and Miller [personal communication] also provides some support for this notion. Unlike the training of voicing distinctions, these researchers have experienced great difficulties in training place distinctions in chinchillas.

In general, then, the findings of Experiment 3 suggest differences in hemispheric responding between neonates and adults. Although some mechanisms may be present at birth that enable the neonate to detect certain acoustic changes, further hemispheric development and linguistic exposure may be necessary before the neonates' responses are comparable to those of adults. A great deal more work is needed in this area. Further research into the acoustic and phonetic dimensions that affect differential hemispheric responding is obviously needed. Cutting (1974) has suggested some directions that this research might take. Research with infants and children could well supplement the research with adults, to isolate acoustic factors that might contribute to differential hemispheric processing and to its development. However, care should be taken in extrapolating from infant data to adult data or from adult to infant data, given the differences in the physiological and cognitive states of the two organisms. Psycholinguists have been criticized for making this overgeneralization in the past (Derwing, 1973), and one would hope that it would not be repeated in the future.

REFERENCES

Barnet, A.B., de Sotillo, M., & Campos, M. (1974) EEG sensory evoked potentials in early infancy malnutrition. Paper presented to the Society for Neuroscience, St. Louis.

Basser, L.S. (1962) Hemiplegia of early onset and the faculty of speech with special reference to the effects of hemispherectomy. *Brain, 85,* 427–460.

Butterfield, E.C., & Cairns, G.F. (1974) Infant reception research. In R.L. Schiefelbusch & L.L. Lloyd (Eds.), *Language perspectives–acquisition, retardation, and intervention.* Maryland: University Park Press.

Cohn, R. (1971) Differential cerebral processing of noise and verbal stimuli. *Science, 172,* 599–601.

Crowell, D.H., Jones, R.H., Kapuniai, L.E., & Nakagawa, J.K. (1973) Unilateral cortical activity in new born humans: An early index of cerebral dominance. *Science, 180,* 205–208.

Cutting, J.E. (1974) Two left-hemisphere mechanisms in speech perception. *Perception & Psychophysics, 16,* 601–612.

Derwing, B.L. (1973) *Transformational grammar as a theory of language acquisition.* New York: Cambridge Univ. Press.

Dorman, M.F., & Hoffman, R. (1972) Short-term habituation of the infant auditory evoked response. *Haskins Laboratories Status Report on Speech Research, SR - 29/30,* 121–124.

Eimas, P.D. (1974) Auditory and linguistic processing of cues for place of articulation by infants. *Perception & Psychophysics, 16,* 513–521.

Eimas, P.D., Siqueland, E.R., Jusczyk, P., & Vigorito, J. (1971) Speech perception in infants. *Science, 171,* 303–306.

Entus, A.K. (1974) Hemispheric asymmetry in processing of dichotically presented speech and nonspeech sounds by infants. Unpublished doctoral dissertation, McGill Univ.

Gazzaniga, M.S. (1970) *The bisected brain.* New York: Appleton.

Geschwind, N. (1965) Disconnexion syndromes in animals and man. *Brain, 88,* 585–644.

Geschwind, N., & Levitsky, W. (1968) Human Brain: Left-right asymmetries in temporal speech region. *Science, 161,* 186–187.

Greenberg, J.H. (Ed.). (1963) *Universals of language.* Cambridge: MIT Press.

Kimura, D. (1961) Cerebral dominance and the perception of verbal stimuli. *Canadian Journal of Psychology, 15,* 166–171.

Kimura, D. (1967) Functional asymmetry of the brain in dichotic listening. *Cortex, 3,* 163–178.

Kuhl, P.K., & Miller, J.D. (1975) Speech perception by the chinchilla: The voiced-voiceless distinction in alveolar plosive consonants. *Science, 190,* 69–72.

Lenneberg, E.H. (1967) *Biological foundation of language.* New York: Wiley.

Lisker, L., & Abramson, A.S. (1964) A cross-language study of voicing in initial stops: Acoustical measurements. *Word, 20,* 384–422.

Macnamara, J. (1972) Cognitive basis of language learning in infants. *Psychological Review, 70,* 1–13.

Milner, B. (1958) Psychological defects produced by temporal lobe excision. *Proceedings of the Association of Research into Nervous Mental Disorders, 36,* 244–257.

Molfese, D.L. (1972) Cerebral asymmetry in infants, children and adults: Auditory evoked responses to speech and music stimuli. Unpublished doctoral dissertation, Pennsylvania State Univ.

Molfese, D.L., Freeman, R.B., & Palermo, D.S. (1975) The ontogeny of brain lateralization for speech and nonspeech stimuli. *Brain & Language, 2,* 356–368.

Newcombe, F. (1969) *Missile wounds of the brain: A study of psychological deficits.* New York: Oxford University Press.

Papçun, G., Krashen, S., Terbeek, D., Remington, R., & Harshman, R. (1974) Is the left hemisphere specialized for speech, language and/or something else? *Journal of the Acoustical Society of America, 55,* 319–327.

Piaget, J. (1970) Piaget's theory. In P. Mussen (Ed.), *Carmichael's handbook of child psychology.* New York: Wiley.

Pisoni, D.B. (1971) On the nature of categorical perception of speech sounds. Unpublished doctoral dissertation, Univ. of Michigan.

Regan, D. (1972) *Evoked potentials in psychology, sensory physiology and clinical medicine.* New York: Wiley.

Ritter, W., Vaughn, H., & Costa, L. (1968) Orienting and habituation to auditory stimuli: A study of short term changes in average evoked responses. *Journal of Electroencephalography and Clinical Neurophysiology, 25,* 550–556.

Rosenzweig, M.R. (1951). Representations of the two ears at the auditory cortex. *American Journal of Physiology, 167,* 147–158.

Shankweiler, D.P., & Studdert-Kennedy, M. (1967) Identification of consonants and vowels presented to the left and right ears. *Quarterly Journal of Experimental Psychology, 19,* 59–63.

Siqueland, E.R., & DeLucia, C.A. (1969) Visual reinforcement of nonutritive sucking in human infants. *Science, 165,* 1144–1146.

Studdert-Kennedy, M., & Shankweiler, D.P. (1970) Hemispheric specialization for speech perception. *Journal of the Acoustical Society of America, 48,* 579–594.

Tezner, D. (1972) Etude anatomique de l'asymetrie droit-gauche du planum temporale sur 100 cerveaux d'adults. Unpublished doctoral dissertation, Universite de Paris.

Wada, J.A., Clark, R., & Hamm, A. (1973) Asymmetry of temporal and frontal speech zones in 100 adult and 100 infant brains. Paper presented to the 10th International Congress of Neurology, Barcelona.

Witelson, S.F., & Pallie, W. (1973). Left hemisphere specialization for language in the newborn: Anatomical evidence for asymmetry. *Brain, 96,* 641–646.

3

Bilateral Alpha Rhythm in Children During Listening and Looking

RONALD A. COLE
NINA CUMMINGS

When humans are relaxed, drowsy, or in meditative states, the EEG typically reveals a predominance of alpha waves having a frequency between 8 and 12 Hz. If a subject in this state is given a problem to solve, the alpha waves are replaced by asynchronous beta waves having a frequency greater than 12 Hz. The percentage of alpha rhythm may thus be used as a rough measure of the amount of ongoing information processing at a particular cortical location. The more alpha rhythm that is present, the less ongoing information processing is assumed to be occurring. Based on our present knowledge of cerebral specialization of function, we should expect to find less alpha rhythm in the left hemisphere during linguistic tasks than during spatial tasks, while the opposite pattern should occur in the right hemisphere.

Morgan, McDonald, and MacDonald (1971) first recorded differences in bilateral EEG alpha activity as a function of cognitive task. They recorded occipital alpha rhythm while subjects answered questions that required either "analytical" processing (e.g., *Add 16 and 18; What is an English word that begins with S and ends with S?*) or questions designed to initiate spatial processing (e.g., *Picture a child swinging on a swing*). The subjects' bilateral EEG was analyzed in terms of the proportion of right- to left-hemisphere alpha rhythm in the two tasks. It was found that relatively less alpha rhythm occurred in the right hemisphere for 16 of 20 subjects under the spatial condition. In a second study, Morgan, MacDonald, and Hilgard (1974) compared the proportion of right- to left-hemisphere occipital alpha during verbal, numerical, spatial, and musical tasks. As in their earlier research, significantly more alpha activity was observed in the right hemisphere during the analytical tasks than during the spatial tasks. In addition, both analytical and spatial tasks produced a general depression of alpha rhythm in both hemispheres.

Galin and his colleagues have independently confirmed these results. Galin and Ornstein (1972) examined the ratio of right to left EEG power during different cognitive tasks. Their measure of power—the integrated raw EEG signal between 1 and 35 Hz—is roughly equivalent to the alpha rhythm measures used in the Morgan *et al.*, studies, since alpha waves are of greater amplitude than beta waves. Thus, an increase in the amount of alpha rhythm in one hemisphere would also produce an increase in the overall power of the integrated EEG for that hemisphere. Galin and Ornstein (1972) examined bilateral EEG in both temporal (T_3, T_4) and parietal (P_3, P_4) lobes for verbal tasks (writing or mentally composing a letter) and spatial tasks (Kohs Block Design and Minnesota Paper Form Board test). The results showed that the ratio of right-hemisphere power to left-hemisphere power was greater on the verbal than on the spatial tasks.

In a second study, Galin and Ellis (1975) replicated and extended their previous results to include evoked potentials. In this experiment the integrated EEG power in the alpha band was recorded from temporal and parietal sites while the subject was either writing or constructing a two-dimensional pattern with colored blocks. During these tasks, subjects were also presented with light flashes every 3 seconds and an evoked response was recorded to each flash. Galin and Ellis report that the alpha power ration Right/Left was higher in the writing task than in the spatial task at all cortical locations for all subjects. In addition, the evoked potential Right/Left power ratio was also higher during the verbal tasks.

The experimental technique used in these experiments represents a novel approach to the study of cerebral specialization during ongoing information processing. The present research was designed as a preliminary investigation of lateralization of cognitive function in 4- to 6-year-old children.

METHOD

Subjects

The entire student population of the Carnegia—Mellon Children's School served as subjects. The majority of children at this school come from upper-middle-class homes. At the time of testing, the children ranged in age from 3.3 to 6.2 years of age. There were 2 3-year-olds (3.3, 3.11), 18 4-year-olds (4.0 to 4.11), 17 5-year-olds (5.0 to 5.11) and 5 6-year-olds (6.0 to 6.2). Hand preference tests conducted at the end of the experiment revealed only 3 of the 42 children to be left handed. The data for the three left handers was excluded from the analysis. In addition, 4 children were unable or unwilling to complete the experimental session, so that the final sample consisted of 35 children between the ages of 3 and 6. Each child was tested individually in a session lasting approximately 25 min.

Stimuli and Apparatus

The stimuli consisted of two short stories and a silent movie. The stories were taken from a children's reader and were suggested by the staff of the children's school. The stories were thought to contain material that would captivate all of the subjects. Each story took approximately 5 min to read and was found to hold the child's attention adequately. The movie was a 5-min color cartoon based on Walt Disney's *101 Dalmations.* The cartoon was shown on a small screen placed 4 feet in front of the child, using a Bell and Howell "Super 8" projector.

The bilateral alpha rhythm was recorded using two Alphaphone Brainwave Analyzers manufactured by Aquarius Electronics. The bandpass filter on each analyzer was set between 8 and 12 Hz, and each analyzer was calibrated before and after the experiment to ensure accuracy. No "drift" was found to occur. EEG was recorded from each hemisphere using a bipolar recording system consisting of three silver-plated surface electrodes. The percentage of alpha rhythm from each hemisphere, integrated over a 2.5-sec interval, was displayed continuously on a meter on the front of the brain wave analyzer. The percentage of alpha rhythm for each hemisphere was monitored by reading these dials at 5-sec intervals during the experiment and recording the percentage value. A Hunter counter–timer with a digital display placed between the two brain wave analyzers signaled the 5-sec intervals.

Procedure

Prior to the week of experimentation, we brought one of the brain wave analyzers and one set of electrodes into the children's school to familiarize the children with the equipment. We placed the electrodes on one of the teachers, on ourselves, and finally let the children try them out. Under our supervision, the children turned the unfamiliar knobs, watched the lights blink, and listened to the noise of brain waves. This familiarization process served to dispel the fear of most children toward the strange equipment and to provide a willingness on their part to participate later in the actual experiment.

Each child, accompanied by a teacher, was tested individually in a familiar laboratory room separated from the classroom. The presence of the teacher as well as an initial game of letting each child play with the digital counter–timer were used to maximize incentive and cooperation. If at this point the child was obviously reluctant to be placed under the electrodes, he/she was eliminated from the experiment. The child was then seated in a chair behind a small desk with his/her back to the brain wave analyzers. The second experimenter then applied the electrodes (Figure 1).

The electrode placement usually took between 1 and 2 min. The child's forehead was first cleaned with alcohol. An elastic terrycloth headband was then placed around his head, as shown in Figure 1. The headband was used to hold the

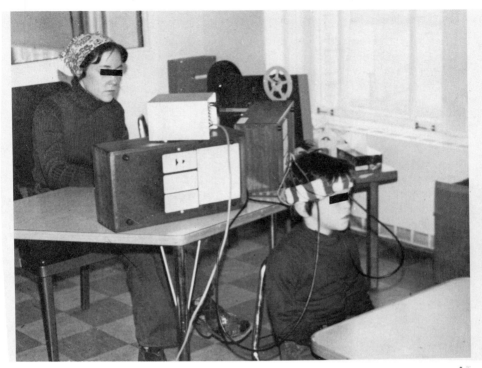

Figure 1. The subject, with electrodes in place beneath the headband, is seated directly in front of the two brain wave analyzers. The Hunter counter—timer is shown on top of the left analyzer. The movie projector is beside the right analyzer.

electrodes in place. Four of the electrodes were placed on the child's forehead: The two ground electrodes were placed at the center of the forehead, while the other two were placed approximately 1 inch above the child's eyebrows. The remaining two electrodes were placed one finger's width above each ear. Although placement was not determined by precise landmarks on the skull, it was approximately the same for all subjects, and was justified by the convenience and ease of the placement procedure. It was immediately apparent by looking at the brain wave analyzer when a good electrode placement had been obtained. Bilateral alpha rhythm was thus recorded between frontal and temporal sites.

The child was then read the first story either by the teacher or by the experimenter. The reader's chair was placed directly in front of the child at eye level. The child was told he would see a cartoon after the story was completed and was allowed to talk and ask questions about the story. The child's second task was to watch the movie. The child was instructed not to talk during the movie. Following the cartoon, the second story was read to the child, and again questions were allowed. The second story was included so that alpha rhythm differences between the stories and the cartoon could not be attributed to a general effect of relaxation over the course of the experiment.

While the child was occupied with the story and the cartoon, one of the experimenters recorded the subject's bilateral alpha rhythm. This experimenter was operating "blind," since he/she did not know which brain wave analyzer was connected to which hemisphere. The experimenter watched the Hunter timer and recorded the percentage of alpha rhythm from one of the analyzers every 5 sec. Since the experimenter alternated between the two dials every 5 sec, alpha activity was recorded at 10-sec intervals from each hemisphere. The first percentage was recorded approximately 30 sec after the story or cartoon began, and recordings were taken at 10-sec intervals from each hemisphere for 4 min. There were thus 24 percentage scores for each hemisphere for each cognitive task. Since these scores were found to be quite stable over the 4-min interval, a mean percentage score was calculated for each hemisphere for each story and for the cartoon.

Following the second story, hand preference was established by placing a crayon and blank sheet of paper in front of the child and asking him/her to write his/her name or draw a picture. In addition, the experimenter asked the child to "play catch" with one of the pillows in the room, and the preferred arm was observed.

RESULTS

The mean percentage of alpha rhythm for the two hemispheres during each story and the Cartoon is presented for the individual subjects in Table 1. The percentage scores were first analyzed using the ratio comparisons employed by previous investigators examining bilateral EEG. Galin and Ornstein (1972) compared the ratio of right to left hemisphere alpha (R/L) for the different tasks; Morgan *et al.* (1971) examined the ratio of right hemisphere alpha to total alpha (R/R + L), while Morgan *et al.* (1974) compared the proportion of R−L/R + L for the different cognitive tasks.

Correlated t-tests comparing Story 1 and the Cartoon reviewed no significant differences for any of these measures. A comparison of the Cartoon and Story 2 revealed significantly more right-hemisphere alpha during the story (consistent with Galin and Ornstein, 1972) for the R/L measure (t_{34} = 2.28, $p < .01$), but no difference was found for either of the other two measures. Thus, five of the six comparisons do not support the results of previous research with adults.

An examination of each hemisphere separately during the different tasks suggests that the type of stimulation presented to the child does affect ongoing EEG activity. As Figure 2 shows, children produce more alpha in the left hemisphere while watching a cartoon than when listening to a story. This effect is as strong for the 4-year-olds as it is for the 6-year-olds. Of the 35 children tested, 28 increased their percentage of left-hemisphere alpha from Story 1 to the Cartoon (t_{34} = 6.7, $p < .01$), while 24 of 35 children produced a decrease in left-hemisphere alpha from

TABLE 1   Mean Percentage of Alpha Rhythm for Each Child under Each Condition

			Left hemisphere			Right hemisphere		
Name	Age at time of testing	Sex	Story 1	Cartoon	Story 2	Story 1	Cartoon	Story 2
1. Dina	3.3	F	20	25	18	29	50	30
2. Joshua	3.11	M	17	22	21	47	49	49
3. Daniel	4.0	M	21	21	19	41	45	44
4. Katy	4.0	F	23	23	22	49	34	39
5. Christina	4.1	F	19	23	18	36	33	32
6. Laurie S.	4.1	F	21	27	21	36	33	30
7. Thaddeus	4.2	M	15	20	22	12	9	19
8. Chris	4.2	M	22	22	21	26	23	23
9. Stephanie	4.2	F	26	25	24	22	22	24
10. Eben	4.4	M	18	25	18	31	35	25
11. Peter A.	4.5	M	15	20	14	37	46	47
12. John	4.6	M	20	21	20	18	17	27
13. Katie	4.8	F	18	19	23	8	19	12
14. Billy	4.11	M	28	35	24	21	29	19
15. Jenny	4.11	F	20	18	30	12	21	14
16. Peter M.	5.0	M	32	37	38	21	24	18
17. Peter B.	5.0	M	16	14	30	19	21	15
18. Lee	5.1	M	17	23	19	21	39	34
19. Laura	5.1	F	17	18	14	25	36	38
20. Ellen	5.2	F	22	21	21	16	12	15
21. Ezra	5.3	M	7	16	16	21	7	23
22. Brian J.	5.4	M	15	26	16	26	42	34
23. Sarah	5.4	F	17	18	16	24	29	29
24. Kevin	5.5	M	16	20	22	16	25	38
25. Blake	5.6	M	17	25	18	24	38	30
26. Amy	5.8	F	12	19	16	26	20	19
27. Greg	5.8	M	13	24	17	7	14	14
28. Barbara	5.10	F	12	19	19	26	33	42
29. Eddy	5.10	M	14	18	18	14	23	33
30. Robert	5.11	M	18	23	18	9	20	22
31. Sandy	6.0	F	15	17	13	18	18	15
32. Mona	6.0	F	8	19	16	21	40	33
33. Bret	6.0	M	15	21	17	1	6	5
34. Jill	6.0	F	11	13	16	12	19	18
35. Julie	6.2	F	13	21	18	27	21	29

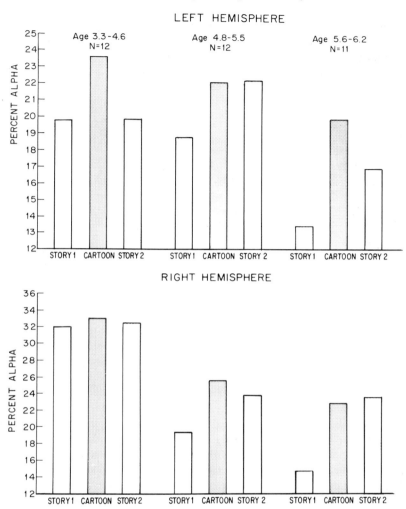

Figure 2. Mean percentage alpha rhythm in each hemisphere for each cognitive task.

the cartoon to the second story ($t_{34} = 2.06, p < .05$). Twenty of the children produced first an increase in left-hemisphere alpha from the first story to the cartoon and then a decrease from the cartoon to the second story ($\chi^2 = 10.54, p < .01$). If we accept the assumption that an increase in alpha rhythm indicates an attenuated level of information processing, the results are consistent with the notion that the left-hemisphere temporal lobe is more involved in ongoing verbal activity than in ongoing visual activity in young children.

It is interesting to note that the pattern of results observed in the left hemisphere was reflected to a lesser extent in the right hemisphere during the different tasks. In general, there was an increase in alpha activity from Story 1 to the Cartoon (t_{34} = 3.54, p < .01), as found in the left hemisphere, but there was no corresponding decrease in alpha rhythm during Story 2.

DISCUSSION

The experiment was intended as a preliminary investigation of the effects of cognitive task on children's bilateral alpha rhythm. As such, we want to stress that the results must be viewed as merely suggestive. While the Alphaphone Brainwave Analyzers had several advantages—such as being portable and easily connected to the subject—they did not provide the desired precision in the collection and analysis of data. Ideally, in an experiment measuring EEG activity, one would like to have a continuous record of the overall alpha density in each hemisphere. A comparison of the area under the waveform in the alpha band in each hemisphere would then provide an accurate measure of the relative amount of alpha in each hemisphere during different cognitive tasks. By contrast, our measure of alpha rhythm was provided by one experimenter reading a dial on a meter at 5-sec intervals (10 sec for each hemisphere). The width of the entire meter was approximately 1.5 inches and the marks on the meter indicating 5% differences in alpha were only about $\frac{1}{8}$ inch apart. To make matters worse, on about one-fifth of the trials the dial on the meter would be moving during the observation period and the experimenter would have to estimate the percentage value. Clearly, our procedure provided only a crude measure of the percentage of alpha rhythm in each hemisphere.

Having described the various deficiencies of our data collection procedure, we would like to assert that the increase in alpha rhythm in the left hemisphere during the cartoon probably represents a real effect. We defend this conclusion on a number of grounds. First, after actually recording the percentage scores during the experiment, it soon became clear to both of us that the dial could be read quickly and accurately. In other words, the experimenters learned a skill, and the feeling was that the readings were made with consistency. Moreover, any variation introduced by the experimenter during the recording procedure should have been randomly distributed across the different tasks. There is no reason to assume that the experimenter, who did not know which machine was connected to which hemisphere, would consistently record higher scores from the brain wave analyzer connected to the left hemisphere during the cartoon. Second, although the size of the increase in left-hemisphere alpha rhythm during the cartoon was quite small—about 4%—the effect was extremely consistent across subjects. Two of every three children produced more left-hemisphere alpha rhythm during the cartoon than during *either* story. Moreover, as Figure 2 reveals, the effect is still obtained—with a single exception—when the children are divided into subgroups according to their age at the time of testings. Thus, the pattern of results observed in the left hemisphere—first an increase in alpha from the Story 1 to the cartoon followed by a decrease in alpha from the cartoon to Story 2—is difficult to explain in terms of experimentally induced artifacts.

In summary, our results suggest that there is an increase in left-hemisphere alpha rhythm—presumably indicating a decrease in information processing in that hemisphere—when 4- to 6-year-old children observe a cartoon, as compared to their left-hemisphere alpha rhythm when listening to a story. We did not detect a similar pattern of results in the right hemisphere.

We conclude that while our results are merely suggestive, the measurement of bilateral alpha rhythm during different cognitive tasks presents an exciting paradigm for examining the cerebral specialization of function during ongoing information processing in both children and adults.

ACKNOWLEDGMENT

We gratefully acknowledge the many hours of assistance provided by the director, Dr. Ann Taylor, and staff of the Carnegie—Mellon University Children's School: Robert Skena, Judy Nathanson, Jean Eubanks, Barbara Ray, and Dorothy Hanna.

REFERENCES

Galin, D., & Ellis, R.R. (1975) Asymmetry in evoked potentials as an index of lateralized cognitive processes: Relation to EEG alpha assymetry. *Neuropsychologia, 13,* 45–50.
Galin, D., & Ornstein, R. (1972) Lateral specialization of cognitive mode: An EEG study. *Psychophysiology, 9,* 412–418.
Morgan, A.H., MacDonald, H., & Hilgard, E.R. (1974) EEG alpha: Lateral assymetry related to task, and hypnotizability. *Psychophysiology, 11,* 275–282.
Morgan, A.H., McDonald, P.J., & MacDonald, H. (1971) Differences in bilateral alpha activity as a function of experimental task, with a note on lateral eye movements and hypnotizability. *Neuropsychologia, 9,* 459–469.

4

Multiple Language Experience and the Development of Cerebral Dominance

RICHARD STARCK, FRED GENESEE,
WALLACE E. LAMBERT, MICHAEL SEITZ

Ever since Broadbent (1954) devised the dichotic listening paradigm, many researchers have used the technique to explore lateralization of cerebral function (e.g., Bryden, 1963; Kimura, 1961, 1964, 1967). Research utilizing the technique has demonstrated that when right-handed human subjects are presented verbal, in contrast to nonverbal, stimuli dichotically, they tend to process more efficiently information received through the right in contrast to the left ear. That is, when verbal stimuli are presented dichotically, subjects tend to recall first and more accurately verbal material presented to their right ear. This pattern of ear asymmetry may be related to anatomical asymmetries in the auditory pathways (Rosenzweig, 1951; Sinha, 1959; Seitz & Mononen, 1974), to asymmetries in acoustical analysis (Porter & Berlin, 1975), and to asymmetries in cortical functions (Kimura, 1961, 1967; Milner, 1958).

Even though current electrophysiological (Molfese, 1972, and Chapter 2, this volume) and anatomical (Witelson & Pallie, 1973) evidence indicates that some cerebral asymmetry is present at or shortly after birth, measures of ear asymmetry in general suggest that the strength of cerebral asymmetry, at least for the processing of linguistic matter, increases with age (Kimura, 1963; Knox & Kimura, 1970; Geffner & Hochberg, 1971) and stabilizes around age 12 (Lenneberg, 1967; Penfield & Robert, 1959; Zangwill, 1960). However, estimates of the age when stability is achieved vary widely from study to study, and it may well be that stability is achieved much earlier than the onset of puberty (Krashen & Harshman, 1972). This variance may be due to differences in experimental measures and, as data from the present study suggest, differences among subjects in types of language experience.

The research of Geffner and Hochberg (1971) indicates that age of onset of cerebral asymmetry may also be influenced by such environmental factors as social class. These researchers report that a group of children from low socioeconomic backgrounds did not demonstrate a right-ear advantage until 7 years of age, whereas a comparison group of children from middle socioeconomic backgrounds demonstrated laterality by age 4. However, it was not clear from their study which characteristics of social class background were responsible for the observed differences.

Using a variation of the standard dichotic technique, Bever (1970) tested two groups of 4.5-year-old boys from New York's Harlem, one that had participated in an "intellectual enrichment" program and a comparison group that had not. At the end of the training period, it was found that children with the enrichment experience demonstrated a significantly stronger right-ear effect than did those in the comparison group. These results supported Bever's original contention that "experimental enrichment" facilitates the development of cerebral asymmetry.

This research led us to test out the generality of Bever's enrichment hypothesis with a highly linguistic form of enrichment provided by "immersion" programs, that is, educational programs that provide instruction and academic activities in a second language from kindergarten on. A series of studies have shown that the immersion experience has no detrimental effects on first language development; at the same time children in these programs develop second language skills far superior to those attained by children in regular second language programs (Lambert & Tucker, 1972; Swain, 1974). In fact, there is some evidence that immersion may favorably affect cognitive development (Bain, 1974; Balkan, 1970; Ben-Zeev, 1972; Cummins & Gulutsan, 1974; Ianco-Worrall, 1972). The experimental children in the present study were attending a "double immersion" program in a Montreal elementary school. In this program, the children, who were all from monolingual English homes, received part of their course instruction in French and part in Hebrew; no instruction was given in English (Genesee, Sheiner, Tucker & Lambert, 1975).

Speculating that multilingual experience might be a strong form of enrichment (Bain, 1974; Balkan, 1970; Ben-Zeev, 1972; Cummins & Gulutsan, 1974; Lambert, 1974; Peal & Lambert, 1962), the working hypothesis for the present study was that children who have had linguistically enriched schooling may develop a more lateralized verbal processing system than comparable children without that form of linguistic enrichment.

METHOD AND PROCEDURE

Subjects

All the children were native speakers of English, and all were of the Jewish faith. Those referred to as "monolingual" attended schools where all course instruction is given in English, and where no other language was used at home. The "trilingual" subjects were attending a school in which course instruction was given exclusively in French and in Hebrew; these children received no formal schooling in English.

There is no reason to believe that students in the double immersion program were selected in any way for language competence. Rather their attendance at this particular school reflected their parents desire to send their children to a parochial school where Hebraic studies were a traditional part of the curriculum. The public school used for comparison purposes did not have an immersion program available for its pupils. All course instruction in the comparison school was in English.

The children were selected from three grades: kindergarten, Grade 1 and Grade 2; the average ages in years and months were 6:2, 7:1, and 8:1 for the monolingual groups, and 6:0, 6:11, and 7:11 for the trilingual groups. There were eight subjects in each monolingual grade—four boys and four girls; in the trilingual grades there were four boys and four girls at the kindergarten level, three boys and five girls at the Grade 1 level, and five boys and three girls at the Grade 2 level.

The three trilingual groups were tested for proficiency in French, Hebrew, and English, and their performance was compared with that of matched samples of children who were studying French as a second language in a traditional Hebrew school (see Genesee *et al.,* 1975). The two groups were found to have the same proficiency in English and Hebrew language skills, but the immersion students were significantly better in all aspects of the French language.

Subjects in the present study were matched in advance for IQ as measured by Raven's Progressive Matrices, Colour Version (1956). Care was taken to ensure that all subjects came from similar socioeconomic backgrounds; using Blishen's (1962) index of socioeconomic status, all subjects came from families falling within the top two categories of the scale, indicating that they were all from upper-middle-class families. Finally, since handedness is strongly correlated with cerebral asymmetry (Goodglass & Quadfasel, 1954; Wada & Rusmussen, 1960) only right-handed children were included in the samples.

Apparatus and Testing Materials

Preparation of Tapes

The method used to prepare the tapes was similar to that described by Mononen (1971). The tape was recorded on a Sony TC-654-4 Quadriadic tape recorder. The stimulus pairs were first matched as closely as possible for intensity and stimulus onset using the Sony tape recorder's input and output VU meters. To further check the synchrony and intensity of the stimulus pairs, they were played through a Tektronix type RM-564 storage oscilloscope. The calibrated storage scope enables one to match the two stimulus words for simultaneous onset of their initial phonemes within 10 msec.

The stimulus words were in English and consisted of various combinations of monosyllabic numbers one through ten, excluding the digit seven. Each digit occurred equally often in each ear. In all there were 15 pairs. The tape consisted of

5 single pairs (e.g., "six" in one channel, "three in the other), 5 double pairs (e.g., "six" and "three" followed by "two" and "nine"), and 5 triple pairs. Thus, a total of 30 words were presented in each ear with a 5-sec space between pairs and a 10-sec space between trials.

Procedure

Headset position was counterbalanced across subjects in the following manner. Half of the children wore the earphones with the right earphone on the right ear and the left earphone on the left ear and the other half wore the earphones in the reverse position. Thus, half of the subjects heard the stimuli recorded in Channel 1 in the right ear and the stimuli recorded in Channel 2 in the left ear, while the reverse was true for the remaining half of the subjects. Volume levels for both channels were equated and set at constant low level.

Subjects were tested individually in a quiet room. They were told that they would hear numbers presented through the earphones, and that at least two different numbers would be played at exactly the same time. In addition, they were informed in advance of the number of pairs they would hear and were asked to repeat what they heard after all members of a set had been presented. They were encouraged to guess if unsure of what they heard. Care was taken to explain the directions in detail in advance. Subjects repeated what they heard within the 10-sec intertrial while the experimenter recorded all responses.

Each subject was given a practice run, consisting of one complete presentation of the stimulus tape and then, after a short rest period, the experimental task began.

RESULTS AND DISCUSSION

Since accuracy and order of recall are both effective measures of ear asymmetry (Broadbent, 1954), analyses of variance were performed for each measure separately. The basic variables in each analysis were *Language Experience* (monolingual, trilingual), *Ear* (right, left), and *Age* (6-, 7-, and 8-year-olds).

Accuracy of Recall

For accuracy of recall, there were two significant main effects (see Table 1): (1) an Ear effect—words arriving at the right ear were identified more accurately than words arriving at the left ear [F (1,42) = 15.12, $p < .01$]; (2) an Age effect—accuracy improved with age [F (2,42) = 10.88, $p < .01$].

There were also two significant interactions: (1) As predicted, there was a significant interaction of Language Experience × Ear, indicating that the trilingual group demonstrated a clear right-ear advantage while the monolingual group did not [F (1,42) = 4.75, $p < .05$]. (2) Finally, there was a significant Age × Ear interaction [F (2,42) = 3.6890, $p < .05$], indicating that although the right ear had a consistent advantage over the left, the magnitude of the advantage decreased with age.

TABLE 1 Mean Left- and Right-Ear Scores for Accuracy of Response: Study 1 (1974)

Language experience	Ear stimulated	Grade K Age 6	Grade 1 Age 7	Grade 2 Age 8	Mean ear scores K + 1 + 2	Mean group scores L + R
Monolingual	Left	19.250	23.125	26.125	22.83	
(N = 24)	Right	22.125	21.500	27.375	23.67	23.25
Trilingual	Left	19.375	22.000	24.500	21.96	
(N = 24)	Right	24.125	23.375	25.250	24.92	23.44
Mean age scores		21.22	23.00	25.81		

Apparently, with age, the child becomes more capable of processing both left- and right-ear information. One would, thus, expect that the ability to repeat accurately both items of a dichotic pair (i.e., double corrects) would increase with age (Porter & Berlin, 1975), and we did in fact find a significant increase in double correct scores with age $[F(2,14) = 11.02, p < .01]$.

Order of Recall

The order of recall analysis for Study 1 also provides evidence for a right-ear advantage (see Table 2). Right-ear stimuli were reported first more often than were left-ear stimuli $[F(1,42) = 8.21, p < .01]$. However, this right-ear advantage is primarily due to trilingual rather than monolingual subjects, as indicated by the Language Experience × Ear interaction $[F(1,42) = 5.53, p < .025]$. No other significant main effects or interactions were found.

In summary, we adopted Broadbent's dichotic listening procedure as a means of measuring the relationship of lateral asymmetry to enriched language experience. Our working hypothesis was that, with factors such as social class background and measured IQ controlled, children with a multilingual experience would demonstrate greater asymmetry than monolingual children. Support for the prediction was

TABLE 2 Mean Number of Times Recall was Initiated with Information Received through Left versus Right Ear: Study 1 (1974)[a]

Language experience	Ear stimulated	Grade K Age 6	Grade 1 Age 7	Grade 2 Age 8	Mean ear scores K + 1 + 2
Monolingual	Left	12.875	14.875	16.125	14.625
(N = 24)	Right	16.000	14.875	13.875	14.917
Trilingual	Left	13.250	12.625	13.500	13.125
(N = 24)	Right	15.750	16.625	15.875	16.083

[a]Left- and right-ear scores do not total to 30 if a subject did not correctly recall at least half of the stimuli presented on any one trial.

provided by both accuracy and order of recall results although our trilingual group of subjects did not show a consistent right-ear advantage at all three age levels. Overall, our findings lend support to Bever's contention that it is possible to influence the development of cerebral asymmetry by providing an enriched learning experience.

Because of the potentially controversial nature of these findings, we felt it was important to substantiate them, if possible, in a follow-up study. Therefore, 1 year later we went back to the same grade levels and retested the kindergarten and Grade 1 pupils who were then in Grades 1 and 2 and added new 6-year-old trilingual and monolingual kindergarten groups, making sure that they were comparable in ethnic and socioeconomic background and Raven IQ scores. Thus, we tested comparable groups of 6-, 7-, and 8-year olds and used exactly the same testing procedure and analyses as in Study 1.

RESULTS: STUDY 2

Accuracy of Recall

For accuracy of recall, three main effects were demonstrated (see Table 3): (1) an Ear effect—words arriving at the right ear were identified more accurately than words arriving at the left ear [F (1,42) = 9.51, $p < .01$]; (2) an Age effect—overall performance of the subjects improved with age [F (2,42) = 31.81, $p < .001$]; (3) a Language effect—trilingual subjects were more accurate than monolingual subjects [F (1,42) = 14.49, $p < .01$]. Unlike the first study, there was no Language Experience X Ear interaction, indicating that the monolinguals showed as much right-ear advantage this time as the trilinguals. No other main effects or interactions were found.

Order of Recall

There was one main effect due to Ear (see Table 4)—items presented to the right ear were reported prior to those presented to the left ear [F (1,42) = 6.77, $p < .05$]. Unlike Study 1, there was no significant Language Experience X Ear interaction, which means that both monolingual and trilingual groups contributed to the observed right-ear order of report advantage.

In summary, the results of the replication are not completely consistent. The variability of results from study to study may be due to the age groups we worked with, to the unreliability of the measures themselves, or to the theoretically more relevant possibility that experiential differences between our groups influence the development of ear asymmetry. Our argument hinges on the general consistency of the trilingual relative to the monolingual subjects. The trilingual subjects, disregarding age-group divisions, demonstrated a consistent pattern of right-ear superiority on both accuracy and order of recall measures in both studies. In contrast, the

TABLE 3   Mean Left and Right Ear Scores for Accuracy of Response Study 2 (1975)

Language experience	Ear stimulated	Grade K Age 6	Grade 1 Age 7	Grade 2 Age 8	Mean ear scores K + 1 + 2	Mean group scores L + R
Monolingual	Left	14.380	17.120	23.500	18.333	
(N = 24)	Right	17.500	20.000	25.750	12.083	19.708
Trilingual	Left	19.620	20.880	25.125	21.875	
(N = 24)	Right	18.380	25.250	28.250	23.958	22.917
Mean age scores		17.469	20.812	25.656		

monolingual subjects did not show a consistent right-ear advantage, giving evidence of it in Study 2 but not in Study 1.

In conclusion, then, the general trends of our findings lend support to the enrichment hypothesis and suggest that the diversified language experiences may have strengthened and helped to stabilize the cerebral asymmetry of our trilingual subjects earlier than that of their monolingual peers, at least insofar as this is reflected in ear asymmetry affects. There are, however, inconsistencies in the data (e.g., the 6-year-old trilinguals in Study 2 go against the general trend for the trilingual subjects as a whole) that qualify the reliability of the outcomes, especially with the youngest age group. Furthermore, the present results pertain only to children from middle-class homes.

On the matter of age, Bever's subjects were almost 2 years younger than our youngest group, and thus their enrichment experiences may have had a relatively stronger impact than the enrichment experience of our subjects. Furthermore, if Krashen and Harshman (1972) are correct in their belief that cerebral lateralization is complete by age 5, then the differences demonstrated between our groups may reflect other types of cognitive enhancement besides those reflected by cerebral laterality per se.

In spite of these inconsistencies in our experiments, bi- or multilingual experiences do seem to help establish more reliable ear asymmetry effects, which are

TABLE 4   Mean Number of Times Recall Was Initiated with Information Received through Left versus Right Ear Study 2 (1975)[a]

Language experience	Ear stimulated	Grade K Age 6	Grade 1 Age 7	Grade 2 Age 8	Mean ear scores K + 1 + 2
Monolingual	Left	14.000	13.875	13.500	13.790
(N = 24)	Right	14.125	15.505	16.375	15.333
Trilingual	Left	11.500	12.375	13.125	12.333
(N = 24)	Right	14.125	16.125	16.500	15.583

[a]Left- and right-ear scores do not total to 30 if a subject did not correctly recall at least half of the stimuli presented on any one trial.

thought to reflect enhanced cerebral asymmetry. Whether or not this helps in the overall development of the child's linguistic processing system is another question. We now need to determine more clearly when the multilingual experiences might have maximum effect. One next step might be to study younger subjects, say 4 years of age, and at the same time to explore alternative means of assessing cerebral asymmetry. These considerations, in fact, have now been incorporated into several ongoing studies.

ACKNOWLEDGMENTS

This research was supported in part by grants from the Canada Council and Defence Research Board of W. E. Lambert and G. R. Tucker. The authors would like to thank Larry Mononen and Josiane Hamers for technical assistance and valuable advice and the School of Human Communication Disorders, McGill University, for the use of their electronic equipment, funded by the Medical Research Council of Canada.

REFERENCES

Bain, B.C. (1974) Bilingualism and cognition: Toward a general theory. In S. Carey (Ed.), *Bilingualism, biculturalism and education.* Edmonton Univ. of Alberta.
Balkan, L. (1970) *Les effets du bilinguisme Francais-Anglais sur les aptitudes intellectuelles.* Bruxelles: Aimau.
Ben-Zeev, S. (1972) The influence of bilingualism on cognitive development and cognitive strategy. Ph.D. abstract, Univ. of Chicago, *Committee on Human Development,* June 10.
Bever, T.G. (1970) Are there psycho-social interactions that maintain the low I.Q. score of the poor? Columbia Univ. mimeo.
Blishen, B.R. (1962) A socioeconomic index for occupations in Canada. *Canadian Review of Sociology and Anthropology, IV* (1), 41–53.
Broadbent, D.E. (1954) The role of auditory localization in attention and memory span. *Journal of Experimental Psychology, 3,* 47.
Bryden, M.P. (1963) Ear preference in auditory perception. *Journal of Experimental Psychology, 65,* 103–105.
Cummins, J.P., & Gulutsan, M. (1974) Some effects of bilingualism on cognitive functioning. In S. Carey (Ed.), *Bilingualism, biculturalism and education.* Edmonton: Univ. of Alberta.
Geffner, D.S., & Hochberg, I. (1971) Ear laterality performance of children from low and middle socioeconomic levels on a verbal dichotic listening task. *Cortex, 3,* 193–203.
Genesee, F., Sheiner, E., Tucker, G.R., & Lambert, W.E. (1976) An experiment in trilingual education. *The Canadian Modern Language Review, 32,* 115–128.
Goodglass, H., & Quadfasel, F.A. (1954) Language laterality in left-handed aphasics. *Brain, 77,* 521–548.
Ianco-Worrall, A.D. (1972) Bilingualism and cognitive development. *Child Development, 43,* 1390–1400.
Kimura, D. (1961a) Some effects of temporal lobe damage on auditory perception. *Canadian Journal of Psychology, 15,* 156–165.
Kimura, D. (1963) Speech lateralization in young children as determined by an auditory test. *Journal of Comparative and Physiological Psychology, 56,* 899–902.

Kimura, D. (1964) Left right differences in the perception of melodies. *Quarterly Journal of Experimental Psychology, 16,* 355–359.

Kimura, D. (1967) Functional asymmetry of the brain in dichotic listening. *Cortex, 3,* 163–178.

Knox, C., & Kimura, D. (1970) Cerebral processing of nonverbal sounds in boys and girls. *Neuropsychologia, 8,* 227–237.

Krashen, S., & Harshman, R. (1972) Lateralization and the critical period. *UCLA Working Papers in Phonetics, 23,* 13–21.

Lambert, W.E. (1974) Cultural and learning as factors in learning and education. In F.E. Aboud & R.D. Meade (Eds.), *Cultural factors in learning and education.* Bellingham: Western Washington State College.

Lambert, W.E., & Tucker, G.R. (1972) *Bilingual education of children: The St. Lambert experiment.* Rowley, Newbury House.

Lenneberg, E.H. (1967) *The biological foundations of language.* New York: Wiley.

Milner, B. (1958) Psychological defects produced by temporal lobe excision. *Proceedings of the; Association for Research into Nervous and Mental Disorders, 36,* 224–257.

Molfese, D.L. (1972) Cerebral asymmetry in infants, children and adults auditory evoked responses to speech and noise stimuli. Unpublished doctoral dissertation, Pennsylvania State Univ.

Mononen, L. (1971) Perceptions on dichotically presented verbal-nonverbal sequences. Unpublished masters' thesis, McGill Univ.

Peal, E., & Lambert, W.E. (1962) The relations of bilingualism to intelligence. *Psychology Monographs, 76,* No. 27, Whole No. 546.

Penfield, W., & Robert, L. (1959) *Speech and brain mechanism.* Princeton, New Jersey: Princeton Univ. Press.

Porter, F.J., & Berlin, C. (1975) On interpreting developmental changes in the dichotic right-ear advantage. *Brain and Language, 2,* 1975, 186–200.

Raven, J.C. (1956) *Coloured progressive matrices: Sets A, Ab, B.* London: Lewis.

Rosenzweig, M.R. (1951) Representation of the two ears at the auditory cortex. *American Journal of Physiology, 167,* 147–158.

Seitz, M., & Mononen, L. (1974) Averaged electroencephalic response (AER) differences between ipsilateral and contralateral hemispheres in a dichotic listening paradigm. Paper presented at the American Speech and Hearing Association Meeting, Las Vegas, Nevada.

Sinha, S.P. (1959) The role of the temporal lobe in hearing. Unpublished Masters' thesis, McGill Univ.

Swain, M. (1974) French immersion programs across Canada. *The Canadian Modern Language Review, 31,* 117–130.

Wada, J., & Rasmussen, T. (1960) Intracarotid injection of sodium amytal for the lateralization of cerebral speech dominance, experimental and clinical observations. *Journal of Neurosurgery, 17,* 266–282.

Witelson, S., & Pallie, W. (1973) Left hemisphere specialization for language in the newborn: Neuroanatomical evidence of asymmetry. *Brain, 96,* 641–646.

Zangwill, O. (1960) *Cerebral dominance and its relation to Psychological function.* Edinburgh: Oliver & Boyd.

5

Visual Field and Cerebral Hemisphere Preferences in Bilinguals

JOSIANE F. HAMERS
WALLACE E. LAMBERT

The concept of cerebral hemispheric dominance for language functions dates back to Broca's (1969) discussion of the association between aphasia and lesions or disease in the left hemisphere. Since that time there has been an accumulation of evidence for shifts of dominance from left to right hemisphere following some lesion to the left in early childhood (Geschwind, 1972; Lenneberg, 1967; Penfield & Roberts, 1969). This neurophysiological evidence for the plasticity of brain functions suggests that there is a critical period for language acquisition during which both hemispheres may be capable of becoming the dominant center for language functions.

Apart from clinical evidence, a number of experimental techniques have been developed to assess cerebral dominance for language. Kimura (1961, 1973) used dichotic listening as a means of demonstrating the asymmetry of the two hemispheres in the auditory perception of verbal material. Bryden (1965) also found that, with right-handed subjects, verbal input data are more readily identified when presented tachistoscopally in the right than in the left visual field.

The relation between cerebral dominance, speech functions, and handedness has been investigated intensively in the past decade (Benton, 1965; Milner, 1962; Zangwill, 1960). From the evidence so far available, it seems clear that right-handedness fairly reliably indicates left-hemisphere dominance for language (Benton, 1965) but left-handedness does not reliably indicate right-hemisphere dominance.

Thus, most available information indicates that language functions are organized or integrated in some way in the dominant, usually the left, cerebral hemisphere.

Nevertheless, subsequent evidence suggests that verbal functions also involve the nondominant hemisphere. For example, Gazzaniga and Sperry (1967) showed that, whereas the expressive aspects of language are apparently confined to the dominant hemisphere, some forms of comprehension of written and spoken words are controlled by the nondominant hemisphere. This leaves open the possibility, then, that verbal recognition may depend on both hemispheres.

Our interest in the topic of cerebral dominance stems from our own work with bilinguals (Hamers & Lambert, 1972, 1974; Lambert, 1969), especially the remarkable ability most bilinguals have of keeping their two languages functionally independent. Most of the clinical observations have been done with monolinguals and amazingly little is known about the cerebral dominance for language in bilinguals. Although there are some clinical reports on bilingual patients who, following a cerebral insult or lesion, lost the use of only one of their languages, the validity of such observations has been questioned by Penfield and Roberts (1959), who argue, from their clinical experience, that a unique brain mechanism likely serves both languages in the case of the bilingual. The investigation of bilingual aphasics by Lambert and Fillenbaum (1959), however, presents a strong argument for differential loss of function in one of a bilingual's languages in the aphasic state; but, even though they proposed that the bilingual's two language systems might have a neurophysiological independence, there was no suggestion that the systems would be necessarily seated in different hemispheres.

The general purpose of the present experiment was to ascertain whether cerebral dominance for one type of verbal activity is located in the same hemisphere for bilinguals regardless of the language used or whether there is some evidence of hemispheric sharing. This is, then, a pilot study limited to a verbal recognition task where speed of recognition of the language of presentation (French or English) is tested using balanced bilinguals. The question is whether or not bilinguals (all right handed) will recognize French and English words equally rapidly when they are presented to one hemisphere as when they are presented to the other.

The rationale behind choosing a language recognition task is the following: When asked to decode verbal stimuli presented to him, the bilingual subject's first step in linguistic processing is to recognize the language of the verbal material presented. This was demonstrated in an experiment by Hamers and Lambert (1974), who found that (a) bilinguals have difficulty decoding verbal material if there are no indications from linguistic or environmental clues as to the language to be used to process the verbal material, and (b) the slightest environmental clue as to which language is the appropriate one for decoding helps the bilingual disambiguate the verbal material and decide on the language to be used for processing. We argue, therefore, that recognition of the linguistic code in which verbal material is presented is either a prerequisite for or the first step in "linguistic processing."

METHOD

Apparatus

The apparatus was similar to that used by Corballis, Miller, and Morgan (1971) in their experiment on interhemispheric matching of visual information. Stimuli were French and English words typed in the center of a clear slide, and presented via a tachistoscope (Scientific Prototype Model GB). A slide projector was fixed on a device that could be moved from a left or a right fixed position, so that each word flashed on the left or on the right from the central fixation point.

The subject was seated in a separate room from the experimenter in front of a 9×9 inch response box provided with two buttons. The subject's hands rested on the box with an index finger on each key. A timer (an Electronic Counter 5212A) connected to the tachistoscope was started by the onset of the slide and stopped whenever one of the keys was pressed. Printouts were available for the elapsed time between stimuli and responses and for the particular keys depressed.

Procedure

The subject was asked simply to press a particular key when an English word appeared on the screen and a different key when a French word appeared. The correspondence between key and language was balanced in the design so that for half of the trials the left key was assigned to English and the right key to French and for the other half of the trials the key—language correspondence was reversed.

Subjects reacted to a total of 140 slides, each with either an English or a French word typed in lowercase letters. Each word was presented either in the left or in the right visual field. There were 35 English words and their French translations; each word appeared twice, once in the left and once in the right visual field. The words were all concrete words with high imagery ratings (Paivio, Yuille, & Madigan, 1968); they were also approximately the same length in their French and English versions. No specific language markers, such as accents in French, were used. The 140 slides (35 English and 35 French words each presented two times) were mixed in a random order with the limitation that half the words would appear first in English and then in French and that half the words would first be presented in the right visual field and then in the left. Each stimulus was exposed for 100 msec, in order to avoid possible eye movements; there was a 2-sec interval between each stimulus word.

In summary, the task required a recognition of the language of presentation. For bilinguals this is something different from differentiating a known code from an unknown one, as would be the case for monolinguals. Instead it calls on the subject who acts as his own control, to categorize words into one or the other of two known codes, with attention given to the relative speed of categorization when the words are presented to contrasting visual fields and presumably contrasting cerebral hemispheres.

Subjects

The subjects were 15 French–English right-handed bilingual adults, all of whom reported that they had normal vision and had no need for correction. They were considered as balanced in their command of French and English if (a) their speed of reaction in a color naming task in French and in English was equivalent (if the difference between their mean reaction time in the two languages exceeded 100 msec they did not qualify); and (b) on a global judgment of their bilingual proficiency they were considered to be native speakers of English by an English-speaking judge and as native speakers of French by a French-speaking judge. Other information about the age of acquisition of the two languages (they had to be fluent in both languages before the age of 10) and about their personal use of the two languages was available, but no attempt was made to select them as compound or coordinate bilinguals (see Lambert, 1969).

The experiment lasted 20 min; subjects had a short rest halfway through, while the slide projector carousel was changed.

RESULTS AND DISCUSSION

Mean reaction times were calculated for each subject for the following subsets: (a) French words appearing in the right visual field, (b) French words appearing in the left visual field, (c) English words appearing in the right visual field, and (d) English words appearing in the left visual field. As errors of language identification were extremely rare (for most subjects there were no errors), the analysis of the results was restricted to the reaction times for correct responses only. A two-way analysis of variance (two levels of language of stimulus, French and English, and two levels of visual field, left and right) was performed. The results are: (a) there is no language of stimulus effect ($F_{1,14}$ = 1.53; n.s.), i.e., subjects identify French words as fast as they do English ones; (b) there is a significant difference between the speed of responding to words given in the left in contrast to the right visual fields ($F_{1,14}$ = 5.01; $p < .05$), meaning that right-handed bilinguals recognize faster the language of a word when presented to the right of the fixation point than they do when it is presented to the left of the fixation point (mean reaction times are 949 and 979 msec); and (c) there is no interaction effect of language of presentation and visual field ($F_{1,14}$ < 1), which means that bilinguals recognize equally fast French or English words presented on the same side. The mean reaction times are given in Table 1.

Of the 15 subjects, 12 responded faster to stimuli presented in the right visual field and 3 responded faster to stimuli presented in the left visual field. To the extent that this difference in speed of responding is attributable to cerebral

TABLE 1 Mean Reaction Times Given to French and English Words
Presented in the Left and the Right Visual Fields

	French words	English words
Left visual field (right hemisphere)	969	990
Right visual field (left hemisphere)	944	954

dominance, the proportion of right-hemisphere dominance appears very high relative to other investigations. Benton (1965) for example, states that several researchers have found about 6% of right-handed subjects who do not show left-cerebral dominance, and Milner (1973) gives 4% as a more accurate estimate.

Two subjects showed a different left—right dominance in French and in English. These subjects processed English words more rapidly when they appeared in the right visual field and showed a slight trend to process French words more rapidly via the left visual field. Three other subjects showed a substantial left—right difference in the processing of one language and almost no left—right difference in processing the other language. These fascinating cases suggest that, with broader sampling, more examples might be found that deviate from the more general "both languages on the same side" pattern. The major outcome, however, is that, these two exceptions aside, this sample of bilinguals showed a cross-language visual field dominance, in the sense that both languages were more efficiently processed on the same side.

This overall outocme, tentative as it is, lends support to Penfield's notion that one hemisphere only is dominant for both languages of the bilingual person. The findings suggest, too, that some general language-independent mechanism may account for performance such on tasks as the language recognition one employed here. But much more research is now needed before we can be certain even that faster recognition from one visual field corresponds unambiguously with cerebral dominance (see Kimura, 1961; Bryden, 1965). We need, then, much larger samples of bilinguals and carefully documented language acquisition histories for each bilingual.

REFERENCES

Benton, A.L. (1965) The problem of cerebral dominance. *Canadian Psychologist, 6,* 332–348.
Broca, P. (1969) Remarques sur le siège de la faculté du langage articulé, suivies d'une observation d'aphémie (1861). In H. Hécaen & J. Dubois (Eds.), *La naissance de la neuropsychologie du langage.* Paris: Flammarion.
Bryden, M.P. (1965) Tachistiscopic recognition, handedness and cerebral dominance. *Neuropsychologia, 3,* 1–8.
Corballis, M.C., Miller, A., & Morgan, M.J. (1971) The role of left-right orientation in

interhemispheric matching of visual information. *Perception and Psychophysics, 10,* 385–388.

Gazzaniga, M.S., & Sperry, R.W. (1967) Language after section of the cerebral commisures. *Brain, 90,* 131–148.

Geschwind, N. (1972) Language and the brain. *Scientific American, 226,* 76–83.

Hamers, J.F., & Lambert, W.E. (1972) Bilingual interdependencies in auditory perception. *Journal of Verbal Learning and Verbal Behavior, 11,* 303–310.

Hamers, J.F., & Lambert, W.E. (1974) Bilingual's reactions to cross-language semantic ambiguity. In S.T. Carey (Ed.), *Bilingualism, biculturalism and education.* Edmonton: Univ. of Alberta, Printing Department.

Kimura, D. (1961) Cerebral dominance and the perception of verbal stimuli. *Canadian Journal of Psychology, 15,* 166–171.

Kimura, D. (1973) The asymmetry of the human brain. *Scientific American, 228,* 70–78.

Lambert, W.E. (1969) Psychological studies of interdependencies of the bilingual's two languages. In J. Puhvel (Ed.), *Substance and structure of language.* Los Angeles: Univ. of California Press.

Lambert, W.E., & Fillenbaum, S. (1959) A pilot study of aphasia among bilinguals. *Canadian Journal of Psychology, 13,* 28–34.

Lenneberg, E. (1967) *Biological foundations of language.* New York: Wiley.

Milner, B. (1962) Laterality effects in audition. In V.B. Mountcastle (Ed.), *Interhemispheric relations and cerebral dominance.* Baltimore: John Hopkins Univ. Press. Pp. 177–195.

Milner, B. (1973) Human brain function. Press conference, A.P.A., Montreal, August 26.

Paivio, A., Yuille, J.C., & Madigan, S. (1968) Concreteness, imagery and meaningfulness values for 925 nouns. *Journal of Experimental Psychology,* Monograph Supplement, *76.*

Penfield, W.P., & Roberts, L.R. (1959) *Speech and brain mechanisms.* London: Oxford Univ. Press.

Zangwill, O.L. (1960) *Cerebral dominance and its relation to psychological function.* London: Oliver & Boyd.

6

Hemispheric Asymmetry in Processing of Dichotically Presented Speech and Nonspeech Stimuli by Infants

ANNE KASMAN ENTUS

It is well known that the two cerebral hemispheres of the adult human brain are functionally asymmetrical. In most persons, the left hemisphere is responsible for verbal skills, while the right hemisphere is specialized for nonverbal tasks (e.g., Milner, 1971). Much of the evidence for differential specialization stems from clinical studies of neurological patients with well-lateralized lesions, a series of patients with surgical interruption of the corpus collosum, and experimental studies of normal individuals by means of various techniques, such as EEG recordings, tachistoscopic stimulation, and dichotic listening.

The dichotic listening procedure is an effective way to demonstrate hemispheric asymmetry with auditory input. Different stimuli are presented simultaneously to each ear and the listener's task is to recall or recognize what he has heard. Such experiments have typically revealed a right-ear superiority for verbal stimuli, such as words, consonants, and digits (e.g., Kimura, 1961; Shankweiler & Studdert-Kennedy, 1967), and a left-ear superiority for auditory patterns such as music (e.g., Kimura, 1964). Because there is evidence that the contralateral auditory pathways from ear to cortex are functionally dominant over the ipsilateral ones (Rosenzweig, 1951), a right-ear advantage for speech stimuli implies a left-hemisphere dominance, and a left-ear advantage for nonspeech sounds reflects right-hemisphere dominance.

Whereas we have substantial evidence regarding cerebral specialization in man, relatively little is known about the course of its development. The most prevalent view has been that lateralization of language emerges somewhere between the ages of 2 and 12, after the child has had some experience with language both as a listener and as a speaker (e.g., Zangwill, 1960). Data from clinical case studies (e.g., Basser, 1962) have shown that damage to the language dominant (left) hemisphere is much less disruptive to acquired language skills in young children than it is in older children and adults. This has led Lenneberg (1967) to postulate that the extent of language impairment reflects the degree to which the affected hemisphere has become specialized for language, implying equipotentiality between the two hemispheres in the early years.

The findings I present here challenge the view that hemispheric asymmetry takes several years to develop and suggest that it is present in early infancy, possibly even at birth. Recent data from several sources have already pointed to this conclusion. For example, it is now known that very young infants discriminate speech in a manner that parallels adult speech perception (e.g., Eimas, Siqueland, Jusczyk, & Vigorito, 1971; Moffitt, 1971; Morse, 1972; Trehub, 1973, 1974). These investigators have shown that by 1 month of age infants are capable of differentiating consonant and vowel contrasts that occur in their own language environment, as well as foreign language contrasts that they had never heard before. Infants make these fine perceptual discriminations in a linguistically relevant manner reflecting capacities which, in adults at least, are thought to depend on functional properties confined to the left hemisphere. Moreover, the presence of left-right morphological asymmetry in cortical areas involved in language processing observed in adult brains (Geschwind & Levitsky, 1968) has now been observed in infant brains as well. Asymmetry of both the temporal planum (Wada, 1973, 1975; Witelson & Pallie, 1973) and the frontal operculum (Wada, 1975) becomes discernible as early as the twenty-ninth gestational week. Finally, there is evidence that in infants, as in adults, auditory evoked responses to speech stimuli are larger when recorded from the left hemisphere, while responses to other sound stimuli are larger when recorded from the right hemisphere (Molfese, 1972).

PROCEDURE

To assess hemispheric specialization in infants, I combined the dichotic listening procedure with the nonnutritive High Amplitude Sucking (HAS) paradigm developed by Siqueland and Delucia (1969) and employed in recent studies of infant speech perception. As used in this study, the paradigm involves the presentation of a dichotic stimulus pair contingent on the infant's sucking. As the infant learns that it is his sucking that determines the stimulus event, his sucking rate typically increases relative to its (noncontingent) baseline level. However with the continued presentation of the same stimulus pair, the sucking rate decreases, presumably as a result of a reduction in the reinforcing properties of the stimuli. When a prespecified decrement criterion (defined as a rate at least one-third below the previous maximum rate) is reached and maintained for two successive minutes, the stimulus in one ear is changed while the other ear continues to receive the original stimulus heard during the preshift (predecrement) phase. The new combination is then presented for 5 min. After a short break, the procedure is repeated, only this time the novel stimulus is presented to the other ear (see Figure 1).

The major departure from the usual implementation of the HAS procedure consists of substituting dichotic stimulation for the standard single stimulus. In the standard use of the paradigm, when the decrement criterion is met, experimental infants are presented with a contrast stimulus while control infants continue to receive the original stimulus for the same length of time. Typically, experimental babies show recovery of sucking whereas control babies' sucking rates remain low. Discrimination of the stimulus change is inferred from the recovery of sucking of experimental babies relative to that of controls. The use of dichotic stimulation provides a means of exploring differences in the recovery of sucking rate as a function of the ear (left versus right) that receives a novel stimulus. If a novel stimulus in one ear leads to greater recovery of sucking than does a novel stimulus in the other ear, we may assume that the hemisphere contralateral to the ear associated with a greater recovery rate is more proficient in dealing with the stimulus in question. Thus, a significant difference between ears in the rate of recovery may be taken to reflect differences in hemispheric processing of the stimulus material.

Each infant was placed in a semireclining infant seat and wore stereophonic headphones (Maico, Model 5488). The experimenter, seated on the infant's right, held a blind Evenflow nipple in the baby's mouth. A Statham (Model P23AA) physiological pressure transducer, attached to the nipple, sent a signal to the DC preamplifier of a Grass poligraph (Model 79), which supplied a graphic record of sucking. A criterion level was set mechanically on the polygraph, and pen deflections beyond this level activated a Sony quadraphonic taperecorder, which

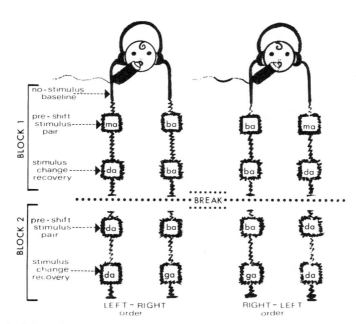

Figure 1. Schematic representation of the experimental procedure showing stimulus sequence and ear order.

presented the stimuli to the infant via the headphones. (The criterion level was adjusted for each infant such that most of the infant's sucks would be of sufficient pressure to activate the sound.) Two pen deflections per second were required for continuous activation of the taperecorder. Criterion sucks were counted by the minute on automatic counters.

STIMULUS MATERIALS

In Experiment 1, the stimuli were the consonant–vowel syllables /ma/, /ba/, /da/, and /ga/, spoken by an adult male voice. The stimuli in Experiment 2 were renditions of the note A (440 Hz) on four instruments—piano, viola, bassoon, and cello.[1] Six dichotic tapes were prepared with the aid of a PDP-11 computer.[2] Each tape consisted of 1000 identical instances of each of the following stimulus pairs: /ma/ and /ba/, /da/ and /ba/, /da/ and /ga/, piano and cello, piano and bassoon, and viola and bassoon. Each pair lasted 500 msec, with a 500-msec interval between pairs. The stimuli were presented at an intensity level judged to be comfortable and clearly audible by adult listeners, which was 76 dB for the syllables and 70 dB re: .0002 dynes/cm^2 for the musical notes as measured by a Grason Stadler sound level meter.

SUBJECTS AND DESIGN

Subjects were recruited through birth announcements in the local newspapers. Of the infants who were brought to the laboratory for testing, a total of 55 were excluded from the study. Factors responsible for subject attrition are summarized in Table 1. There were 48 babies (24 boys and 24 girls) in each experiment, with an overlap of 16 (8 males and 8 females) who participated in both. Both sexes were subdivided into two age groups, under 75 days (young) and over 75 days (old), with mean ages of 50.1 and 100.0 days, respectively, in Experiment 1, and 43.3 and 96.8 days, respectively, in Experiment 2. Half the infants heard the first change in the left ear and the second in the right ear; the order was reversed for the other half.

---

[1] The speech stimuli were recorded in a broadcast studio on an Ampex Mono tape recorder (Model 351) with a Gates console, full-track reel-to-reel at 7½ inches per second. The music stimuli were prepared in the Music Department, McGill University. The note played on the cello was plucked on the harmonic.

[2] Two computer programs were used in preparing the dichotic tapes. The first was used to transfer the original stimuli onto Dec tape and to determine that the duration of each was exactly 500 msec. The secon was used to line up the onset of each dichotic pair and record it on a quadrasonic Sony tape recorder at 7½ inches per second.

TABLE 1 Subject Attrition: Subjects Excluded from the Study, by Age and Factors Responsible for Subject Attrition

	Young	Old	Total
	N	N	N (%)
Excessive crying	5	35	40 (73)
Failure to complete both blocks	0	9	0 (16)
Deep sleep	1	2	3 (5)
Failure to reach the decrement criterion	0	1	1 (2)
Failure to emit sucks	0	1	1 (2)
Equipment failure	0	1	1 (2)
Total	6	49	55 (100)

TABLE 2 Summary of Significant F Ratios in the Analyses of Variance in Postshift Recovery Scores

Experiment	Effect	Means (%)	F	df	P
Speech	Ears (left–right)	Left ear = 59.9 Right ear = 71.5	9.24	1/40	.01
	Minutes (1 to 5)	1 = 59.5 2 = 67.4 3 = 68.0 4 = 70.0 5 = 63.8	4.49	4/40	.01
Music	Ears (left–right)	Left ear = 71.0 Right ear = 58.4	17.72	1/40	.001
	Minutes (1 to 5)	1 = 59.2 2 = 65.6 3 = 66.5 4 = 67.8 5 = 64.4	3.06	4/40	.05
	Age (young–old)	Young = 70.0 Old = 59.4	10.66	1/40	.01
Speech and music ($N = 16$)	Stimuli (speech–music)	Speech = 66.4 Music = 59.6	4.90	1/14	.05
	Ear × stimuli interaction	Speech Left ear = 55.9 Right ear = 76.8 Music Left ear = 66.1 Right ear = 53.1	23.90	1/14	.001

The data for each infant consisted of recorded numbers of sucks per minute, expressed as a percentage of the maximum preshift sucking rate.

Results

Analyses of variance on the last 5 min preceding stimulus change (preshift) revealed no significant differences as a function of which ear was to receive a novel stimulus. Analyses of variance of the postshift recovery scores were undertaken to determine the effects of ears, minutes, age, sex, and order (left–right versus right–left). Significant analysis of variance effects are summarized in Table 2. In both experiments there was a significant difference in recovery scores between ears. Recovery of sucking was greater in response to a stimulus change in the right ear (right ear mean = 71.5, left ear mean = 55.9) in the speech experiment, while in the music experiment greater recovery occurred following a stimulus change in the left ear (right ear mean = 58.4, left ear mean = 71.0). The clear finding, therefore, was that the speech stimuli resulted in a right-ear advantage, and the music stimuli in a left-ear advantage. The other significant effect obtained in both experiments was due to minutes, with the sucking rate in the first minute being significantly lower than in the next four (see Figure 2).

The only other significant effect was that of age in the music experiment (young = 70.0, old = 59.4). Young infants showed overall greater recovery of sucking than did the older infants, suggesting that the music stimuli were less reinforcing for the older infants (see Figure 3). None of the remaining main effects, nor any interactions with ears, approached conventional levels of significance.

A separate analysis of variance was performed on the postshift recovery scores of the 16 infants who participated in both experiments. This analysis revealed that the overall mean recovery scores were greater to speech stimuli than to music stimuli (speech = 66.4, music = 59.6), reflecting the greater reinforcing value of the speech stimuli. The other significant effect was the ear X stimulus type interaction, with the recovery rate being greater to a stimulus change in the right ear with speech (right ear mean = 76.8, left ear mean = 55.9) and greater in the left ear with music (right ear mean = 53.1, left ear mean = 66.1). This within-subject observation confirms the difference observed between subjects in the speech and music experiments (see Figure 4).

In the speech experiment, 34 of 48 infants (71%) showed a right-ear superiority; and in the music experiment, 38 of 48 infants (79%) showed a left-ear superiority. These proportions are in keeping with those reported for dichotic listening studies with children (e.g. Bryden & Allard, 1973) and Lenneberg's (1967) observation that 30% of young children show aphasia after injury to the right hemisphere. Of the 16 infants who participated in both experiments, 13 showed a right-ear advantage for speech and 16 showed a left-ear advantage for music (see Figure 5).

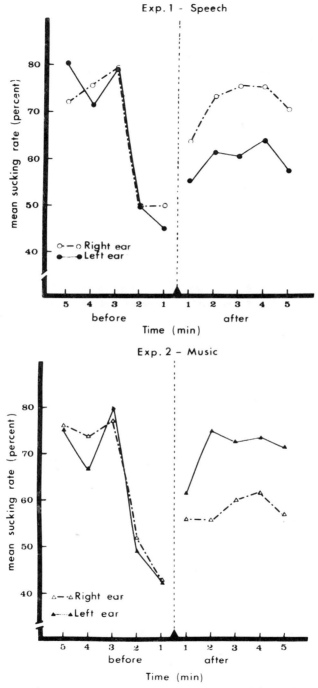

Figure 2. Mean number of sucks per minute, as a percentage of the maximum predecrement sucking rate, for 5 min before and after the decrement criterion in Experiment 1 (speech) and Experiment 2 (music).

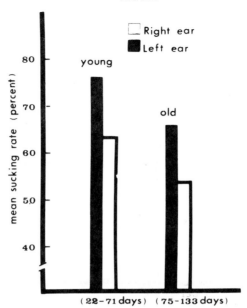

Figure 3. Mean postdecrement sucking rates of young and old infants in Experiment 2 (music).

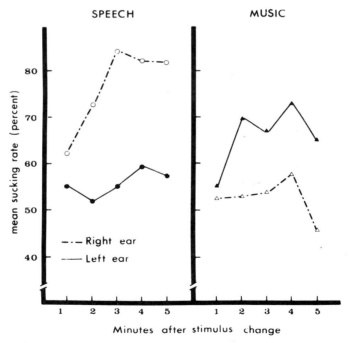

Figure 4. Mean number of sucks per minute, as a percentage of the maximum predecrement sucking rate, for 5 min after the decrement criterion of 16 infants who participated in both experiments.

PATTERN OF EAR DIFFERENCES

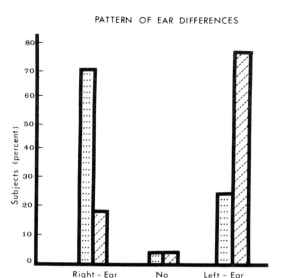

Figure 5. Proportion of infants displaying ear asymmetry in the speech and music experiments.

DISCUSSION

These results indicate that infants between the ages of 22 and 140 days display the typical adult pattern of lateral asymmetry for dichotically presented speech and nonspeech stimuli. Functional asymmetries thus appear to be present at a very early age, possibly even at birth. One conclusion to be drawn from this is that the equipotentiality of the infant brain, whereby one side can readily take over the functions of the other, must be attributed to plasticity, rather than to a lack of hemispheric specialization.

To formulate a description that takes into account all of the available data, we might borrow the concepts of *prospective significance, prospective potency,* and *determination,* as applied to a rather similar situation that exists in embryology. In the early development of the embryo the prospective significance of a given embryonic zone is the specific tissue into which it differentiates in the normal course of development. The prospective potency of that zone is the set of tissues into which it could develop should injury elsewhere so demand. As normal ontogenesis proceeds, determination occurs, at which time the embryonic region loses prospective potency and achieves prospective significance (Balinsky, 1970).

Similarly, in the development of functional hemispheric asymmetry, the prospective significance of each hemisphere might be to mediate specific functions (in most persons this means, for instance, that the prospective significance of the left hemisphere is to be responsible for verbal skills). In the event of injury to one hemisphere, the intact hemisphere may have the prospective potency to mediate functions normally subserved by the damaged region, provided that the damage occurs prior to determination, that is before prospective significance has been achieved. This description encompasses the results of the present study as well as the clinical data on which the equipotentiality hypothesis is based. The present results agree with the available neuroanatomical and physiological evidence in suggesting that hemispheric asymmetry is part of man's biological endowment and that it is functional by 3 weeks of age.

ACKNOWLEDGMENTS

This research was supported by Grant No. 9425-10 to Michael C. Corballis from the Defence Research Board of Canada and a grant from the Faculty of Graduate Studies and Research McGill University. The author acknowledges the use of the computer-based laboratory of the McGill University Department of Psychology, supported by the National Research Council of Canada, the FCAC program of the Quebec Ministry of Education, and the McGill University Graduate Faculty.

REFERENCES

Balinsky, B.I. (1970) *An introduction to embryology.* (3rd ed.) Philadelphia: Saunders.
Basser, L.S. (1962) Hemiplegia of early onset and the faculty of speech with special reference to the effects of hemispherectomy. *Brain, 85,* 427–460.
Bryden, M.P., & Allard, F. (1973) Dichotic Listening and the development of linguistic processes. Research Report *No. 44,* Univ. of Waterloo.
Eimas, P.D., Siqueland, E.R., Jusczyk, P. & Vigorito, J. (1971) Speech perception in infants. *Science, 171,* 303–306.
Geschwind, N. & Levitsky, W. (1968) Human brain: Left-right asymmetries in temporal speech region. *Science, 161,* 186–187.
Kimura, D. (1961) Cerebral dominance and the perception of verbal stimuli. *Canadian Journal of Psychology, 15,* 156–165.
Kimura, D. (1964) Left-right differences in the perception of melodies. *Journal of Experimental Psychology, 16,* 355–358.
Lenneberg, E.H. (1967) *Biological foundations of language.* New York: Wiley.
Milner, B. (1971) Interhemispheric differences in the localization of psychological processes in man. *British Medical Bulletin, 27*(3), 272–277.
Moffitt, A.R. (1971) Consonant cue perception by twenty to twenty-four week old infants. *Child Development, 42,* 717–731.
Molfese, D. (1972) Cerebral asymmetry in infants, children and adults: Auditory evoked responses to speech and noise stimuli. Presented at 84th Annual meeting of the Acoustical Society of America, Miami, Florida.
Morse, P.A. (1972) The discrimination of speech and nonspeech stimuli in early infancy. *Journal of Experimental Child Psychology, 14,* 477–492.
Rosenzweig, M.R. (1951) Representation of the two ears at the auditory cortex. *American Journal of Physiology, 167,* 147–158.
Shankweiler, D.P., & Studdert-Kennedy, M. (1967) Identification of consonants and vowels presented to left and right ears. *Quarterly Journal of Psychology, 19,* 59–63.

Siqueland, E.R., & DeLucia, C.A. (1969) Visual reinforcement of nonnutritive sucking in human infants. *Science, 165,* 1144–1146.

Trehub, S.E. (1973) Infants' sensitivity to vowel and tonal contrasts. *Developmental Psychology, 9,* 91–96.

Trehub, S.E. (1974) Natural syllabic and polisyllabic sound discrimination abilities in infants. Paper presented at meetings of the American Speech and Hearing Association, Las Vegas, Nevada.

Wada, J. (1973) Interhemispheric sharing and shift of cerebral speech function. Presented at the 4th (New York, 1969) and 10th (Barcelona, 1973) International Congress of Neurology.

Wada, J., Clark, R. & Hamm, A. (1975) Cerebral hemispheric asymmetry in humans. *Archives of Neurology, 32,* 239–246.

Witelson, S.F., & Pallie, W. (1973) Left hemisphere specialization for language in the newborn; neuroanatomical evidence of asymmetry. *Brain Research, 96,* 641–646.

Zangwill, O. (1960) *Cerebral dominance and its relation to psychological function.* Edinburg: Oliver and Boyd.

7

Acoustic Problems in Dichotic Listening Tasks

CHARLES I. BERLIN
JOHN K. CULLEN, JR.

Dichotic listening tasks, in which competing signals are presented to both ears, are currently being used to study central auditory perception in children and adults. One of the major purposes of this chapter is to clarify some of the underlying variables that must be understood if results are to be meaningfully interpreted.

The acoustic signals used in dichotics are of many forms, covering pure tones, nonsense syllables, words, or sentences, depending upon the central process being studied. We shall attempt to develop the subsequent sections of this chapter around principles applicable to dichotic speech perception. However, the reader should recognize that control of level, frequency response, subject hearing screening, and so on are generally pertinent to dichotic experiments in which signals other than speech are employed.

CONTROL OF ACOUSTIC VARIABLES

Not surprisingly, signal level and signal-to-noise (S/N) ratio affect performance in dichotic experiments much as these factors affect performance in monaural or binaural perception tasks. However, in dichotic tasks, investigators are often interested in between-ear performance differences as well. In dichotic speech tasks, for example, the difference in right-ear and left-ear performance (so-called right-ear advantage, or REA) is often the primary dependent variable.

It is difficult to set criteria as to what constitutes "normal" REA. However, if experimenters consider acoustic factors irrelevant and present stimuli at levels that have varying effects on the accuracy of recall, they magnify the difficulties of interpretation. Many researchers have presented their tapes at "comfort level" without regard for the absolute sound pressure measurements or the relationship of the consonant-to-vowel energies in their stimuli; few studies specify the S/N ratio of the tapes used, the nature of the temporal asynchrony, or the monaural intelligibility of the signals without dichotic competition. We would therefore address ourselves to these factors first.

Intensity

The type of speech material and the level at which it is given determines the absolute stimulus intelligibility as well as the total number of correct tokens perceived. Within certain limits, the relative advantage of one ear over the other remains the same, independent of absolute level. However, if there are small asymmetries either between channels or in the peripheral auditory system of a listener, the level at which the test is given may affect this advantage materially.

Figure 1 demonstrates the result of manipulating intensity in one channel, while the opposite channel is held at 80 dB sound pressure level (SPL). The right-ear superiority is maintained for as much as a 10-dB difference near 80 dB. However, if the pivotal sound pressure is near 50 dB SPL, this is not the case (Figure 2). The right-ear superiority is maintained only so long as the difference between the channels does not exceed 5 dB. This highlights the importance of channel balance, as well as absolute intensity, in presenting dichotic signals. Thus, methodology must include procedures to assure repeatable calibration of absolute levels and channel balance. One method of accomplishing calibration, as well as complete audio system check-out, is to place a tone of known frequency and voltage on the lead portion of experimental tapes. If the amplitude of this tone is adjusted to have a fixed, known relationship to the recorded amplitude of the stimuli, overall system calibration and balance can be achieved by playback through subject earphones to

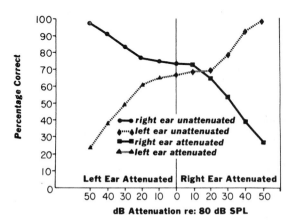

Figure 1. Dichotic right-ear advantage with attenuation of signals to one or the other ear. Unattenuated ear received signals at 80 dB SPL.

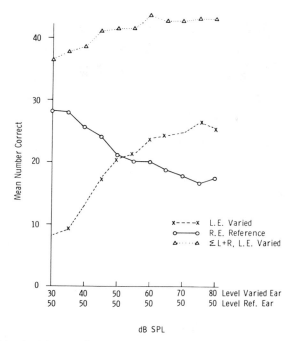

Figure 2. Dichotic right-ear advantage with change of left-ear performance as a function of intensity above and below the 50 dB SPL point.

an artificial ear and a sound level meter. Given the fixed relationship between stimulus amplitude and the calibration signal, an investigator can specify the level of the stimuli in decibels SPL. Even with an "ideal" calibration system such as the artificial ear and sound level meter, caution must be exercised to ensure that levels are repeatable. First, sound measuring devices are calibrated in effective, or root-mean-square (rms) units, and the rms value of a sinusoidal calibration signal and a speech signal are not the same even though they may have the same peak-to-peak value. If equivalent rms levels are used for calibration, the peak, and peak-to-peak values of the vocalic portion of the speech wave will, in general, be greater than that of the calibration signal. This is illustrated in Figure 3 where the rms value of a 750-Hz calibration tone has been equated to the average rms value for a number of consonant–vowel (CV) stimuli. Note also that the rms value of a CV token varies depending upon the consonant and the vowel, as seen in Figure 3. One technique to avoid the obvious ambiguity inherent in the rms values of sinusoids and various speech signals is to adopt the operational criterion of equating the vowel (or vocalic) segments of each stimulus on a peak-to-peak basis, and to set the amplitude of the calibration signal equal to this value. Figure 4 shows an example of this technique using a 1000-Hz calibration signal and several CV tokens.

In using sound level meters and artificial ears, it should be remembered that the standard 6-cubic centimeter coupler is not suitable to sound intensity measures

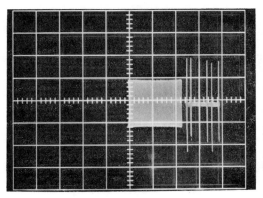

Figure 3. 1000-Hz cal tone (solid rectangular oscillograph) followed by vowel peaks. Tone and vowels. set at identical rms values.

with all earphones. Accurate intensity measures can be obtained only with tele-phone-type receivers, or earphones similar to standard audiometric earphones equipped with circular ear cushions similar to the MX41/AR. Circumaural enclo-sures, or earphones with oddly-shaped ear cushions usually cannot be calibrated directly with an artificial ear unless the coupling plate is modified.

Artificial ears and sound level equipment are relatively expensive instruments often not available to a laboratory. There are several techniques that, while not giving signal level in units of sound intensity, can be used to obtain channel balance and assure consistency in presentation level from subject to subject. Probably the most readily instrumented technique is to use an audio frequency voltmeter to measure the voltage developed by the calibration signal across earphone terminals.

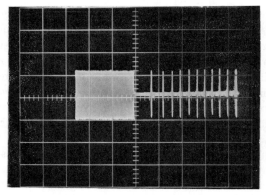

Figure 4. 1000-Hz cal tone (solid rectangular oscillograph) followed by vowel peaks. Tones and vowels now have equal peak-to-peak amplitudes but will appear to be different when viewed through voltmeters or VU meters.

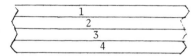

Figure 7. Schematic of a piece of recording tape with four possible tracks along which information can be recorded.

In addition, poor track alignment for audio tapes is often a source of unwanted noise.

Two-channel tapes (so-called stereo tapes) may be recorded in a variety of formats. A quarter-inch tape may be divided into four potential tracks, as shown in Figure 7. Some recorders use Tracks 1 and 2 for the first channel, and Tracks 3 and 4 for the second channel. These recorders are called "half-track recorders," meaning that approximately one-half the width of the tape is used for the information in each channel. Other recorders are "quarter-track recorders," in which either Tracks 1 and 3 or 1 and 4 are used as separate channels. A dichotic tape recorded on a half-track machine is usually compatible with a quarter-track playback device in which Tracks 1 and 4 are used, albeit with a decreased S/N ratio. However, if one uses a 1–3 playback model, two problems will ensue: First, the S/N ratios will be poor, as in a 1–4 configuration; second, and more important, channel separation will suffer. Under certain conditions, the contents of Track 3 may appear in both channels. In addition, signal intensity may be differentially affected because of head alignment relative to the recorded information tracks. Similar problems will be encountered if one attempts to play back tapes recorded quarter-track on a half-track instrument.

Frequency Bandwidth

Figure 8 shows the effects of reducing frequency bandwidth by low-pass filtering. The abscissa shows upper cutoff frequency and the ordinate, percentage correct. A 1000-cycle difference in bandpass between channels can obscure a REA. For each comparable filter condition, however, the right ear outperforms the left. Therefore, channel frequency response must be matched if ear advantage data are to be interpretable.

Time Relationships

Many older forms of dichotic tests have been arranged so that the onsets of the signals *appear* to the ear to be simultaneous (e.g., Katz, 1962; Kimura, 1961). There has been research to show that the largest REA's for nonsense syllables occur when signal onsets are precisely simultaneous oscillographically (Hannah, 1971). It is important to recognize that REA, while reflecting linguistic factors carried by the acoustic signal, also depends upon temporal factors. For example, in most auditory theory one expects the leading signal in a pair to be better received. However, in

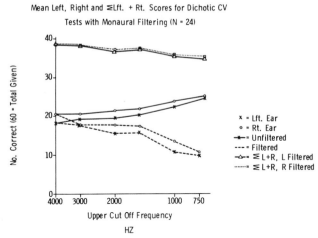

Figure 8. Dichotic listening results when one ear is filtered and the other ear receives unfiltered speech at a 4000-Hz upper frequency bandpass (from Cullen *et al.*, 1974).

dichotic listening it is the *trailing* signal that is better perceived within certain temporal ranges (Studdert-Kennedy, Shankweiler, & Schulman, 1970; Berlin, Lowe-Bell, Cullen, Thompson, & Loovis, 1973b). Figure 9 shows these results in normals. The left ear performs as well as the right ear when the message to the left ear arrives

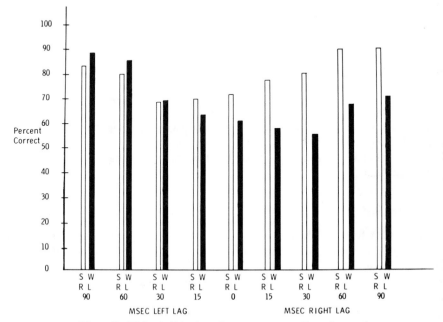

Figure 9. Dichotic listening when messages are time staggered.

30 to 60 msec *after* the message to the right ear. This phenomenon has also been found in children (Mirabile, 1975).

The beginning user of dichotic speech materials should also appreciate that the frequency response of a VU meter is adequate only for a continuous sine wave. The transient nature of speech is such that VU meters will not read the same way for speech as they do for pure tones. It is important to recognize that for a dichotic tape in which the onsets of CV pairs or digits are oscillographically simultaneous, the onsets will not necessarily appear to be simultaneous when viewed on VU meters.

Phase

There is no direct evidence of an interaction between phase and performance on dichotic speech perception tasks. One possible exception comes from the work of Bertelson and Tisseyre (1972), who show that an advantage accrues to a speech signal that "appears" to come from the right hemispace. Thus, one might project that giving a slight phase lead to the signal presented to an ear would tend to give an ear advantage.

NONACOUSTIC FACTORS

Phonetic Effects

Numerous studies have investigated errors and performance as a function of the phonetic dimensions of the dichotic stimuli presented (see, for example, Pisoni & McNabb, 1974; Studdert-Kennedy & Shankweiler, 1970; Studdert-Kennedy, Shankweiler, & Pisoni, 1972). In some cases, these interactions can operate to obliterate ear advantage effects when adequate counterbalancing is not observed. For example, in simultaneous syllable presentations, the voiceless stops /p, t/ or /k/ are usually better perceived than the voiced stops /b, d/ or /g/ (Berlin *et al.*, 1973b; Lowe, Cullen, Berlin, Thompson, & Willett, 1970). The voiceless–over-voiced preponderance is so strong that if one were consistently to put a voiceless CV in the left ear in competition with a voiced CV in the right ear, there would invariably be a left-ear advantage.

Subject Variables

Reliability

The dichotic REA is ordinarily a very reliable phenomenon within groups; however, considerable variability can be seen within and between subjects. Figure 10 shows the results of dichotic listening tests repeated over an 8-week period (Porter, Troendle, & Berlin, 1976). For the group, the total number of correct

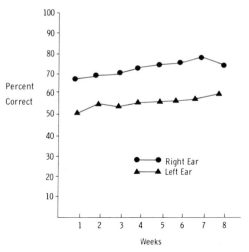

Figure 10. Group performance on dichotic tests over an 8-week period.

tokens perceived goes up, but the right—left ear differences remain statistically the same. Individual subjects fall into three basic types:

1. Strongly right-eared—these stay strongly right eared throughout an experiment.
2. Weakly right-eared—these subjects sometimes show a REA, sometimes show no ear advantage, and other times a weak left-ear advantage.
3. Moderately left-eared—these subjects fluctuate in their ear advantage and occasionally show no ear advantage; however, they never show *right*-ear advantages.

Age and Sex

In our dichotic CV paradigm, subjects are usually asked to respond to *both* syllables. Thus, the subject can get one syllable right, both syllables right, or both syllables wrong. When these data are analyzed for so-called single correct trials and double correct trials, a unique series of effects can be observed: From 5 through 15 years of age, the right—left ear differences remain the same. However, normal subjects show gradually improving double correct trial scores (Berlin, Hughes, Lowe-Bell, & Berlin, 1973a). While there is some argument in the literature as to the interpretation of this REA with respect to age (Porter & Berlin, 1975; Satz, Bakker, Goebel, and Van der Vlugt, 1975), there is no disagreement that the total correct score seems to improve as a function of age.

Differences in REA as a function of sex have been examined by Kimura (1963) and Knox and Kimura (1970). Although, in these developmental studies, females show a higher overall performance level than do males of comparable age up to about 11 years, when overall performance reaches adult levels, the sex differences are not significant. Since the magnitude of the REA is dependent on performance level, it would be difficult to evaluate sex-related REA differences anyway, because subject performance levels are rarely equated.

Patient Data

In studying children with such learning disabilities as dyslexia and/or central auditory problems (Sobotka, 1973; Tobey, Cullen, & Rampp, 1976), the REAs for single-correct trials are like those of normals, but the double-correct trial score is much lower. If dichotic listening in this paradigm is to have any clinical utility, it may show up in the total-correct score obtained by the individual subject. In normal subjects, about 65% to 80% of all possible syllables are correctly identified in a dichotic CV task. In subjects with brain lesions (such as temporal lobectomes, hemispherectomes, etc.) the total score rarely exceeds 50% of all syllables after correction for guessing. While this is not the place to review, in detail, data on patients with circumscribed brain lesions, it should also be noted that patients with specific lesions in the temporal lobe and/or corpus callosum do not show a lag effect. These data are clarified elsewhere (Berlin, Cullen, Lowe-Bell, & Berlin, 1974) and are cited here only to show that one CV generally interferes with the perception of the other CV in the opposite ear during dichotic listening, provided the two auditory pathways, in fact, converge on a final common pathway. A "disconnection," after temporal lobectomy, hemispherectomy, or corpus callosum section, releases one channel from interference by the other and generally produces a high score in one ear and an extremely low score in the other.

STIMULUS VARIABLES

CVs versus Digits

Sobotka (1973) found that scores for both normal and dyslexic subjects are different for dichotic CV tests and dichotic digits tests. Some of the subjects were right eared for digits and left-eared for CVs, and vice versa. Still others showed *large* ear advantages for one stimulus and *small* ear differences for the other, with no systematic trend for either type of stimulus. It appears that these two tasks are not necessarily reflecting the same neural processes (Porter & Berlin, 1975). Thus, it is inappropriate to ask whether digits or CVs are "better" as dichotic stimuli.

Scoring of Dichotic Tasks

Underlying the interpretation of *dichotic* tests is the assumption that they are, in fact, testing left-hemispheric language dominance. How one scores left-hemispheric dominance is moot; as yet we know of no satisfactory way to take dichotic listening scores and project "strength of lateralization of language function" onto them. Many investigators measure the absolute right–left differences for REA. Others use an "index" such as right minus left divided by total performance

(Studdert-Kennedy & Shankweiler, 1970), yet others use the construct of the ϕ correlation coefficient in an attempt to remove performance level effects from right–left differences (Kuhn, 1973).

All "hybrid" measures are still based on ear differences arising from the one-item correct trials, the correct item being assignable to the right or left ear. As such, transforms of the data provide no better measure or more insight into left-hemispheric dominance for language.

Synthetic versus Natural CVs

Most of the effects we have discussed have been observed with either natural or synthetic speech. In one experiment (Lowe *et al.*, 1970) we presented the same CVs with both natural and synthetic speech to the same listeners and found essentially no differences in REAs. Each type of stimulus has its unique advantages with respect to subject performance—with synthetic speech one can specify, a priori, the acoustic characteristics of the signals; with natural speech it must be done a posteriori by analysis. However, synthetic speech is not always uniformly intelligible to all listeners, especially young children, and therefore performance levels can be affected.

SUMMARY

It should be obvious from the foregoing discussion that there are many factors other than hemispheric specialization or brain dysfunction which affect overall dichotic performance and ear advantages. The results of dichotic tests must therefore be interpreted carefully in light of these factors. *Thus, the following premises, common to many experiments, should be questioned:*

1. Dichotic speech listening always reveals the dominance of the left hemisphere *proportional to the size of the REA.*
2. The absence of a difference in ear scores is, in some way, pathological, while a large and consistent REA is "normal."
3. All dichotic speech tests are alike and give common results proportional to the underlying left-hemispheric asymmetry for speech.

ACKNOWLEDGMENTS

Supported in part by funds obtained from National Institutes of Health, USPHS Program Project Grant No. NS-11647, and National Institute of General Medical Sciences, Special Fellowship 5 FO3 GM52343. Necessary laboratory facilities were provided through a grant from The Kresge Foundation.

REFERENCES

Berlin, C.I., Cullen, J.K., Jr., Lowe-Bell, S.S., & Berlin, H. (1974) Speech perception after hemispherectomy and temporal lobectomy. *Proceedings of Speech Communication Seminar,* Speech Transmission Laboratory (Pub.), Stockholm, Sweden, Pp. 9–15.

Berlin, C.I., Hughes, L.F., Lowe-Bell, S.S., & Berlin, H.L. (1973a) Dichotic right ear advantage in children 5 to 13. *Cortex, 9*(4), 393–401.

Berlin, C.I., Lowe-Bell, S.S., Cullen, J.K., Jr., Thompson, C.L., & Loovis, C.F. (1973b) Dichotic speech perception: An interpretation of right-ear advantage and temporal offset effects. *Journal of the Acoustical Society of America, 53*(3), 699–709.

Bertelson, P., & Tisseyre, F. (1972) Lateral asymmetry in the perceived sequence of speech and nonspeech stimuli. *Perceptual Psychophysiology, 11,* 356–362.

Cullen, J.K., Jr., Thompson, C.L., Hughes, L.F., Berlin, C.I., & Samson, D.S. (1974) The effects of varied acoustic parameters on performance in dichotic speech perception tasks. *Brain and Language, 1,* 307–322.

Hannah, J.E. (1971) Phonetic and temporal titration of the dichotic right ear effect. Unpublished doctoral dissertation, Department of Speech, Louisiana State Univ., Baton Rouge, Louisiana.

Katz, J. (1962). The use of staggered spondaic words for assessing the integrity of the central auditory system. *Journal of Auditory Research, 5,* 327–337.

Kimura, D. (1961) Cerebral dominance and the perception of verbal stimuli. *Canadian Journal of Psychology, 15,* 166–171.

Kimura, D. (1963) Speech lateralization in young children as determined by an auditory test. *Journal of Comparative and Physiological Psychology, 56,* 899–902.

Knox, C., & Kimura, D. (1970) Cerebral processing of nonverbal sounds in boys and girls. *Neuropsychologia, 8,* 227–237.

Kuhn, G.M. (1973) The phi coefficient as an index of ear differences in dichotic listening. *Cortex, 9*(4), 450–457.

Lowe, S.S., Cullen, J.K., Jr., Berlin, C.I., Thompson, C.L., & Willett, M.E. (1970) Perception of simultaneous dichotic and monotic monosyllables. *Journal of Speech and Hearing Research, 13*(4), 812–822.

Mirabile, P.J. (1975) Dichotic lag effect and right-ear advantage in children 7 to 15. Unpublished master's thesis, Univ. of New Orleans, Department of Psychology, New Orleans, Louisiana.

Pisoni, D.B., & McNabb, S.D. (1974) On dichotic interactions of speech sounds and the processing of phonetic features. *Brain and Language, 1*(4), 351–362.

Porter, R.J., Jr., & Berlin, C.I. (1975) On interpreting developmental changes in the dichotic right-ear advantage. *Brain and language, 2,* 186–200.

Porter, R.J., Jr., Troendle, R., and Berlin, C.I. Effects of practice on the perception of dichotically presented stop-consonant vowel syllables. *Journal of the Acoustical Society of America, 59*(3): 679–682, 1976.

Satz, P., Bakker, D.J., Goebel, R., & Van der Vlugt, H. (1975) Developmental parameters of the ear asymmetry: A multivariant approach. *Brain and Language, 2,* 171–185.

Sobotka, K. (1973) Neuropsychological and neurophysiological correlates of reading disability. Unpublished master's thesis, University of New Orleans, Department of Psychology, New Orleans, Louisiana.

Studdert-Kennedy, M., & Shankweiler, D. (1970) Hemispheric specialization of speech perception. *Journal of the Acoustical Society of America, 48,* 579–594.

Studdert-Kennedy, M., Shankweiler, D., & Pisoni, D.B. (1972) Auditory and phonetic processes in speech perception: Evidence from a dichotic study. *Cognitive Psychology, 3,* 455–466.

Studdert-Kennedy, M., Shankweiler, D., & Schulman, S. (1970) Opposed effects of a delayed channel on perception of dichotically and monotically presented CV syllables. *Journal of the Acoustical Society of America, 48,* 599–602.

Tobey, E.A., Cullen, J.K., Jr., & Rampp, D.L. (1976) Performance of children with auditory-processing disorders on a dichotic, stop-vowel identification task. Paper presented at the Fourth Annual Meeting of the International Neurospcyhology Society, Toronto, Ontario, Canada, February 1976. Submitted for publication, *Journal of Speech and Hearing Research.*

Part II

Cerebral Specialization for Language in Brain-damaged Patients

WHAT IS IT THAT IS LATERALIZED?

It is well accepted that the left hemisphere is more adept at linguistic functioning than the right. Language is presented primarily in the left cerebral hemisphere in most right-handed people. But, what aspects of language dispose to left lateralization and are there language functions for which the right hemisphere is better?

Acoustic Variables

Input does not have to be linguistic in order to produce a left-hemisphere preference. Backward speech produces a right-ear advantage, REA (Kimura & Folb, 1968). Such a stimulus is easily recognized as speech by adults and therefore may produce a REA through association, that is, speech noises may come to be left laterlized because of their association with language (cf. Bartholomeus, 1974a, b). However, this cannot be said of neonates, who also show a greater left-hemisphere response for speech sounds (Molfese, 1972). There would appear to be some acoustic factor producing the asymmetry. Investigations as to specific acoustic factors involve simple features, such as the presence of transitions and bandwidth (Chapter 2), and interactions dependent on the subject's knowledge of the speaker's characteristics, such as vocal tract size (Darwin, 1971). Although the left hemisphere may be dealing with speech, the right hemisphere does show some ability in dealing with acoustic factors but not phonological information (Zurif & Ramier, 1972). Other linguistically relevant cues, such as the emotional tone of a sentence, may even be right lateralized (Haggard & Parkinson, 1971). Similarly, Ades (1974) credits the right hemisphere with some speech-processing abilities.

Not all speech stimuli produce a REA, however, Van Lancker and Fromkin (1973) found knowledge of the language was needed to produce a REA for Thai tone words. Bartholomeus (1974b) found sung material likewise failed to produce a REA, whereas the same material spoken did. It would appear that both linguistic and acoustic factors are involved.

Psycholinguistic Variables

The most widely accepted division of hemisphere abilities is with reference to linguistic versus spatial characteristics (Head 1926; Witelson, 1974; Ingram, 1975; Chapters 8 and 10, this volume). Similarly, the left ear (right hemisphere) shows an advantage over the right for nonlinguistic environmental sounds (Knox & Kimura, 1970), whereas the reverse is so for language stimuli (Kimura, 1961).

Other psychological factors in language behavior are also of interest. For example, it could be that communicative skills are left lateralized, thereby accounting for similar lateralization of language skills. Kimura (1976), for example, suggests that "the left hemisphere is particular well adapted, not for symbolic function *per se*, but for the execution of some categories of motor activity which happened to lend themselves readily to communication." However, there are many vehicles for communication, and a symbolic visual system has been taught to aphasics with some degree of success (Hughes, 1974; Glass, Gazzaniga, & Premack, 1973).

The left hemisphere has also been credited with superiority over the right in the processing of syntax, an integral part of language (Chapter 8; Zurif & Sait, 1970). The isolated right hemisphere of split-brain patients shows little or no syntactic capability (Gazzaniga & Hillyard, 1971). Similarly, auditory sequencing has been found to be relatively more disturbed by left-hemisphere damage that also produces aphasia (Albert, 1972).

Related to this, and closely tied into the processing—on either the input or output side—of linguistic material, is the highly sophisticated ability to detect and control rhythms. An acute sense of timing is absolutely necessary for the acquisition and production of speech (Chapter 20). Efron (1963) pointed out that it was precisely this sort of ability with which aphasics have trouble. More recently, Robinson and Solomon (1974) found a right-ear advantage for rhythms in normal subjects.

The right hemisphere is by no means devoid of the prerequisite skills for language. Zaidel (in press) found that the right hemisphere in split-brain patients is capable of a fair degree of semantic interpretation, showing average auditory vocabulary of 11.5 years old. On the other hand, no syntactic abilities are credited to the right (Gazzaniga & Hillyard, 1971), as already mentioned.

Although the right hemisphere is unable to read, presumably because of its lack of ability to produce or manipulate phonological sequences (Gazzaniga, 1970), aphasics whose language uses an ideographic writing system show a mixed syndrome. For example, Yamadori (1975) presents a case of a Japanaese patient with left-hemisphere damage who had lost the ability to read Kana, a phonographic system, but could still read Kanji, the ideographic writing system. Presumably, different skills are utilized in reading the latter because of the visuo-spatial nature of the Kanji system. Apparently, it is not language per se that is left laterlized, but certain skills requisite to linguistic performance, which are represented primarily in the left. In certain cases, alternate skills can be employed (e.g., Glass et al., 1973) to achieve similar ends.

REFERENCES

Ades, A.E. (1974) Bilateral component in speech perception? *Journal of the Acoustic Society of America, 56,* 610–616.

Albert, M.L. (1972) Auditory sequencing and left cerebral dominance for language. *Neuropsychologia, 10,* 245–248.

Bartholomeus, B. (1974a) Dichotic singer and speaker recognition. *Bulletin of the Psychonomic Society, 2,* 407–408.

Bartholomeus, B. (1974b) Effects of task requirements on ear superiority for sung speech. *Cortex, 10,* 215–223.

Darwin, C.J. (1971) Ear differences in the recall of fricatives and vowels. *Quarterly Journal of Experimental Psychology, 23,* 46–62.

Efron, R. (1963) Temporal perception, aphasia and déjà vu. *Brain, 86,* 403–424.

Gazzaniga, M.S. (1970) *The Bisected Brain.* New York: Appleton.

Gazzaniga, M.S., & Hillyard, S.A. (1971) Language and speech capacity of the right hemisphere. *Neuropsychologia, 9,* 273–280.

Glass, A.V., Gazzaniga, M.S., & Premack, D. (1973) Artificial language training in global aphasics. *Neuropsychologia, 11,* 95–103.

Haggard, M.P., & Parkinson, A.M. (1971) Stimulus and task factors as determinants of ear advantages. *Quarterly Journal of Experimental Psychology, 23,* 168–177.

Head, H. (1926) *Aphasia and kindred disorders of speech.* New York: Cambridge Univ. Press.

Hughes, J. (1974) Acquisition of a non-vocal "language" by aphasic children. *Cognition, 3,* 41–55.

Ingram, D. (1975) Motor asymmetries in young children. *Neuropsychologia, 13,* 95–102.

Kimura, D. (1961) Cerebral dominance and the perception of verbal stimuli. *Canadian Journal of Psychology, 15,* 166–171.

Kimura, D. (1976) The neural basis of language qua gesture. In H. Whitaker & H.A. Whitaker (Eds.), *Studies in neurolinguistics.* Volume 2. New York: Academic.

Kimura, D., & Folb, S. (1968) Neural processing of backwards speech sounds. *Science, 161,* 395–396.

Knox, C., & Kimura, D. (1970) Cerebral processing of nonverbal sounds in boys and girls. *Neuropsychologia, 8,* 227–237.

Molfese, D.L. (1972) Cerebral asymmetry in infants, children and adults: Auditory evoked responses to speech and music stimuli. Unpublished doctoral dissertation, Pennsylvania State Univ.

Robinson, G.M., & Solomon, D.J. (1974) Rhythm is processed by the speech hemisphere. *Journal of Experimental Psychology, 102,* 508–511.

Van Lancker, D., & Fromkin, V.A. (1973) Hemispheric specialization for pitch and "tone": Evidence from Thai. *Journal of Phonetics, 1,* 101–109.

Witelson, S.F. (1974) Hemispheric specialization for linguistic and non-linguistic tactual perception using a dichotomous stimulation technique. *Cortex, 10,* 3–17.

Yamadori, A. (1975) Ideogram reading in alexia. *Brain, 98,* 231–238.

Zaidel, E. (in press) Auditory vocabulary of the right hemisphere following brain bisection or hemidecortication. *Cortex.*

Zurif, E.B., & Ramier, A.M. (1972) Some effects of unilateral brain damage on the perception of dichotically presented phoneme sequences and digits. *Neuropsychologia, 10,* 103–110.

Zurif, E.B., & Sait, P.E. (1970) The role of syntax in dichotic listening. *Neuropsychologia, 8,* 239–244.

8

Hemispheric Equipotentiality and Language Acquisition

MAUREEN DENNIS
HARRY A. WHITAKER

THE EQUIPOTENTIALITY HYPOTHESIS

Hemispheric equipotentiality refers to a supposed equivalence of the two cerebral hemispheres for basic language capacity. Language lateralization is held to develop from an equipotential state existing in the first 2 years of life. The condition for hemispheric equivalence is that language shall not have lateralized; a progressive loss of the equipotential characteristic is assumed to occur as linguistic skills come under the control of one side of the brain. Equipotentiality has taken two different forms: one based on proposals about the anatomical features of the two hemispheres, the other on suppositions about language behavior.

Early casts of the equipotentiality hypothesis stressed the anatomic symmetry of the hemispheres as the reason for their innate functional equivalence in language. The fact that the two brain halves seemed to be mirror images of each other was to Marie (1922) a compelling reason for supposing their similar latent linguistic capacity.

> The inborn centers which we know (and they are not numerous) are always bilateral and very clearly symmetrical. The motor centers of the limbs, the centers of vision, have their location in each of the two hemispheres in symmetrical regions.... How can we admit the existence of an inborn center for speech which would be neither bilateral nor symmetrical [p. 180]?

Central to this first form of the equipotentiality hypothesis is a statement about the anatomical characteristics of the brain. Accordingly, neuroanatomy will confirm or disconfirm it. The evidence does not support a view of physical hemispheric identity: There are structural left—right asymmetries in the anatomical and vascular features of the language-processing cerebral regions at birth and in adulthood

(Geschwind & Levitsky, 1968; Teszner, Tzavaras, Gruner & Hécaen, 1972; LeMay & Culebras, 1972; Matsubara, 1960; Wada, 1974; Witelson & Pallie, 1973).

In accepting the structural identity of the two hemispheres, Marie realized that he had not explained why the left hemisphere rather than the right was so often the language-dominant one. He offered this suggestion:

> Far from possessing a center of speech at birth, each individual must, by his own effort, create one; and it is in the left parieto-temporal zone that this occurs. Why? Perhaps simply because the nerve elements of the left hemisphere develop a little before those of the right hemisphere [p. 181].

Arguing strongly for anatomic symmetry, Marie nevertheless postulated a hemispheric asymmetry in developmental rates.

Later authors have dissociated anatomy and function in a reverse direction, accepting structural differences but denying functional asymmetries in the two hemispheres. Lenneberg (1971), for example, doubts the relevance of fiber architecture to language capacities, suggesting that the association between the two remains to be established. In this manner, it is possible to assert hemispheric equivalence for language functions while admitting to the facts of anatomic asymmetry: Regardless of their structural differences, the left and right hemispheres are similarly good language substrates. Since the second form of equipotentiality is cast in behavioral and maturational terms, it must be assessed by the adequacy with which it accounts for observed language behavior. To evaluate this cast of the hypothesis, it is necessary to trace and appraise the observations traditionally held to support the identity of latent linguistic capacities in the two hemispheres.

LANGUAGE FUNCTIONS AFTER EARLY LATERALIZED CEREBRAL DAMAGE

The classical evidence for the claim that cortical specialization for language does not exist at birth has been the apparent lack of association between laterality of early cerebral pathology and language status. The history of these observations is old.

As early as 1868, Cotard observed that individuals who were hemiplegic from infancy might not show aphasia even though their whole left hemisphere was atrophied. Note that Cotard has viewed the language of infantile hemiplegics in terms of the presence or absence of adult aphasia. But equipotentiality postulates an equivalence of language skills, not just a similar lack of aphasic signs, in the two infant hemispheres. The issue, then, is not whether nonaphasic right infantile hemiplegics exist but whether right- and left-sided cases are similarly liable to disordered language. The incidence of language disturbances as a function of laterality of infantile hemiplegia is shown in Table 1 for Cotard and later nineteenth-century researchers. Impaired language is associated significantly more often with left- than with right-hemisphere damage. Twentieth century studies

TABLE 1 Language Disorder as a Function of Laterality of Childhood Hemiplegia: Nineteenth Century

	N language disordered/N cases (%)	N language disordered right hemiplegics/N right hemiplegics (%)	N language disordered left hemiplegics/N left hemiplegics (%)
Cotard (1868)	9/23 (38.1)	8/13 (61.5)	1/10 (10.0)
Gaudard (1884)	33/80 (41.3)	25/55 (45.4)	8/25 (32.0)
Bernhardt (1885)	11/18 (61.1)	11/14 (78.6)	0/4 (0.0)
Lovett (1888)	7/26 (26.9)	3/13 (23.1)	4/13 (30.8)
Wallenberg (1886)[a]	62/160 (38.8)	45/94 (47.9)	17/66 (25.8)
Osler (1888)	13/120 (10.8)	12/68 (17.6)	1/52 (1.9)
Sachs and Peterson (1890)	17/105 (16.2)	10/52 (19.2)	7/53 (13.2)
Wulff (1890)	8/24 (33.3)	6/9 (66.7)	2/15 (13.3)
Freud and Rie (1891)	10/35 (28.6)	7/23 (30.4)	3/12 (25.0)

[a]Wallenberg's review includes selected cases from Cotard (1868).

(Table 2), with the exception of Basser (1962), produced a similar set of results: The likelihood of language disturbances resulting from infantile damage to one cerebral hemisphere is greater with left than with right lesions. In infancy, the two hemispheres are not equally at risk for disordered language.

Hemispheric equipotentiality is alleged to hold until the onset of speech: Only after the age of 2 is it claimed that right and left lesions are unequally disruptive of language (Lenneberg, 1969). It is therefore important to demonstrate that the lateralized early lesion effects on language in Tables 1 and 2 do not occur only in cases with appreciable language development before the cerebral insult. Annett (1973) considered language in right and left infantile hemiplegics who incurred damage before 13 months of age. Left-sided cerebral insult more frequently resulted in language impairments ($N = 50$, disordered language in 32.0%) than did right-sided injury ($N = 41$, disordered language in 10.1%). Even before speech has developed, the two hemispheres are not equally prone to a disruption of language by lateralized cerebral insult.

Although early left and right lesions appear to have different effects on language, right-hemisphere damage does cause reported language disturbances significantly more often in infantile than in adult cases (Russell & Espir, 1961). Does the

TABLE 2 Language Disorder as a Function of Laterality of Childhood Hemiplegia: Twentieth Century

	N language disordered/N cases (%)	N language disordered right hemiplegics/N right hemiplegics (%)	N language disordered left hemiplegics/N left hemiplegics (%)
Dunsdon	39/64	31/34	8/30
(1952)	(61.0)	(91.2)	(37.5)
Basser	34/102	16/48	18/54
(1962)	(33.3)	(33.3)	(33.3)
Ingram	12/75	11/44	1/31
(1964)	(16.0)	(25.0)	(0.03)
Bishop	9/17	5/7	1/8
(1967)	(53.0)	(71.4)	(12.5)
Annett	31/108	24/59	7/49
(1973)	(28.7)	(40.7)	(14.9)

language impairment produced by early right-hemisphere injury differ in degree or in kind from that following early left-hemisphere damage? Bishop (1967) found that dysarthric conditions occurred in 52.9% and 53.8%, respectively, of left and right infantile hemiplegics, but that right hemiplegics showed also a relative delay in reaching some speech milestones. These data suggest two important conclusions. They indicate, first, that one effect of early left-hemisphere damage may be delayed language acquisition. The language delay relates especially to the acquisition of simple syntax: In comparison to those with left-sided paralysis, right hemiplegics are delayed in acquiring word combinations (Bishop, 1967; Hood & Perlstein, 1955) but not single words (Basser, 1962; Bishop, 1967; Hood & Perlstein, 1955). Bishop's data suggest, second, that articulatory defects may follow early damage to either hemisphere, but that only in the left hemisphere do these articulatory problems correlate with other language disorders. Either perinatal hemisphere, it appears, is prone to impaired speech output; the left is additionally at risk for language delays. The number of articulatory, linguistic, and articulatory-plus-linguistic impairments in the cases represented in Tables 1 and 2 is uncertain, since most authors do not make these particular distinctions. It is important to explore more systematically and with larger numbers of cases the kind, as well as the number, of language defects following early right-hemisphere injury. At present, it is not possible to decide whether the incidence of bona fide language impairments in the right-hemisphere damaged cases in Tables 1 and 2 is significantly greater than that in comparable right-lesioned adults.

With early cerebral damage of sufficient severity to produce hemiplegia, the assumption is that the undamaged hemisphere subserves speech and language. The extent of such functional reorganization, however, is difficult to measure, and to varying degrees the damaged hemisphere may continue to shape language. Decortication of the diseased cerebral tissue provides the assurance that speech and language functions are subserved by the more intact hemisphere. Early reports suggested that language status was not related to the laterality of the hemidecortication (Basser, 1962; McFie, 1961). While these data indicated that either hemisphere could provide the substrate for some language functions, they did not give unequivocal support to hemispheric equipotentiality. The criteria for language disturbance did not always include measures of language acquisition as well as later linguistic functioning. The lack of adultlike linguistic impairments in hemidecorticate infantile hemiplegics is not evidence for hemispheric equipotentiality unless it can also be shown that early left-hemisphere damage has no detrimental effects on language acquisition. Where measures of acquisition were used, the relevant dimension was not always assessed. Basser (1962), for example, measured only age at first word(s) and did not consider the acquisition of word combinations. Many language functions were not assessed in early investigations of the effects of hemidecortication on language. Certain linguistic abilities are in fact inferior in the isolated right hemisphere of hemidecorticate infantile hemiplegics. That is, the understanding of some syntactic forms is more highly developed in hemidecorticates possessing the left brain half (Dennis & Kohn, 1975). Discrimination of syntax in the residual right hemisphere is inferior in two ways to that of the left: The adult rate of proficiency is lower, and the age at which nonrandom performance is attained is higher. Thus, both the mature level of this language function and the rate of its acquisition are different in right- as compared with left-hemidecorticate infantile hemiplegics. A third difficulty of interpretation with early studies comes about because of an observed relationship between language status and intelligence level. Infantile hemiplegics, whether right or left, with IQ scores below 70 show some language problems (Bishop, 1967). The intelligence level of the hemidecorticates in the Basser and McFie studies varies widely, (e.g., 64.9% and 56.0%, respectively, of Basser's right and left infantile hemiplegics have IQ scores below 79), making assessment of the incidence of true language problems difficult. The association between lesion laterality and linguistic ability varies with intelligence; it cannot be considered independently of IQ level. What must next be considered, then, is the interrelationship between side of early brain damage, language capacity, and intelligence.

INTELLIGENCE, LANGUAGE, AND EARLY LESION LATERALITY

Right and left infantile hemiplegics do not differ in overall intelligence (Annett, 1973; Hammill & Irwin, 1966; Reed & Reitan, 1969), nor is there a selective association between Verbal IQ and right hemiplegia or Performance IQ and left hemiplegia (Annett, 1973; Basser, 1962; Carlson, Netley, Hendrick & Prichard, 1968; McFie, 1961; Reed & Reitan, 1969).

The significance of the lack of lateralized IQ results in infantile hemiplegics must be tempered by the fact that IQ measures do not reliably predict lesion laterality in cases of cerebral injury sustained in adulthood. The association between adult left-hemisphere lesions and low Verbal IQ, on the one hand, and right-hemisphere lesions and depressed Performance IQ, on the other, has been both asserted (e.g., Kløve & Reitan, 1958; Reitan, 1955) and denied (Smith, 1965). The discrepancy in these results arises in part from variations in the degree of chronicity of the lesions. When the brain damage is acute, Verbal–Performance IQ differentials are predictive of lesion laterality; when the cerebral injury is chronic, they are not (Fitzhugh, Fitzhugh & Reitan, 1962). The acuteness of the adult lesion appears to be a more potent predictor of IQ score configurations than is lesion laterality. Such findings are highly pertinent to interpretation of the IQ scores of infantile hemiplegics. Early brain lesions are by definition chronic—a subject must be at least 5.5-years old before being measurable on the WISC or WAIS, and is usually much older. The absence of lateralized IQ deficits after infantile damage may relate as much to the length of time the lesion has existed as to the point in development when it was sustained.

Still another qualification of the meaning of intelligence scores in infantile hemiplegics comes from the observed association between Verbal IQ and adult aphasia. Reitan (1960) found that Verbal IQ measures are lowered by aphasia, rather than by left-hemisphere damage as such (a finding consistent with the acuteness-of-lesion data). To the extent that the Verbal IQ measure is sensitive to adult aphasic conditions, it need not also reflect the syntactic impairments and delayed language acquisition that characterize right infantile hemiplegics (Bishop, 1967; Dennis & Kohn, 1975; Dunsdon, 1952; Hood & Perlstein, 1955).

The patterning of Verbal and Performance IQ scores expresses certain distributional properties of the measuring instrument as well as the characteristics of the subjects tested. As Full Scale IQ increases, the proportion of individuals with a higher Verbal than Performance IQ increases; as Full Scale IQ decreases, a greater number of people show higher Performance than Verbal IQ (Matarazzo, 1972). The relationship between Verbal and Performance IQ itself changes as a function of overall intelligence level. It is not possible to judge the significance of a Verbal–Performance configuration without reference to the level of general intelligence. When intelligence scores in an investigation vary widely, the pattern of Verbal–Performance IQ may reflect more about these metric features of the test than about the attributes of the subjects. Verbal and Performance IQ scores in normal subjects are most similar at average levels of intelligence. Consequently, atypical IQ configurations are more likely to express subject, and not test, properties in individuals of near-average general intelligence.

For some authors, a variant of the intelligence score, rather than the score itself, has the clearest relationship to left-hemisphere lesions incurred in adulthood. The following are some of the measures used to identify left from right adult lesions: vocabulary-scaled score (Parsons, Vega & Burns, 1969); the mean of the scaled scores for information, comprehension, similarities, and vocabulary (Lansdell, 1968); a "verbal comprehension quotient" (Tellegen & Briggs, 1967); and a quantified pattern analysis (Simpson & Vega, 1971). Do these measures select left from right injury in nonretarded individuals with early and demonstrably unilateral cerebral damage, that is, hemidecorticate infantile hemiplegics with onset of pathology under 1 year of age and Full Scale IQ above 70? As Table 3 shows, none of the variant verbal IQ measures provides a clear separation between left and right early injury.

Intelligence scores might nevertheless be considered meaningfully related to language skills, were such an association demonstrable, that is, if Verbal IQ predicted language status in infantile hemiplegics of adequate general intelligence. But it does not. Language impairments or delays are more common in right than in left hemiplegics, even when IQ is controlled (Annett, 1973; Bishop, 1967). The syntactic competence of the seven subjects tested (Table 3) is related to the laterality of the lesion (Dennis & Kohn, 1975), even though their verbal IQ scores and verbal IQ variant scores are not. It is perhaps not surprising that syntactic impairments would not be reflected in verbal IQ measures, since there is no subtest in the WISC or WAIS that directly assesses the knowledge of language structure. It is also not remarkable that verbal IQ fails to indicate whether or not language acquisition was retarded at a stage of development earlier than that at which verbal IQ was measured. What remains to be studied is whether verbal IQ measures (on instruments such as the Wechsler Preschool and Primary Scale of Intelligence) made at ages when acqustion is obviously delayed would be lower in right than in left infantile hemiplegics.

The interpretative qualifications outlined are not meant to question the validity of IQ measures in cases of early brain damage but, rather, to suggest that the age at

TABLE 3 Verbal IQ and Verbal IQ Variant Measures in Left and Right Hemidecorticates Differing in Syntactic Comprehension[a]

Measure	Left hemidecorticates				Right hemidecorticates			
	VB	DW	KK	LC	RN	SZ	PK	CB
Verbal IQ[b]	85	91	87	78	86	79	95	83
Vocabulary-scaled score	9	7	7	6	8	6	11	8
Mean scaled score (SS) for information, comprehension, similarities, and vocabulary	8.5	8.5	8.0	6.3	8.0	6.3	9.3	6.8
Verbal comprehension quotient[c]	92	91	89	80	88	78	96	82
Pattern analysis (number of left-hemisphere signs)[d]	4	1	1	4	2	3	3	6

[a]Histories and performance on syntactic tests are described in Dennis and Kohn (1975) for all subjects except SZ, whose history is in Kohn and Dennis (1974).

[b]Depending on age at testing, some subjects were tested on the WISC, some on the WAIS.

[c]Verbal comprehension quotient = [(SS information + SS comprehension + SS similarities + SS vocabulary) × 1.4 (WAIS) or 1.5 (WISC) + 44 (WAIS) or 40 (WISC)] (Tellegen & Briggs, 1967).

[d]Left-hemisphere signs: vocabulary > comprehension; vocabulary > arithmetic; vocabulary > similarities; picture completion > arithmetic; picture completion > similarities; picture arrangement > arithmetic (Simpson & Vega, 1971).

which the lesion is sustained may not be the factor producing different score configurations in early- and late-lesioned cases. IQ score patterning also reflects the metric properties of the intelligence test distribution, the acuteness of the lesion, the presence of aphasia, and, undoubtedly, other factors as well. As a consequence, verbal IQ measures in nonretarded infantile hemiplegics predict neither how rapidly nor how well language develops. What the intelligence test results do show is that either hemisphere can provide the substrate for verbal cognitive skills; but, demonstrably, we cannot infer from these findings a hemispheric equipotentiality for language.

LANGUAGE ACQUISITION IN ONLY A RIGHT OR A LEFT HEMISPHERE: A TEST CASE FOR EQUIPOTENTIALITY

What kind of evidence would confirm the hypothesis that the two hemispheres are equally good substrates for language? The test case would be if the level of language capacity possible in a right hemisphere under ideal developmental conditions were equal to that of a left hemisphere. Two organisms would be needed, one born with only a left, another with only a right, hemisphere. At no time must either have been twin-brained. The language acquisition process itself would need to proceed without cortical malfunction. In short, what would be assessed would be the level of linguistic development in each separate hemisphere. Under such conditions, how rapidly and how well could each hemisphere acquire language?

The three children studied here do represent test cases for equipotentiality. Each possesses only a right or a left hemisphere. Surgical removal of one brain half antedated the beginning of speech, so acquisition of speech and language has involved only one hemisphere. The children were diagnosed at birth as cases of Sturge—Weber—Dimitri syndrome. The seizures that began soon after birth were resistant to anticonvulsive medication, so one hemisphere was surgically removed. The histological examination of the resected brain tissue revealed the small pathological changes characteristic of Sturge—Weber—Dimitri syndrome. There were microscopic foci of calcification in the cortex itself, and angiomatoses of the meninges of most of the lobes of the brain. The hemispherectomy proved effective in stopping the seizures. None of the children has had seizures during the period of language acquisition, so relatively normal educational progression has been possible. In subject MW, the right hemisphere (RH) was removed; in subjects SM and CA, the left hemisphere (LH). All the children are of normal and comparable levels of intelligence (Verbal IQ: MW 96, SM 94, CA 91; Performance IQ: MW 92, SM 87, CA 108; Full Scale IQ: MW 93, SM 90, CA 99). Detailed descriptions of the medical histories are in Dennis and Whitaker (1976).

How has language developed in each isolated hemisphere by the age of 9? Performance on the Illinois Test of Psycholinguistic Abilities (ITPA) (Kirk, McCarthy, & Kirk, 1968) is shown in Table 4. The test provides measures of different language processes (comprehension, association, expression) in different

TABLE 4   Language Development in Right and Left Hemidecorticates[a]

Subtest	MW (RH) 9:5[b]	SM (LH) 9:4[b]	CA (LH) 9:5[b]
Auditory reception			
Psycholinguistic age	AN[c]	8:10	8:4
Scaled score	37	34	32
Visual reception			
Psycholinguistic age	7:9	8:10	8:10
Scaled score	31	35	35
Auditory association			
Psycholinguistic age	10:1	7:11	7:8
Scaled score	39	29	28
Visual association			
Psycholinguistic age	5:3	7:7	6:6
Scaled score	20	31	27
Verbal expression			
Psycholinguistic age	7:8	6:10	6:0
Scaled score	32	29	26
Manual expression			
Psycholinguistic age	8:4	6:9	7:2
Scaled score	34	29	30
Grammatical closure			
Psycholinguistic age	9:8	8:10	7:0
Scaled score	37	34	22
Visual closure			
Psycholinguistic age	4:8	7:0	6:6
Scaled score	15	27	25
Auditory memory			
Psycholinguistic age	6:0	6:10	7:7
Scaled score	29	31	33
Visual memory			
Psycholinguistic age	8:4	7:10	8:4
Scaled score	35	34	35
Composite Psycholinguistic Age	7:8	7:9	7:3
Mean scaled score	30.9	31.3	29.3

[a]As measured on the Illinois Test of Psycholinguistic Abilities (Kirk, McCarthy, & Kirk, 1968).
[b]Chronological age.
[c]Above the norms for the test, i.e., psycholinguistic age above 10:4.

modalities (auditory, manual, visual). The scores are expressed as both age equivalences and standard scores.

The configuration of subtest performance is different in the three hemidecorticates, although their overall psycholinguistic ages are comparable. Each child shows considerable within-test variation. MW's auditory comprehension is above the norms for the test (i.e., above 10:4), while his visual receptive skill is below his chronological age. Since the auditory score is at ceiling, the scale score difference

fails to reach statistical significance. For the associative tests, the difference between MW's auditory and visual skills is dramatic: the psycholinguistic age and the
scale scores for the two are significantly different. The second striking dissociation
of modalities shown by MW is between grammatical and visual completion. His
acquisition of automatic habits for handling syntax and grammatical inflections is
slightly above his chronological age, but visual closure is at a low level of development. Auditory memory is poorer than visual memory, but not significantly so.
Manual and verbal expressive skills are at comparable levels of development.

Dissociation of modalities in the receptive and associative processes is not
evident in either of the left hemidecorticates: Auditory and visual reception, and
auditory and visual association, are similarly developed. SM is more proficient at
grammatical than at visual closure, but CA is not. Neither left hemidecorticate
shows any difference between the two modalities expression and memory.

Some of the low scores on the test perhaps reflect the limiting physical disability
suffered by all three children. Their evident embarrassment at performing bilateral
motor movement with a hemiparesis probably caused a general lowering of their
manual expression scores. Nevertheless, the right hemidecorticate differs from the
left hemidecorticates on tests of visual closure, where it might have been expected
that a hemianopsia would lower scores uniformly.

The level of development of other functions appears also to depend on the
laterality of the hemidecortication. MW is superior to SM and CA in the auditory
channels for comprehension and association; SM and CA exceed MW in the ability
to understand and associate visual stimuli. Some of the ITPA subtests, it should be
stressed, are linguistic only by a stipulative definition. Visual closure, for example,
is a classical test of right-hemisphere function (e.g., DeRenzi & Spinnler, 1966).
Evidently, the total ITPA score measures more than purely linguistic functions. The
configuration of ITPA performance of the three hemidecorticates reflects a right-
hemisphere superiority for visuo-spatial tasks (Kohn & Dennis, 1974) as well as a
greater left-hemisphere proficiency at auditory language.

Auditory comprehension was explored more fully in the Token Test (Table 5).
This test measures the ability to execute a variety of complex verbal commands
varying in information and in syntactic complexity. In Parts 1 to 4, the adjectival
content of the noun phrases increases systematically although the commands are
syntactically the same. Part 5 introduces a variety of different verbs and noun phrase
structures into the predicates, thereby complicating the syntax of the commands.

Only MW is able to maintain proficient performance in the face of the increased
syntactic demands of Part 5, although all the hemidecorticate children can manage
the informational complexity of Parts 1 to 4. Were the left hemidecorticate
impairment one of global inability to handle complex verbal material or of immediate memory, performance could be expected to be most debilitated on those
commands with the greatest information load. But it appears to be syntactic rather
than informational complexity that degrades the scores of SM and CA. The two left
hemidecorticates but not MW, for example, had difficulty in utilizing the syntactic
information conveyed by words like *when, after,* and *before,* and in analyzing

examples of overt instrumentals (Whitaker & Noll, 1972), especially those in which the surface word order was not the same as the temporal order of the action. The defect of SM and CA on the Token Test appeared to be one of syntax at least as much as content. Developmental dysphasics, by contrast, are disordered on the Token Test in proportion to the informational complexity of the command; when syntactic complexity is increased but information level reduced, their performance actually improves (Tallal, 1975).

In relation to the left, the isolated right hemisphere appears to acquire certain components of auditory language less well, especially the ability to respond to the structural or syntactic aspects of heard utterances (see also Dennis & Kohn, 1975). These findings parallel the earlier reports of delayed acquisition of word combinations, but not of single words, in right infantile hemiplegics (Bishop, 1967; Hood & Perlstein, 1955).

Posing the equipotentiality question in terms of the presence or absence of adultlike aphasias produces false negative evidence for the influence of laterality of early lesion on linguistic functions. The effects of early left hemisphere injury on language seem to be expressed as delayed acquisition of word relationships, rather than as adult aphasic syndromes. It is not surprising that this should be so. Infantile damage disrupts a volatile, developing system, and what is most obviously altered is the ongoing course of this development. A full right-hemisphere control of language, as in left hemidecorticate infantile hemiplegics, causes difficulties with language structure even in adulthood.

Hemispheric equipotentiality does appear to make an untenable supposition about the brain because it neither explains nor predicts at least two facts about language—that the two perinatal hemispheres are not equally at risk for language delay or disorder and that they are not equivalent substrates for language acquisition.

TABLE: 5 Comprehension of Complex Commands in Right and Left Hemidecorticates[a]

Test	MW (RH) 9:4[b]	SM (LH) 8:0[b]	CA (LH) 8:0[b]
Part 1 (Touch the red circle)	100.0	100.0	100.0
Part 2 (Touch the small red circle	100.0	90.0	100.0
Part 3 (Touch the yellow circle and the red rectangle)	100.0	100.0	100.0
Part 4 (Touch the small blue circle and the large green circle)	90.0	70.0	100.0
Part 5 (Touch the yellow circle with the blue rectangle, etc.)	90.9	63.6	77.3
Total score	95.2	80.6	91.9

[a]As measured by the percentage of correct scores on the Token Test (De Renzi and Vignolo, 1962).
[b]Chronological age.

ACKNOWLEDGMENT

This research was supported by a Hospital for Sick Children Fellowship and an Ontario Mental Health Foundation Scholarship to the first author. We thank Dr. E.B. Hendrick for permission to test the patients, and Dr. J. Arbit and Dr. C. Netley for providing some of the intelligence test scores. Dr. B. Kohn, Dr. C.A. Wiegel-Crump, and O.A. Selnes generously helped with the translations.

REFERENCES

Annett, M. (1973) Laterality of childhood hemiplegia and the growth of speech and intelligence. *Cortex, 9,* 4–33.
Basser, L.S. (1962) Hemiplegia of early onset and the faculty of speech with special reference to the effects of hemispherectomy. *Brain, 85,* 427–460.
Bernhardt, M. (1885) Ueber die spastiche cerebral paralyse im Kindersalter (Hemiplegia spastica infantilis), nebst einem Excurse ueber "Aphasie bei Kindern". *Archiv für pathologische Anatomie und für Klinische Medicin, 102,* 26–80.
Bishop, N. (1967) Speech in the hemiplegic child. In *Proceedings of the 8th Medical and Educational Conference of the Australian Cerebral Palsy Association.* Melbourne, Victoria: Tooronga Press. Pp. 141–153.
Carlson, J., Netley, C., Hendrick, E.B., & Prichard, J. (1968) A reexamination of intellectual disabilities in hemispherectomized patients. *Transactions of the American Neurological Association, 93,* 198–201.
Cotard, J. (1868) Etude sur l'atrophie cérébrale. Thèse pour le doctorat en Medecine. Paris: A. Parent.
Dennis, M., & Kohn, B. (1975) Comprehension of syntax in infantile hemiplegics after cerebral hemidecortication: Left hemisphere superiority. *Brain and Language, 2,* 475–486.
Dennis, M., & Whitaker, H.A. (1976) Language acquisition following hemidecortication: Linguistic superiority of the left over the right hemisphere. *Brain and Language, 3,* 404–433.
DeRenzi, E., & Spinnler, H. (1966) Visual recognition in patients with unilateral cerebral disease. *Journal of Nervous and Mental Disease, 142,* 515–525.
DeRenzi, E., & Vignolo, L. (1962) The Token Test: a sensitive test to detest receptive disturbances in aphasics. *Brain, 85,* 665–678.
Dunsdon, M.I. (1952) *The educability of cerebral palsied children.* London: Newnes.
Fitzhugh, K.B., Fitzhugh, L.C., & Reitan, R.M. (1962) Wechsler-Bellevue comparisons in groups with "chronic" and "current" lateralized and diffuse brain lesions. *Journal of Consulting Psychology, 26,* 306–310.
Freud, S., & Rie (1891) cited in Freud, S. (1897). *Infantile cerebral paralysis.* Trans. L. Russin. (1968) Coral Gables, Florida: Univ. of Miami Press.
Gaudard (1884) cited in Freud, S. (1897). *Infantile cerebral paralysis.* Trans. L. Russin, 1968. Coral Gables, Florida: Univ. of Miami Press.
Geschwind, N., & Levitsky, W. (1968) Human brain: Left-right asymmetries in temporal speech region. *Science, 161,* 186–187.
Hammill, D., & Irwin, O.C. (1966) IQ differences of right and left spastic hemiplegic children. *Perceptual and Motor Skills, 22,* 193–194.
Hood, P.N., & Perlstein, M.A. (1955) Infantile spastic hemiplegia. II. Laterality of involvement. *American Journal of Physical Medicine, 34,* 457–466.
Ingram, T.T.S. (1964) *Paediatric aspects of cerebral palsy.* Edinburgh: E & S Livingstone.

Kirk, S.A., McCarthy, J.J., & Kirk, W.D. (1968) *Examiner's manual: Illinois test of psycholinguistic abilities.* Urbana, Illinois: Univ. of Illinois Press.

Kløve, H., & Reitan, R.M. (1958) Effect of dysphasia and distortion on Wechsler-Bellevue results. *Archives of Neurology and Psychiatry, 80,* 708–813.

Kohn, B., & Dennis, M. (1974) Selective impairments of visuo-spatial abilities in infantile hemiplegics after right hemidecortication. *Neuropsychologia, 12,* 505–512.

Lansdell, H. (1968) The use of factor scores from the Wechsler-Bellevue scale of intelligence in assessing patients with temporal lobe removals. *Cortex, 4,* 257–268.

LeMay, M., & Culebras, A. (1972) Human brain—morphologic differences in the hemispheres demonstrable by carotid arteriography. *New England Journal of Medicine, 287,* 168–170.

Lenneberg, E. (1969) On explaining language. *Science, 164,* 635–643.

Lenneberg, E. (1971) Of language knowledge, apes and brains. *Journal of Psycholinguistic Research, 1,* 1–29.

Lovett, R. (1888) A clinical consideration of sixty cases of cerebral paralysis in children. *Boston Medical and Surgical Journal, 118,* 641–646.

Marie, P. (1922) Existe-t-il dans le cerveau humain des centres innés ou préformés de langage? *La Presse Medicale, 17,* 117–181.

Matarazzo, J.D. (1972) *Wechsler's measurement and appraisal of adult intelligence.* Baltimore: Williams and Wilkins.

Matsubara, T. (1960) An observation on cerebral phlebograms with special reference to the changes in the superficial veins. *Nagoya Journal of Medical Science, 23,* 86–94.

McFie, J. (1961) The effects of hemispherectomy on intellectual functioning in cases of infantile hemiplegia. *Journal of Neurology, Neurosurgery, and Psychiatry, 24,* 240–249.

Osler, W. (1888) The cerebral palsies of children. *The Medical News, 53,* 29–35.

Parsons, O.A., Vega, A., & Burns, J. (1969) Different psychological effects of lateralized brain damage. *Journal of Consulting and Clinical Psychology, 33,* 551–557.

Reed, J.C., & Reitan, R.M. (1969) Verbal and performance differences among brain-injured children with lateralized motor deficits. *Perceptual and Motor Skills, 29,* 747–752.

Reitan, R.M. (1955) Certain differential effects of left and right cerebral lesions in human adults. *Journal of Comparative and Physiological Psychology, 48,* 474–477.

Reitan, R.M. (1960) The significance of dysphasia for intelligence and adaptive abilities. *Journal of Psychology, 50,* 355–376.

Russell, R., & Espir, M. (1961) *Traumatic aphasia.* New York: Oxford Univ. Press.

Sachs, B., & Peterson, F. (1890) A study of cerebral palsies of early life, based upon an analysis of one hundred and forty cases. *Journal of Nervous and Mental Disease, 17,* 295–332.

Simpson, C.D., & Vega, A. (1971) Unilateral brain damage and patterns of age-corrected WAIS subtest scores. *Journal of Clinical Psychology, 27,* 204–208.

Smith, A. (1965) Verbal and nonverbal test performances of patients with "acute" lateralized brain lesions (tumors). *Journal of Nervous and Mental Disease, 141,* 515–523.

Tallah, P. (1975) Perceptual and linguistic factors in the language impairment of developmental dysphasics: An experimental investigation with the Token Test. *Cortex, 9,* 196–205.

Tellegen, A., & Briggs, P.F. (1967) Old wine in new skins: Grouping Wechsler subtests into new scales. *Journal of Consulting Psychology, 31,* 499–506.

Teszner, D., Tzavaras, A., Gruner, J., & Hécaen, H. (1972) L' asymétrie droite-gauche du planum temporale. A propos de l'étude anatomique de 100 cerveaux. *Revue Neurologique, 126,* 444–449.

Wada, J.A. (1974) Morphologic asymmetry of human cerebral hemispheres: Temporal and frontal speech zones in 100 adult and 100 infant brains. *Neurology, 24,* 349.

Witelson, S., & Pallie, W. (1973) Left hemisphere specialization for language in the newborn: Neuroanatomical evidence of asymmetry. *Brain, 96,* 641–646.

Wallenberg, A. (1886) Ein Beitrag zur Lehre von den cerebralen Kinderlähmungen. *Jahrbuch für Kinderheilkunde, 24,* 384–439.

Whitaker, H., & Noll, D. (1972) Some linguistic parameters of the Token Test. *Neuropsychologia, 10,* 395–404.

Wulff, D. (1890) Cerebrale Kinderlähmung und Geistesschwäche. *Neurologisches Centralblatt, 9,* 343–344.

9

Language Deficits and Cross-Modal Sensory Perception

LINDA CHAPANIS

THEORIES OF CROSS-MODAL PERCEPTUAL LEARNING

There are two general groups of theories proposed to explain cross-modal effects relevant to perceptual learning. One general group is that of integration theories. The other group emphasizes the "unity" of the senses.

Integration Theories

Integration theories use developmental data as evidence and suggest that cross-modal equivalence and transfer are abilities learned as a child develops. Early theories of perceptual learning were based on the conviction that some modes of sensory experience are dependent on others for their meaning. These theories suggest that the sensory modalities are originally separate and specific and that they become integrated during the course of development by association with a common response. Experiments by Birch and Lefford (1963) have attempted to demonstrate this theory. Their study shows developmental curves for intermodal matching for children from ages 5 to 11. Although correct matching increased with age, it cannot be explained by saying that intersensory integration is responsible, since, as Gibson (1969) points out, intramodal matching improves with age as well.

A mediation theory of cross-modal transfer, which asserts that transfer is carried verbally, is said to have support by virtue of data showing that transfer increases with age. There are equivocal studies with animals, however, some showing that animals are unable to carry out transfer fasks (Burton & Ettlinger, 1960; Ettlinger, 1960), others showing positive results (Wilson & Shaffer, 1963). Verbalization may possibly facilitate transfer in children, but it is probably not an essential factor (Blank & Bridger, 1964).

Piaget has presented a mediation theory of cross-modal transfer which is based on the finding that transfer increases with age. A representative schema is built up by systematic exploratory activity. Cross-modal transfer is made possible by the sensorimotor schema, which is a "referent" common to two modalities.

Unity Theories

The opposite point of view from the integration theories stresses what has been referred to as the "unity of the senses" (Hayek, 1952). Gibson (1969) suggests that cross-modal effects stem from the learning of invariant "higher-order" information that is "amodal" or "supramodal". Gibson suggests that it is this supramodal information of a higher order that is responded to with increasing frequency as a child develops. Perhaps, as Gibson suggests, cross-modal transfer of discrimination may turn out to be dependent on the supramodal features common to a number of modes of stimulation. If this is true, the research question in work with language-impaired children might profitably be: "Are there deficits in the development of these children regarding their abilities to detect invariant features common to a number of different modes of stimulation?"

CROSS-MODAL THEORY AND NEUROLOGICAL DEVELOPMENT

It has been shown that the parietal lobe is one of the areas of the brain slowest to develop and myelinate (Geschwind, 1965a,b). As one of the "association areas" it has been believed to be the crossroads for many fiber tracts. Subsequently, it has been taken as the literal representation of cross-modal functions. If the fiber tracts cross at this point, then cognitive skills requiring the "integration" of two sensory modalities must occur here. Visual signals about a given target must combine with auditory signals relating to it in this area of the brain. Since it is believed that this region has a late maturation cytoarchitectonically, often in late childhood (Geschwind, 1965a,b), one might expect a parallel development of the cognitive functions it presumably serves. It is interesting in this regard that Ettlinger (1973) has found infants capable of making cross-modal connections.

CROSS-MODAL PERCEPTION AND LANGUAGE DEFICITS IN CHILDREN

On auditory-visual matching-to-sample tasks which were used to study children with reading disabilities (Birch & Belmont, 1964) and brain damage (Birch & Belmont, 1965), it was found that the children were markedly poorer on such tasks compared to normal controls. Conclusions drawn from these studies were based on the belief that a selective intersensory deficit in certain groups had been revealed by the auditory—visual task. The Birch and Belmont studies assumed that intersensory tasks would be intrinsically more difficult than intrasensory tasks, that is, they assumed that more mistakes would occur on intersensory tasks than on intrasensory tasks. However, when Rudel and Teuber (1971) ran intrasensory controls, it was found that intramodal performance in brain-damaged children was as impaired as cross-modal performance. It appears, then, that *selective* intersensory deficits have not been conclusively demonstrated to occur in patients with certain kinds of cognitive deficits.

There is an additional difficulty with the Birch—Belmont sensory integration theory which arises from the results of studies that deal with the symmetry of cross-modal sequences. The order of presentation of the modalities in cross-modal tasks should make no difference if it is only the integration between modalities that is of importance. This is not the case, however, because Rudel and Teuber (1971) have found significant aymmetries in performance by normal children where the easier task appeared to be the one having a visual standard. No asymmetries were found in brain-damaged children, however, which suggested that the brain-damaged children might not derive as much information from ordinary (simultaneous) visual stimuli as do normal children. Rudel and Teuber postulated that brain-damaged children may therefore have difficulty with the "simultaneous apprehension of sensory information [p. 397]."

Freides (1974) points out that some conditions are associated with modal, rather than with cross-modal, deficits. Selective deficits in one sensory modality in brain-damaged children have not been substantiated, however. Deutsch and Schumer (1970) demonstrated significant differences between brain-damaged children and controls in *each* sensory modality. The results of studies of dyslexic children, though, are conflicting. Reading-disabled children have been found to have selective visual deficits, selective auditory deficits, both of these, and neither of these (Freides, 1974). A study by Corkin (1974) of reading disorders in children suggests that the deficit in this disorder may be part of a "more general deficit in serial organization that cuts across sensory modalities and stimulus materials [p. 353]."

CROSS-MODAL PERCEPTION AND LANGUAGE DEFICITS IN ADULTS

Integration Theories

Geschwind (1965a,b, 1970) has proposed a sensory integration theory to explain language deficits that result from cortical lesions in adults. A reading deficit, for example, is explained by a patient's inability to integrate auditory and visual information. According to Geschwind, this sensory deficit may reflect very specifically the location of the lesion producing it. For example, a lesion in the angular gyrus may "disconnect" the auditory association area from the visual association area and thereby produce a reading deficit.

Geschwind's approach has stimulated a number of attempts to establish correlations between cross-modal functions in general and the neuroanatomical locations that presumably mediate these functions. An example of such a study is that of Butters and Brody (1968), who found that left-hemisphere parietal lobe patients were impaired on auditory–visual, visual–tactual, and tactual–visual matching tasks. However, these same patients also showed deficits on tactual–tactual matching tasks. They might have shown impairment on the other two intramodal matches as well, if they had been tested on those. In another study, Butters, Barton, and Brody (1970) found similar results for patients with severe right-hemisphere parietal damage. However, it was noted that failures of the patients on the auditory-visual task were associated with an inability to decode the auditory patterned stimulus, rather than with a failure in cross-modal association.

Language and Cross-Modal Functions

In a review of cross-modality studies, Ettlinger (1973) reported that apes are capable of making cross-modal matches. Moreover, infants below the age of 12 months have demonstrated sensory equivalence between touch and vision (Ettlinger, 1973). It appears then, on the basis of the data for apes and infants, that language itself is not a necessary prerequisite for cross-modal matching. There is evidence that, in adults, cross-modal matching may be disrupted in those cases where language is disturbed as well as in those cases where it is not disturbed. For example, Belmont, Birch, and Belmont (1968) tested auditory-visual cross-modal matching in brain-damaged patients with and without language disturbance and in a control group of non–brain-damaged patients. No real difference was found in performance between brain-damaged patients with and without language disturbance, although brain-damaged patients as a whole performed more poorly than did the control group. This test, however, used the auditory-visual matching-to-sample technique of Birch and Belmont (1964), which confounds temporal and spatial stimuli. If these are separated, there is some reason to believe that differences in performance can be obtained. This is duscussed further in the next section.

Cross-Modal Functions and Cerebral Localization

Both right- and left-hemisphere damaged patients have been shown to be impaired on cross-modal tasks (Butters & Brody, 1968; Butters *et al.,* 1970; Belmont *et al.,* 1968). In these studies, however, temporal and spatial tasks were confounded.

If temporal and spatial factors are teased apart, the relative degree of deficit resulting from either left- or right-sided lesions may be determined. Efron (1963) has reported data that suggest the left hemisphere may be important for "temporal processing." Numerous other investigators have suggested that the right hemisphere may be important for "spatial abilities" (Hecaen, 1969; McFie, 1969; Miller, 1972; Piercy, 1964; Williams, 1970). In his work with split-brain patients Gazzaniga (1972) has also demonstrated a right-hemisphere superiority for spatial information. Carmon and Benton (1969), in a study of tactile perception of direction, demonstrated that patients with lesions of the right hemisphere perform much more poorly than do patients with left-sided lesions. Fontenot and Benton (1971) have concluded as well, on the basis of a study of perception of direction, that the right hemisphere plays an important role in mediating spatial perception not only in the tactile but in the visual and auditory modalities too. On the other hand, Pohl, Butters, and Goodglass (1972) have found that right-field superiority (implicating functions in the left hemisphere) can be demonstrated by giving a spatial task to normal adults.

Conclusions

In summary, the assumptions underlying the theory of sensory integration are twofold. First, brain damage can interfere with cross-modal functions, leaving intramodal functions unimpaired. Second, since it is *integration* between the modalities that is important, it should make no difference in which modality tasks are presented first. Studies of children and adults have disconfirmed these assumptions and shown that cross-modal tasks are not necessarily more difficult than intramodal tasks and that reversed modality sequences are not necessarily equivalent in difficulty.

The theory has not been adequately tested because studies with brain-damaged patients have not made the proper comparisons between intra- and cross-modal abilities and because equivalent tasks have not been used within as well as between all modalities. As a result, it is not clear what role cross-modal abilities per se play in various cognitive deficits; nor has a clear relationship between neuroanatomical location and "pure" cross-modal integration been established.

LANGUAGE DEFICITS AND SUPRAMODAL FUNCTIONS

Goodglass, Barton, and Kaplan (1968) tested auditory, visual, and olfactory modality functions in aphasic patients and found that there were no differences in performance between any of the modalities when the patients were asked to name objects presented to them. This suggested that a modality nonspecific process (a supramodal process) may intervene between stimulus presentation and meaning.

This concept of a supramodal basis for the disturbance in aphasia is reflected in a variety of studies. DeRenzi, Faglioni, Scotti, and Spinnler (1972) have viewed the impairment in associating color with form in aphasia as an aspect of a more general disorder of conceptualization that was not dependent on the language disorder but associated with it. Spinner and Vignolo (1966) have suggested that a "semantic-associative" disorder, rather than an "acoustic-discriminative" defect, may explain the impaired recognition of meaningful sounds. Sarno, Swisher, and Sarno (1969), in a study of a congenitally deaf man, found that the aphasic disturbances were composed of deficits analogous to those seen in hearing aphasics, which suggests that the congenitally deaf encode and decode language by the same fundamental processes as do those with normal hearing. A defect in auditory processing as such could not have been responsible for the aphasia in this deaf man.

CROSS-MODAL PERCEPTION AND SUPRAMODAL SKILLS: AN INVESTIGATION

Can language deficits occurring in patients with structural neurological damage be shown to be supramodal, that is, the result of disturbances in brain function unrelated to modalities per se?

This question has some affirmative answers based on studies using tasks presented within various modalities. However, it has not been answered for the conditions where tasks are presented *across* as well as within sensory modalities, using tasks that can be said to be equivalent in all sensory modalities. To be truly equivalent in different sensory modalities, a task must be defined by a characteristic such as time or rhythm which can be handled by any modality. In the past, however, attempts to use the parameter of time have confounded it with space. For example, auditory (tapped) rhythms have been matched to visual rhythms (dots printed on cards). The visual rhythms in this case have lost their purely temporal character by being displayed in space on a card. The use of flashes of light might have circumvented the problem of confounding time with space. In cases where flashes of light *have* been used, either the necessary intramodal controls have not been used in studies of cross-modal matching or the studies have been limited to only two modalities rather than using three (vision, touch, and hearing).

Can hemispheric locus of lesion be shown to affect performance on cross-modal tasks when tasks are either purely temporal or purely spatial?

On the basis of studies done so far one might expect left-hemisphere damaged patients to do more poorly on cross-modal tasks that are temporal, and right-hemisphere damaged patients to do more poorly on tasks that are spatial.

Method and Results

In an attempt to answer the above two questions, a study was carried out by this investigator (Chapanis, 1974) in which three sets of matching tasks were devised. One set of matching tasks was purely temporal. Another set was purely spatial. A third set was a combination of temporal and spatial. The tasks that were purely temporal or purely spatial were nonverbal. The tasks that were a combination of temporal and spatial had a nonverbal part and a verbal part. All tasks were presented to eight left- and eight right-hemisphere damaged stroke patients and eight non—brain-damaged controls. Of the eight left-hemisphere patients, five were aphasic. Anteriorly located and posteriorly located lesions were distributed throughout each of the brain-damaged groups.

The Nonverbal Tasks

Temporal Task. In the purely temporal task, the subject had to match a temporal pattern in one modality to a temporal pattern in the same or a different modality. The temporal patterns were four discrete stimuli—four flashes of light, four auditory "beeps," or four taps to the fingertip of the hand ipsilateral to the side of the lesion. (This hand was used during all tasks in the study because the contralateral hand varied considerably in degree of motor and sensory involvement among the patients in both groups.) The administration of the stimuli was programmed by equipment designed specifically for the study.

Each pattern had one of three possible rhythms:

Rhythm I: . . . .
Rhythm II: . . . .
Rhythm III: . . . .

Each rhythm consisted of two short interstimulus intervals (each 250 msec) and one long interstimulus interval (750 msec). The temporal patterns were given both sequentially and simultaneously, to control for memory effects. When they were given sequentially, there was a 2-sec pause between the patterns. When they were given simultaneously, both patterns began and ended at the same time.

The subject's task, which was to match a pattern presented in one modality (visual, auditory, or tactile) to a pattern presented in the same or a different modality, required him to produce a same—different judgment about the pair of patterns. All subjects were given examples of the task before the series was run, and in those cases (among the aphasics) where a verbal response could not be understood, or was not reliable, a nonverbal response, such as nodding the head, was used. If a reliable nonverbal response could not be found, the patient was not included in the study.

On this temporal task, control subjects never made any errors. Moreover, it can be seen from Figure 1 that errors were made in all intramodal (A–A, V–V, T–T) and all cross-modal (A–V, V–A, A–T, T–A, V–T, T–V) combinations. However, comparisons within modality combinations revealed no significant differences. This was true for all patients. An analysis of variance on the number of errors made by left-hemisphere and right-hemisphere patients on this task shows that the location of lesion has a significant effect on the number of errors made. Right-hemisphere patients made significantly more errors ($df = 1,14$; $F = 22.64$; $p < .001$) than did left-hemisphere patients on all modality combinations. There was no difference in the errors made in the sequential and simultaneous presentations.

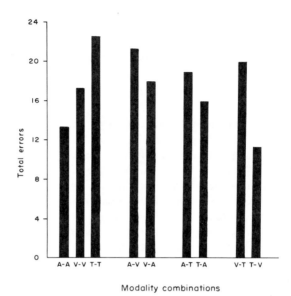

Modality combinations

Figure 1. Errors made on sequential and simultaneous temporal patterns by 8 left- and 8 right-hemisphere stroke patients. Controls made no errors and are not included. A = Auditory, V = Visual, T = Tactile. (Total possible errors for each bar: 64.)

Combined Temporal and Spatial Tasks

TEMPORAL PATTERN COMPARED TO
VISUAL–SPATIAL ANALOGUE

In this task, the patient had to compare a temporal pattern in one sense modality to a visual–spatial analogue of the same or a different pattern. The visual–spatial analogue was constructed by arranging thumbacks on a piece of corkboard. The spaces between the tacks corresponded to, or mimicked, the pause between flashes of light, auditory beeps, or taps to the fingertip. All possible pairings of temporal patterns in all three modalities were tested with all visual–spatial analogues. After every presentation, in the intramodal and cross-modal tasks, the subjects had to say same or different. The results showed that there were no differences between modality combinations on this task. However, the *order of presentation* of the stimuli had a significant effect ($df = 1,70; F = 12.75; p < .005$) on the number of errors made by both groups of patients. The most striking aspect of the data is that there are many more errors made when the spatial layout is presented first and is followed by the temporal pattern. When the temporal pattern is presented first and is followed by the spatial layout, patients made fewer errors. This order effect occurred regardless of whether the temporal patterns were auditory, visual, or tactile. There were no differences between right- and left-hemisphere groups on this task, and control subjects never made any errors.

TEMPORAL PATTERNS COMPARED TO HAPTIC–SPATIAL
ANALOGUE

In this task, the patient had to compare a temporal pattern in one sense modality to a haptic–spatial analogue of the same or different pattern. The haptic–spatial analogue consisted of the same thumbtack layouts described earlier. The difference between this task and the previous one was in the way the tacks were presented. As a haptic[1] analogue, the tack array was concealed by a curtain; the patient ran his fingers over the tacks. He compared that pattern to a temporal pattern presented as flashes of light or auditory beeps. After every presentation a same–different judgment was obtained. An analysis of errors made on this task revealed no significant differences among modality combinations and no differences between right- and left-hemisphere groups. Once again, control subjects never made any errors.

Spatial Task. In this task the subject had to compare a visual–spatial analogue of a temporal pattern to a haptic analogue of the same or different pattern. The visual and haptic analogues consisted of the same thumbtack layouts described in the preceding two tasks. The subject had to make comparisons and give same–different judgments for visual–visual, haptic–haptic, haptic–visual, and visual–haptic patterns. An analysis of variance on the number of errors made by the right- and left-hemisphere groups showed a significant difference in the number of errors made ($df = 1,14; F = 8.64, p < .025$). The right-hemisphere group made more than twice as many errors as the left-hemisphere group. There were no differences, however, between any of the modality combinations, and controls performed perfectly.

Discussion of Results on the Nonverbal Tasks. What has been shown with these nonverbal tasks is that brain-damaged patients do about the same on cross-modal and intramodal matches when the stimuli are equivalent. This is true regardless of the side of a patient's lesion. In other words, when the stimuli are purely temporal, or purely spatial, brain-damaged patients do as poorly on intramodal tasks as they do on cross-modal tasks. However, when the stimuli *combine* temporal and spatial parameters, differences in performance on cross-modal and intramodal matches appear. These differences occur when purely temporal auditory, visual, or tactile patterns are compared with their visual–spatial analogues, and are related to the *order* of presentation of the analogues (visual first or spatial first). Such differences do not appear when purely temporal auditory or visual patterns are compared with haptic–spatial analogues.

The differences obtained here between left- and right hemisphere patients show how important it is to separate the temporal from the spatial characteristics of the stimuli. When the task is purely temporal, patients with right-hemisphere lesions do

---

[1] The term *haptic* is used here because the subject moves his hand actively over the display. This is in contrast to the *tactile* presentation of temporal patterns described earlier, where the subject sits passively and is tapped.

much more poorly than patients with left-hemisphere lesions. This is contrary to what might have been expected on the basis of studies done so far. When the task is purely spatial, the right-hemisphere group again does more poorly than the left hemisphere group. However, when the tasks combine temporal and spatial parameters, there are no differences between the two groups of patients.

The Verbal Task

What happens when a task combines *linguistic* as well as temporal and spatial factors?

To study this, a task was devised in which the subject was presented a trio of letters in one of three modalities—visual, auditory, or tactile—and asked to compare the order of letters in that trio to the order of the same three letters presented either in the same modality or a different modality. As shown in Figure 2, the letters are the same within each pair, but the *sequence* of the letters may be the same or different. Five letters were chosen for this task, from which nine trios were constructed. The letters chosen were J, L, D, S, and R. An auditory—auditory presentation was carried out in the following way. The three letters were said aloud at a speed of about one letter per second, with a pause of a second between letters. There was a pause of two seconds, and those letters were said again, either in the same order, or in a different order. The patient was then asked to give a same—different judgment about the orders of the two sets of letters. So, for example, the patient would hear DSJ—DSJ for a *same* match, and DSJ—JDS for a *different* match.

For visual and tactile presentations, letters $\frac{1}{4}$ inch wide and about 3 inches high were constructed out of tagboard. For intramodal visual presentation, the letters were held up, one letter at a time, for about 2 sec per letter, in front of the patient. After a pause of about 2 sec, these letters were held up again, either in the same or in a different order. For the tactile—tactile presentation (actually haptic) a letter was placed in the patient's hand out of his view and he was allowed to feel it for about 2 sec. Again, there was a pause of about 2 sec between the presentation of each trio of letters. The same general procedure was used for the cross-modal presentations. So, for example, in an auditory—visual presentation the letters were said aloud first, and, after a 2-sec pause, the tagboard letters were held up one at a time in the patient's field of view. All intramodal and cross-modal combinations of the letter sequences were tested. After every presenation, in both the intramodal and the cross-modal tasks, the patient had to make a same—different judgment.

Examples of Letter Task

Modality combination	Same	Different
A–A	DSJ–DSJ	DSJ–JDS
A–V	RJL–RJL	RJL–LJR

Figure 2. Examples of letter-sequencing task.

IN THE EARLY DAYS OF THIS COUNTRY THE
FUNCTIONS OF GOVERNMENT WERE FEW IN NUMBER. MOST
OF THESE FUNCTIONS WERE CARRIED OUT BY LOCAL
TOWN AND COUNTRY OFFICIALS, WHILE CENTRALIZED
AUTHORITY WAS DISTRUSTED. THE GROWTH OF INDUSTRY
AND OF BIG CITIES HAS SO CHANGED THE SITUATION
THAT THE FARMER OF TODAY IS CONCERNED WITH . . . . .

LOCAL AFFAIRS ABOVE ALL

THE PRICE OF LUMBER

THE ACTIONS OF THE GOVERNMENT

THE AUTHORITY OF TOWN OFFICIALS

Figure 3. Sample of reading material from the Goodglass and Kaplan aphasia test. (From Goodglass, H. and Kaplan, E., *The assessment of aphasia and related disorders,* © 1972, Lea & Febiger, Philadelphia. Reprinted by permission of the publisher.)

Discussion of Results on the Verbal Task.   The results show that there were no differences between any modality combinations on this task. The most dramatic aspect of these data is evident when one looks at the data for individual patients. Among the patients, one could be classified as a classical sensory aphasic, that is, she could understand no spoken language, and she also spoke in jargon. Despite these deficits, her reading ability was remarkably preserved. There is a short test of auditory receptive language abilities called the Token Test, where the patient is given commands, and must respond nonverbally. When this patient *listened* to the commands, she got 25 correct out of a total of 80, or 31%. When she *read* the commands, she got 68 correct out of 80, or 85%. Figure 3 shows a sample of other material that the patient was asked to read. This was taken from the Goodglass and Kaplan aphasia test. The task required the patient to point to the multiple-choice answer that would best complete the last sentence of the paragraph. The sensory aphasic patient performed correctly on this extremely complex written passage. Yet

Patient # 2: Sensory aphasia

Modality sequence	Errors
A–A	1
V–V	1
T–T	0
A–V	0
V–A	1
A–T	2
T–A	1
V–T	0
T–V	2

Figure 4. Errors made on letter-sequencing task by a sensory aphasic patient.

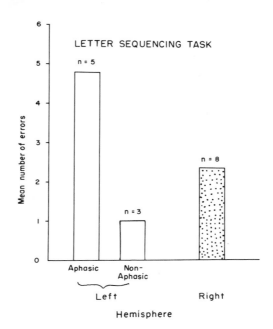

Figure 5. Mean number of errors made on letter-sequencing task by aphasic and nonaphasic left-hemisphere lesion patients, and by right-hemisphere lesion patients.

it was almost impossible for her to respond correctly to oral commands or questions that were only a few words in length.

On the letter-sequencing task, this patient's mistakes were distributed among the intramodal and cross-modal combinations. Figure 4 shows that she made mistakes on those pairs that involved auditory presentations *as well as* those that did not. This was also true of a patient classified as a Broca's aphasic, where auditory comprehension was reasonably intact but production of speech was impaired.

What are the results for this linguistic task looked at in terms of left- and right-hemisphere groups? A Krushkal–Wallis (Siegel, 1956) one-way analysis of variance by ranks performed on the total number of errors made by the left-hemisphere group, the right-hemisphere group, and controls on the letter-sequencing task shows that differences among the groups are significant ($p < .01$). The same test performed on the aphasic left-hemisphere group ($N = 5$), the nonaphasic left-hemisphere group ($N = 3$) and the right-hemisphere group is not significant ($.10 < p < .20$), although, as Figure 5 shows, the mean number of errors produced by the aphasic group exceeds that of both nonaphasic groups.

Summary

The linguistic task described above necessarily involved both temporal and spatial factors. The task was temporal in that the letters were presented sequentially. However, temporal and spatial factors were confounded in those combinations that involved audition, which has to be temporal, and either vision or touch, where stimuli were necessarily spatial. Despite these differences between the linguistic tasks and the nonverbal tasks, the single most important conclusion is that the findings resulting from the linguistic task confirm those from the nonverbal tasks. To sum up, deficits caused by either left- or right-sided lesions on the simple tasks used here are *not* modality specific. This is true for both linguistic and nonlinguistic tasks. Moreover, there are no demonstrable differences between left- and right-hemisphere groups on verbal tasks and on those nonverbal tasks that combined temporal and spatial factors. Differences between the left- and right-hemisphere groups can be demonstrated only when the temporal and spatial characteristics of the stimuli are deliberately separated.

How might these results contribute to understanding developmental issues? Dyslexic children have been studied from a perceptual point of view in a variety of ways. A few of the studies applying sensory integration theory have been discussed here. Benton (1962) suggests that perceptual difficulties may be found in poor readers (and some of these difficulties may indeed be modality specific) but that reading problems in older children are probably more likely to be associated with dysfunction in some aspect of verbal mediation. Based on the data reported here on adult patients both with and without language deficits who show *supramodal* rather than modality-specific deficits, it may be profitable to approach some developmental language deficits from this point of view as well.

REFERENCES

Belmont, L., Birch, H.G., & Belmont, I. (1968) Auditory-visual intersensory processing and verbal mediation. *Journal of Nervous and Mental Disease, 147,* 562–569.

Benton, A. (1962) Dyslexia in relation to form perception and directional sense. In J. Money (Ed.), *Reading disability: Progress and research needs in dyslexia.* Baltimore: Johns Hopkins Univ. Press.

Birch, H.G., & Belmont, L. (1964) Auditory-visual integration in normal and retarded readers. *American Journal of Orthopsychiatry, 34,* 852–861.

Birch, H.G., & Belmont, L. (1965) Auditory-visual integration in brain damaged and normal children. *Developmental Medicine and Child Neurology, 7,* 135–144.

Birch, H.G., & Lefford, A. (1963) Intersensory development in children. *Monographs of the Society of Research in Child Development, 28,*(5), Serial No. 89.

Blank, M, and Bridger, W.H. (1964) Cross-modal transfer in nursery school children. *Journal of Comparative Physiology and Psychology, 58,* 272–282.

Burton, D., & Ettlinger, G. (1960) Cross-modal transfer of training in monkeys. *Nature, 186,* 1071–1072.

Butters, N., Barton, M., & Brody, B. (1970) Role of the right parietal lobe in the mediation of cross-modal associations and reversible operations in space. *Cortex, 6*(2), 174–190.

Butters, N., & Brody, B. (1968) The role of the left parietal lobe in the mediation of intra and cross-modal association. *Cortex, 4*(4), 328–343.

Carmon, A., & Benton, A.L. (1969) Tactile perception of direction and number in patients with unilateral cerebral disease. *Neurology, 19,* 525–532.

Chapanis, L. (1974) Intramodial and cross-modal pattern perception in stroke patients. Unpublished doctoral dissertation, Cornell Univ.

Corkin, S. (1974) Serial ordering deficits in inferior readers. *Neuropsychologia, 12,* 347–354.

DeRenzi, E., Faglioni, P., Scotti, G., & Spinnler, H. (1972) Impairment in associating colour to form, concomitant with aphasia. *Brain, 95,* 293–304.

Deutsch, C., & Schumer, F. (1967) *Brain damaged children: A modality oriented exploration of performance.* Final report to the Vocational Rehabilitation Administration, Department of Health, Education, and Welfare, Washington, D.C. 20201. Institute for Developmental Studies, School of Education, New York Univ., November, 1967.

Efron, R. (1963) Temporal perception, aphasia, and deja vu. *Brain, 86,* 403–424.

Ettlinger, G. (1960) Cross-modal transfer of training in monkeys. *Behaviour, 16,* 56–65.

Ettlinger, G. (1973) The transfer of information between sense modalities: A neuropsychological review. In P. Zippel (Ed.), *Memory and a transfer of information.* New York: Plenum.

Fontenot, D.J., & Benton, A.L. (1971) Tactile perception of direction in relation to hemispheric locus of lesion. *Neuropsychologia, 9,* 83–88.

Freides, D. (1974) Human information processing and sensory modality. *Psychological Bulletin, 81*(5), 284–310.

Gazzaniga, M. (1972) One brain—two minds? *American Scientist, 60,* 311–317.

Geschwind, N. (1965a) Disconnexion syndromes in animals and man. Part I. *Brain, 88,* 237–294.

Geschwind, N. (1965b) Disconnexion syndromes in animals and man. Part II. *Brain, 88,* 585–644.

Geschwind, N. (1970) The organization of language and the brain. *Science, 170,* 940–944.

Gibson, E.J. (1969) *Principles of perceptual learning and development.* New York: Appleton.

Goodglass, H., Barton, M., & Kaplan, E. (1968) Sensory modality and object naming in aphasia. *Journal of Speech and Hearing Research, 11*(3), 488–496.

Goodglass, H. & Kaplan, E. (1972) *The assessment of aphasia and related disorders.* Philadelphia: Lea & Febiger.

Hayek, F.A. (1952) *The sensory order.* Chicago: Univ. of Chicago Press.

Hécaen, H. (1969) Aphasic, apraxic, and agnosic syndromes in right and left hemisphere lesions. *Handbook of Clinical Neurology, 4,* 291–311.

McFie, J. (1969) The diagnostic significance of disorders of higher nervous activity. *Handbook of Clinical Neurology, 4,* 1–12.

Miller, E. (1972) *Clinical neuropsychology.* Middlesex, England: Penguin.

Piercy, M. (1964) The effects of cerebral lesions on intellectual function: A review of current research trends. *British Journal of Psychiatry, 110,* 310–352.

Pohl, E., Butters, N., & Goodglass, H. (1972) Spatial discrimination systems and cerebral lateralization. *Cortex, 8,* 305–314.

Rudel, R., & Teuber, H. (1971) Pattern recognition within and across sensory modalities in normal and brain-injured children. *Neuropsychologia, 9,* 389–399.

Sarno, J., Swisher, L., & Sarno, M. (1969) Aphasia in a congenitally deaf man. *Cortex, 5,* 398–414.

Siegel, S. (1956) *Nonparametric statistics.* New York: McGraw-Hill.

Spinner, H., & Vignolo, L.A. (1966) Impaired recognition of meaningful sounds in aphasia. *Cortex, 2,* 337–348.

Williams, M. (1970) *Brain damage and the mind.* Middlesex, England: Penguin.

Wilson, W., & Shaffer, O. (1963) Intermodality transfer of specific discriminations in the monkey. *Nature, 197,* 107.

10

Electroencephalographic Testing of Cerebral Specialization in Normal and Congenitally Deaf Children: A Preliminary Report

HELEN NEVILLE

Hemispheric specialization refers to the fact that man's two cerebral hemispheres are not functionally equipotential. There are many studies showing the functional asymmetries of the two hemispheres of the human adult. These studies often show a language deficit after trauma to the left hemisphere and deficits in certain nonverbal skills after right-hemisphere trauma. Consistent with these findings are the many psychological studies of normal subjects showing better perception and recall of verbal material presented to the right visual field and right ear (Bryden, 1965; Kimura, 1967; Hines, Satz, Schell, & Schmidlin, 1969; McKeever & Huling, 1971); and better perception and recall of certain nonverbal material presented to the left visual field and left ear (Curry, 1967; Durnford & Kimura, 1971). A number of studies have reported electroencephalographic asymmetries between the hemispheres which are consistent with the concept of functional specialization. These studies have reported greater evoked potential amplitude from the left hemisphere than the right hemisphere upon the presentation of verbal material (Wood, Goff, & Day, 1971; Wood, 1975) and auditory evoked potential predominance of the right hemisphere in other task situations (Dustman & Beck, 1974; Vella, Butler, & Glass, 1972). The present investigation was designed to see if cerebral specialization of function reflects the development of particular behavioral abilities. The question was: Does cerebral specialization develop in parallel with general, *nonverbal* cognitive skills, or must *verbal* comprehension and production have developed before cerebral specialization is evident?

In *Biological Foundations of Language* (1967), and in other papers (e.g., 1971), Lenneberg conjectured that hemispheric asymmetries would develop in the absence of normal language acquisition if the development of nonverbal cognitive skills was normal. This prediction is consistent with Lenneberg's view that perceptual, mathematical, and language abilities have a common neurological correlate. Conceivably, this correlate could be the development of hemispheric specialization of function.

In contrast, others have suggested that cerebral specialization occurs with the acquisition of speech, and that the functional lateralization of verbal skills might precede the lateralization of nonverbal skills (e.g., Bever, 1970, 1974; Gazzaniga, 1970). Still others suggest that functional cerebral specialization is present from birth (see Chapter 14). One way of approaching this question is to compare hemispheric specialization in normal children with hemispheric specialization in children who have failed to acquire speech production and speech comprehension but have normal nonverbal skills.

METHOD

Subjects

Electroencephalographic and behavioral hemispheric asymmetries were studied in 16 normal children aged 9 to 13 years, and 15 congenitally deaf children of the same age range. The deaf children had normal nonverbal IQs, ranging from 93 to 140 on the Wechsler scale. None of these deaf children could speak, according to the reports of their teachers and according to a series of simple tests given by the author. They attended a school for the deaf that did not encourage the use of sign language, but this, of course, does not rule out the possibility that the children knew some signs. (In fact, some of the deaf children reported that they signed when they were at home; these were typically children of congenitally deaf parents. We will return to this point later.) The deaf children had all been diagnosed by their physicians and by the school physician as having hereditary sensorineural deafness, which resulted in 90 or greater decibel loss binaurally over the speech range of frequencies (i.e., 500–1500 Hz). None of the children had any history of other neurological disorder.

Stimuli

The stimuli were line drawings of common objects projected for 10 msec to the left or right visual field. These stimuli ranged from $3°$ to $7°$ of visual angle in width, and from $3°$ to $7°30'$ in height. All projected pictures began $2°$ of visual angle to the left or right of the fixation point. Each of 32 different pictures was projected randomly to each visual field once per session. These line drawings were chosen as stimuli because Olson (1973, unpublished study) found superior left visual field (i.e., right hemisphere) recognition of these in normal children.

Procedure

Task instructions were given verbally (normal subjects) or in pantomime (deaf subjects). Eye position was monitored at the beginning of each trial, both directly and from an electrode placed on the nasion to ensure that subjects were looking at the fixation point at the time of stimulus presentation. Two seconds after presentation of each slide (to allow for evoked potential collection) the child was shown a card and asked to choose, by pointing, one picture out of five which he thought was a picture of the same object he had just seen depicted on the screen. This did not constitute a physical match because, while the objects depicted were the same, the pictures were different (e.g., an open umbrella was to be matched to a closed one). Each child received a score of percentage of correct recognition for stimuli presented to the left visual field and for stimuli presented to the right visual field. Each child was tested in two sessions, one week apart, which were identical except for the counterbalancing order of stimuli.

Recording and Analysis

Evoked potential and behavioral measures of hemispheric asymmetry were obtained simultaneously. Monopolar visual evoked potentials (VEP) were recorded from posterior temporal regions of the left and right hemispheres—T_5 and T_6 in the 10-20 system (Jasper, 1958) referenced to the linked earlobes. An active electrode was also placed on the nasion to ensure that evoked potentials were not contaminated by eye movements. Evoked potentials from the two hemispheres were averaged separately from the two sessions, over left and right field presentations, and separately over correct and incorrect responses. Only the results from VEPs on trials on which the child responded *correctly* are presented here. Each VEP from each child was digitized separately, and independent analyses of variance were performed for the latency and amplitude of each of the peaks. The most prominent feature of the VEPs from all subjects was a large negative wave peaking around 400 msec after stimulus onset (N400). A sharp positive wave at about 270 msec typically preceded this wave (P270) and a slow positivity usually followed it (P970). The VEP in Figure 1 is labeled for these peaks. N400 was designated as the highest negative wave occurring between 300 and 500 msec, P270 as the most positive peak immediately preceding and at the base of N400, and P970 as the most positive point following N400.[1] The amplitudes of these components were measured in two ways (1) from baseline to peak, with 200 msec of the average prestimulus EEG tracing serving as baseline (base—N400; base—P970) and (2) from

---

[1] P970 could not be estimated for three hearing and two deaf subjects.

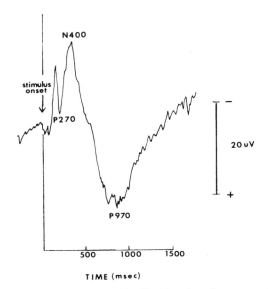

Figure 1. Components of the VEP to the line drawings from normal and deaf children (subject DF).

peak to peak (P270–N400; N400–P970). These different amplitude measures were taken to see how consistent different VEP components were in reflecting hemispheric asymmetries. The latencies of the peaks also were analyzed in view of the hypothesized commissural transfer of information arriving initially at the nonspecialized hemisphere. Such a factor might be expected to produce VEP differences in latency such as were found in an earlier study of auditory evoked potential asymmetries (Neville, 1974). The latencies of the three peaks were taken to be the times of maximum positivity or negativity.

RESULTS

Behavioral Data

There was a very small tendency for better recognition of line drawings presented to the left visual field, for both hearing and deaf children. This effect was not significant either for the hearing subjects (in contrast to the study by Olson, mentioned earlier) or for the deaf subjects. Left-field superiority was shown by 57% of all the children, while 6% of hearing subjects and 14% of deaf subjects showed no difference between the fields. The two groups of children performed at approximately the same level of accuracy on the task (mean percentage of correct responses: hearing subjects, 77; deaf subjects, 81).

Evoked Potentials

Hearing Children

The hearing children showed a strong asymmetry between the hemispheres. For all three peaks, the latencies of the right-hemisphere VEP peaks were earlier than the left-hemisphere VEP peaks, and amplitudes were larger in right- than in left-hemisphere VEPs. These results were found in both sessions, but only the data from Session 1 are presented here. The mean latency differences between the hemispheres for peaks P270, N400, and P970 were 32.8, 31.5, and 29.2 msec, respectively. This difference was significant for P270 and N400 [F for hemisphere main effect (df 1,15) = 8.05, $p < .02$; F (df 1,15) = 5.83, $p < .03$, respectively], while the P970 difference was not significant. For these three latency measures, on average 75% of normal children showed right-hemisphere peaks occurring earlier than left-hemisphere peaks. The amplitude differences between the hemispheres all showed right-hemisphere VEP larger than left-hemisphere VEP, with an average difference of 3.2 μV. These differences were significant for the N400–P970 [F (df 1,12) = 5.1, $p < .03$] and base-N400 [F (df 1,15) = 4.67, $p < .04$] measures and at

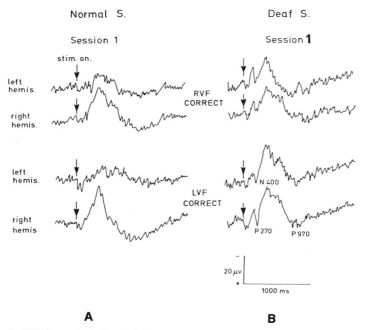

Figure 2. VEP from the left and right hemispheres of one normal hearing child (JC) and one deaf child (MH), Session 1, according to visual field of stimulus presentation. All VEP are averages of about 30 different pictures, correctly recognized by the subject.

the 6% level for the P270–N400 measure $[F (df\ 1,15) = 3.94]$. On average, in 74% of subjects these three VEP components were larger from the right than from the left hemisphere. Section A of Figure 2 shows the VEPs from the two hemispheres of one hearing subject from Session 1, averaged according to left and right visual field presentations. These data suggest that the perception of the pictures was mediated more by the right than by the left hemisphere in these children.

Deaf Children

The deaf subjects did not show these asymmetries. Section B of Figure 2 shows VEPs from the two hemispheres of one deaf subject. The VEPs from the left and right hemispheres tended to be similar in latency and amplitude. The deaf subjects' VEPs tended to reflect anatomical features of the visual projection system: Left visual field presentations resulted in larger right-hemisphere responses and right visual field presentations resulted in larger left-hemisphere responses [Hemisphere × Visual Field interaction for amplitude N400–P970 $(df\ 1, 12) = 9.75, p < .007$; for base–P970, $F (df\ 1, 12) = 5.0, p < .04$). These Hemisphere × Field interactions suggest that the pictures were indeed initially projected to the appropriate hemisphere; the lack of significant hemisphere main effects suggests that neither hemisphere was dominant during the perception of these pictures.

Hearing and Deaf Subjects Compared

Whereas the VEPs from the deaf group did not show the significant asymmetries indicative of hemispheric specialization, they did show some *tendency* toward *left hemisphere* predominance (i.e., opposite to that of the hearing subjects). Table 1 shows the mean VEP component amplitudes from the left and right hemispheres and the differences between the hemispheres for the hearing and deaf subjects. These data, which show the right-hemisphere VEPs to be significantly larger than the left-hemisphere VEPs in the hearing children, and left-hemisphere VEPs to be nonsignificantly larger than the right-hemisphere VEP, in the deaf children, are plotted in Figure 3. The interaction effects [Group (Hearing–Deaf) × Hemisphere] were significant for amplitude measures P270–N400 and base–N400 $[F (df\ 1,29) =$

TABLE 1 Session 1: Mean Microvolts Amplitude for Left Hemisphere (LH) and Right Hemisphere (RH)

	P270–N400	N400–P970	base–N400
Normal subjects			
LH	15.6	22.5	12.1
RH	18.0	26.9	14.9
Difference (RH − LH)	+2.4	+4.4	+2.8
Deaf subjects			
LH	15.1	26.3	13.4
RH	12.9	25.6	12.2
Difference (RH − LH)	−2.2	−0.7	−1.2

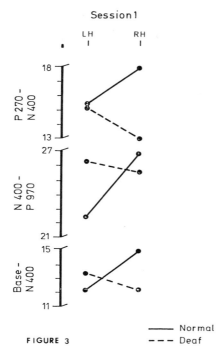

FIGURE 3

Figure 3. Mean microvolts amplitude of left and right hemisphere for three VEP peaks from 16 normal-hearing and 15 deaf children.

7.46, $p < .01$; F (df 1,29) = 5.0, p < .03]. This interaction effect also approached significance for N400–P970 [F (df 1,24) = 2.9, $p = .09$].

Hearing, Signing Deaf, and Nonsigning Deaf Subjects Compared

In view of the unexpected and puzzling tendency for the deaf group to show VEP asymmetries opposite to those of the hearing group, the deaf subjects were divided into two subgroups. As mentioned earlier, each child was asked how, when he was at home, he communicated with his parents. Eight children indicated that they communicated in sign language with their parents (signers) and seven indicated that they communicated with their parents just as they did with the experimenter— largely by pantomime (nonsigners). This breakdown was attempted in order to investigate the possible relation between knowing a language (sign *or* verbal) and the development of cerebral specialization. The VEP amplitude data showed that the *right*-hemisphere VEPs were larger than the left-hemisphere VEPs for hearing subjects, but that the *left*-hemisphere VEPs were larger than the right-hemisphere VEPs for signers; nonsigners showed no asymmetries, or inconsistent and small ones. These data, from Session 1, are plotted in Figure 4. The Three-Group (Hearing, Signers, and Nonsigners) × Hemisphere interaction was significant for P270–N400 [F (df 2,28) = 5.23, $p < .01$] and at the 7% level for

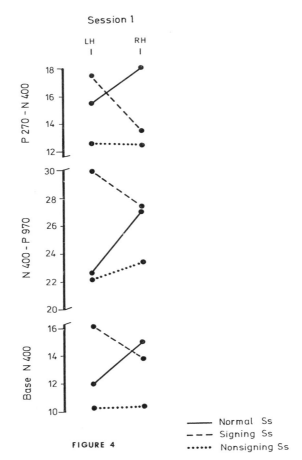

FIGURE 4

——— Normal Ss
– – – Signing Ss
•••••• Nonsigning Ss

Figure 4. Mean microvolts amplitude of left and right hemisphere for three VEP peaks from 16 normal-hearing, 8 signing deaf, and 7 nonsigning deaf children.

base–N400 [F (df 2,28) = 2.87]. The interaction effect showing opposite asymmetries for signing and hearing subjects [Group (Signing–Hearing) × Hemisphere] was significant for P270–N400 [F (df 1,22) = 9.99, $p < .005$] and base–N400 [F (df 1,22) = 4.79, $p < .03$], and at the 7% level for N400–P970 [F (df 1,18) = 3.52]. Thus, this analysis suggests that the tendency for left-hemisphere predominance noted in the deaf group was contributed virtually entirely by the signing subjects in the group.

Correlations between Behavioral and Electrographic Asymmetries

Correlations were performed in an attempt to relate the evoked potential asymmetry to the (nonsignificant) behavioral asymmetry. This involved correlating the VEP asymmetry (difference scores between the hemispheres for the VEP components) with the difference in percentage recognition between the hemifields. These showed, for hearing subjects, Session 1, a significant positive correlation ($r = .54$, $p < .02$) between the VEP asymmetry of the latency of P270 and the difference in percentage recognition of the pictures presented to the left and right visual fields (i.e., the greater the difference in milliseconds by which the right-hemisphere peak P270 preceded the left-hemisphere peak P270, the greater the difference in percentage recognition for the left than the right visual field). Also, within the deaf group, signing children showed a right visual field effect (consistent with the left-hemisphere EP predominance) twice as frequently as did nonsigning children. In Session 2, for example, five of six deaf children who showed a right visual field effect were signers.

DISCUSSION

These data show electroencephalographic hemispheric specialization in normal hearing children aged 9 to 13 years. VEPs collected during perception of line drawings were larger and the components peaked earlier from the right hemisphere than the left hemisphere. The behavioral task did not produce the expected significant left visual field advantage, but the small behavioral asymmetry in that direction did correlate with one measure of VEP asymmetry. The data suggest that the right hemisphere of the hearing children was somehow predominant in this task situation.

The data from the deaf group *as a whole* did not show significant differences between the hemispheres. One might have predicted that the deaf children would show the normal children's pattern of results in the perception of these pictures, which need not be mediated verbally. It was predicted that the deaf children would show hemispheric asymmetries, in view of the fact that they are of normal nonverbal intelligence, and in spite of the fact that they could not speak.

Furthermore, the deaf children of this group who *sign* (but do not speak), did show evidence of cerebral specialization, whereas the nonsigning deaf children did not. Moreover, the data show that the electroencephalographic and behavioral asymmetries of the signers are opposite in direction to those of the normal hearing children. This result may suggest that the deaf signers acquired their sign language much as normal children acquire verbal language—with left-hemisphere specialization playing a role. However, because their language may be characterized as visual–spatial, "spatial" tasks in which normal children show right hemisphere specialization (like the task in this study) may be mediated by the left, or spatial–language, hemisphere in signing children. Alternatively, perhaps the signing children have developed a right-hemisphere specialization for their sign language, leaving the left hemisphere somehow predominant for other, nonlanguage stimuli like those in the present study. To separate these two hypotheses, we are now studying congenitally deaf children who sign both at home and at school. Pictures and signs will be presented in a paradigm similar to the present one. Thus, the question of right- or left-hemispheric specialization for sign language may be resolved. Also, it will be interesting to see the pattern of results with visually presented written words as stimuli.

The question remains as to why the nonsigners did not show specialization. These nonsigning deaf children do, of course, manage to communicate with one another, and with hearing people. They do this with a combination of finger spelling, some signs, and a great deal of gesturing and pantomime. Only if one defines language to be a system of elements with internal structure and hierarchical syntactic organization—which American Sign Language shows (Bellugi & Klima, 1975)—may these nonsigning children be characterized as languageless. That is, although they can communicate, they lack a formal language. The present results, then, suggest the following hypothesis: The acquisition of and hemispheric specialization for formal language (whether verbal or sign) must precede hemispheric specialization for certain nonlanguage tasks (such as the picture recognition task in this study). This hypothesis is currently being tested, by studying congenitally deaf children before and after the acquisition of sign language.

The difference between the signers and nonsigners seen in this study may have resulted not only from the different language experiences of the two groups of children. It may be, for example, that because the signers had deaf parents they would have been recognized as deaf earlier than the deaf children of hearing parents. This factor may conceivably have resulted in different developmental histories. Also, although all of these deaf children had been diagnosed as hereditarily deaf, one is more certain of this diagnosis for the deaf children with deaf parents, than for those with hearing parents, and these latter children may have some other, albeit undetected, neurological abnormality (although the signers and nonsigners had similar IQs).

The data from this study show opposite patterns of hemispheric asymmetries for children whose formal language was acquired by the auditory mode (hearing subjects) and by the visual mode (signing subjects). Children without a formal language did not show hemispheric asymmetries. These findings suggest that the developmental course of cerebral specialization may depend on the fact and mode of acquisition of a formal language system.

ACKNOWLEDGMENTS

I am indebted to the late Professor Eric Lenneberg for guidance throughout all phase of this research. I gratefully acknowledge the assistance given by Dr. Sam Sutton in the instrumentation of the work. This research was partially supported by grants IT01 MH 13894-01 and 1 R03 MH 23268-01 from the National Institute of Health awarded to Dr. Lenneberg.

REFERENCES

Bellugi, U., & Klima, E. (1975) Aspects of sign language and its structure. In J.F. Kavanagh & J.E. Cutting (Eds.), *The role of speech in language.* Cambridge, Massachusetts: MIT Press.

Bever, T.G. (1970) The nature of cerebral dominance in speech behavior of the child and adult. In Huxley & Ingram (Eds.), *Mechanisms of language development.* New York: Academic Press.

Bever, T.G. (1974) The relation of language development to cognitive development. In E.H. Lenneberg (Ed.), *Language and brain: Development aspects.* Neurosciences Research Program Bulletin *12,* No. 4.

Bryden, M.P. (1965) Tachistoscopic recognition, handedness and cerebral dominance. *Neuropsychologia, 3,* 1–8.

Curry, F. (1967) A comparison of left-handed and right-handed subjects on verbal and nonverbal dichotic listening tasks. *Cortex, 3,* 343–352.

Durnford, M., & Kimura, D. (1971) Right hemisphere specialization for depth perception reflected in visual field differences. *Nature, 231,* 395–398.

Dustman, R.E., & Beck, E.C. (1974) The evoked response: Its use in evaluating brain function of children and young adults. Prepublication manuscript.

Gazzaniga, M.S. (1970) *The bisected brain,* New York: Appleton.

Hines, D., Satz, P., Schell, B., & Schmidlin, S. (1969) Differential recall of digits in the left and right visual half-fields under free and fixed order of recall. *Neuropsychologia, 7,* 13–22.

Jasper, H.H. (1958) The ten-twenty electrode system of the international federation. *Electroencephalography and Clinical Neurophysiology, 10,* 371–375.

Kimura, D. (1964) Left-right differences in the perception of melodies. *Quarterly Journal of Experimental Psychology, 14,* 355–358.

Kimura, D. (1966) Dual functional asymmetry of the brain in visual perception. *Neuropsychologia, 4,* 275–285.

Kimura, D. (1967) Functional asymmetry of the brain in dichotic listening. *Cortex, 3,* 163–178.

Knox, C., & Kimura, D. (1968) Cerebral processing of nonverbal sounds in boys and girls. *Neuropsychologia, 6,* 1–11.

Lenneberg, E. (1967) *Biological foundations of language.* New York: Wiley.

Lenneberg, E. (1971) Of language knowledge, apes and brains. *Journal of Psycholinguistic Research, 1,* 1.

McKeever, W.F., & Huling, M.P. (1971) Lateral dominance and tachistoscopic word recognition performance obtained with simultaneous bilateral input. *Neuropsychologia, 9,* 15–20.

Neville, H. (1974) Electrographic correlates of lateral asymmetry in the processing of verbal and nonverbal auditory stimuli. *Journal of Psycholinguistic Research, 3,* 151–163.

Olson, M. (1973) Laterality differences in tachistoscopic picture recognition in children. Unpublished manuscript.

Rizzolatti, G., Umilta, C., & Berlucci, G. (1971) Opposite superiorities of the right and left cerebral hemispheres in discriminative reaction time to physiognomical and alphabetical material. *Brain, 94,* 431–442.

Vella, E.J., Butler, S.R., & Glass, A. (1972) Electrical correlates of right hemisphere function. *Nature, 236,* 125–126.

Wood, C.C. (1975) Auditory and phonetic levels of processing in speech perception: Neurophysiological and information-processing analysis. *Journal of Experimental Psychology: Human Perception and Performance, 104,* 1, 3–20.

Wood, C.C., Goff, W.R., & Day, R.S. (1971) Auditory evoked potentials during speech perception. *Science, 173,* 1248–1251.

11

Dichotic Listening of Callosal Agenesis and Turner's Syndrome Patients

C. NETLEY

Dichotic listening results are often asymmetric in the sense that better recall is found for material presented to one ear than for material presented to the other ear (Kimura, 1961a). It is usually argued that this difference is due to the differential access of the two ears' projection systems to the specialized functions of the two cerebral hemispheres.[1] On this basis, the higher right-ear report scores for verbal material are ascribed to the right ear's advantage over the left in tapping the functions of the verbal left hemisphere (Kimura, 1961b). The evidence for this proposition has usually come from examinations of either neurologically normal individuals of various ages or adult neurological patients who have been without lesions until maturity or close to the age of maturity (Milner, Taylor, & Sperry, 1968). Both sorts of individuals are, by virtue of their normal developmental histories, likely to possess the usual hemispheric specialization—the left hemisphere processing verbal material and the right hemisphere processing nonverbal or spatial material. As a result, dichotic listening data with both normals and the neurologically impaired may be fairly easily accounted for in terms of a developed, physiological system permitting access to a specialized hemispheric function, or alternatively, to the disruption of this, either centrally or somewhere along the projection route (Kimura, 1967).

Several questions can be asked about these concepts. First, how do ear asymmetries, and by implication the central cognitive functions presumed to underlie

[1] An alternative explanation in terms of attentional factors has been offered by Kinsbourne (1970), but whether this really competes with the older one is a moot point (Kimura & Durnford, 1974).

dichotic listening phenomena, develop? Do these depend on some kind of antaga-
nistic competitive action between the hemispheres (Levy, 1969) or are these
processes independent of interactions between the two neural structures? A second
question is, How may we account for the quite significant individual differences in
indices of hemispheric specialization? Dichotic listening performance for example,
is related to handedness (Zurif & Bryden, 1969), sex (Bryden, 1970), and cognitive
characteristics (McGlone & Davidson, 1973). Bryden (1975) has also shown that
hereditary factors may be responsible for some individual differences in dichotic
parameters.

The experiments described here were carried out with two types of patients. The
first type, those with defined neurological lesions, were thought to be relevant to
the question of how hemispheric specialization, as indicated by dichotic listening,
develops. The second type, those with abnormalities in sex chromosome complement, were considered, for reasons to be mentioned later, relevant to the question
of individual differences in the same parameters. The two studies are presented
separately.

STUDY 1: PATIENTS WITH NEUROLOGICAL LESIONS

The subjects were 10 patients with hemispherectomies and 4 with agenesis of the
corpus callosum. Controls were also included in the study. Before describing the
methods and results, it is probably worthwhile to outline in fairly general terms
how dichotically presented verbal material might be processed by these three kinds
of subjects.

The normals, of course, possess two intact cerebral hemispheres and are able, via
the corpus callosum, to exchange information between these neural structures.
Each hemisphere is probably characterized by a relative advantage for certain kinds
of tasks and a disadvantage for others, a crude division of these being that one is
verbal and the other spatial. The usual right-ear dichotic advantage for verbal
material found in normals is then most easily accounted for in terms of that ear's
greater access to the left hemisphere's verbal processing system, whereas the left ear
must depend either on the ipsilateral route (Kimura, 1967) or the corpus callosum
(Springer & Gazzaniga, 1975).

Hemispherectomized subjects present quite a different system. They have only
one hemisphere, and all cognitive functions, both verbal and nonverbal, are carried
out by that hemisphere regardless of whether it is the left or right. Data exist (Kohn
& Dennis, 1974; Dennis & Kohn, 1975) which clearly suggest that the upper limits
of development for the left and right hemispheres are not the same for verbal and
spatial tasks. These findings indicate that the isolated right hemisphere, for example, is less competent than the isolated left hemisphere at verbal tasks (the reverse
being true for spatial tasks). Nevertheless, left hemispherectomized patients may be
able to talk and may be capable of a considerable variety of verbal functions
(Carlson, Netley, Hendrick, & Prichard, 1968), so that even the "inappropriate"

hemisphere is capable of some tasks ordinarily done by the other. With such patients, dichotic listening cannot depend on the corpus callosum, and individual left- and right-ear sources have to be mediated by contralateral and ipsilateral ear routes only.

The third group, those with agenesis of the corpus callosum, are complicated, for several reasons. These patients may be totally without callosal tracts, with dichotic processing being dependent on the same ipsilateral and contralateral routes as in hemispherectomized patients. However, the agenesis may be partial (Ettlinger, Blakemore, Milner, & Wilson, 1972) and may imply the possibility of some interhemispheric communication of an attenuated kind. Finally, callosal agenesis patients may not develop the usual verbal—spatial hemispheric specialization, so that their dichotic performance might be processed by a different system than either normals or hemispherectomized subjects. If agenesis patients are characterized by a relative cortical bilaterality for verbal and spatial functions, their dichotic listening scores would be expected to show less asymmetry than other subjects. Bryden and Zurif (1970) described a callosal agenesis patient with a smaller than usual asymmetry on a verbal dichotic task, a finding which is consistent with the view that speech mechanisms were relatively bilateral in this individual. The contrary studies of Ettlinger and his associates (1972, 1974) are inconclusive, since their callosal agenesis subjects had quite significant cortical lesions likely to override dichotic laterality effects.

Two obvious hypotheses suggest themselves in considering the dichotic listening results of normals and of acallosal and hemispherectomized patients. The first is that ear asymmetries in these groups will depend on the relative integrity of the callosal fibers and their ability to provide interhemispheric communication. Under this hypothesis, ear asymmetries would be largest for the hemispherectomized subjects, next largest for the callosal agenesis subjects, and smallest for normals. The second hypothesis concerns the degree to which verbal functions are represented in the two cerebral hemispheres: The agenesis patients would be expected to show smaller asymmetries than either normal or hemispherectomized subjects. The principal objective of the study presented here was to evaluate the validity of these two possibilities.

Our assessment method was the same for all subjects. Each was tested individually by means of 12 dichotically presented digit triads, with an intertriad interval of 10 sec available for response. The presentation rate was two digits per second. Subjects were simply told to recall as many digits as possible. Earphones were reversed after the initial presentation of the 12-triad series, and a second presentation series was then given.

Our callosal agenesis subjects were selected according to the following criteria:

1. Clear radiological evidence for the congenital absence of the corpus callosum
2. No demonstrated cortical damage or focal neurological signs
3. Normal EEG
4. Average or higher than average IQ

Of 20 cases screened for study, 2 cases satisfied all criteria and a third satisfied all criteria except that the evidence for callosal agenesis was considered probable rather than certain. A fourth patient was also included, although she had a lower than average IQ (WISC verbal IQ: 58; performance IQ: 44) and a possible right-hemisphere cystic lesion.

The 10 hemispherectomized subjects represented 7 left and 3 right removals. They were predominantly cases of congenital or infantile hemiplegia and have been described elsewhere (Carlson *et al.,* 1968; Netley, 1972).

A control group of 9 subjects was also tested. The group consisted of 4 hydrocephalic patients and 5 neurologically normal subjects. The IQ levels and ages at testing of the control group were comparable to those of the agenesis subjects.

The dichotic data for all subjects were tabulated in terms of the number of correct responses for the left and right channels. The sum of these was similar for the control and agenesis groups and exceeded that of the less intelligent hemispherectomy subjects. Table 1 presents these data.

The parameter of most interest was the degree of ear asymmetry shown by the subjects. Ear asymmetry was defined simply as the absolute difference between left and right ear report scores. Figure 1 presents the findings for the three groups.

Median tests (Siegel, 1956, pp. 111−116) resulted in significant differences in ear asymmetries between the agenesis subjects and controls ($p < .05$) and between the agenesis and hemispherectomy subjects ($p < .05$). The control and hemispherectomy groups did not differ significantly.

These findings suggest that when an individual is characterized from birth by a neural system where interhemispheric information transfer may occur or where intrahemispheric information transfer constitutes the only possible organization, then dichotic scores are asymmetric. If neither of these conditions hold, ear scores are essentially equal. This implies that the development of hemispheric specialization may depend on interhemispheric information exchange, possibly of a competitive, antagonistic kind.

A further indication of the correctness of these suggestions is found in an examination of the dichotic results of hemispherectomy patients when they are divided into congenital injury and later injury cases. This author reported (Netley, 1972) that the ear asymmetries in congenital injury cases were less than in later injury cases. It can be argued that congenital injury cases were entirely restricted to intrahemispheric information transfer, while later injury cases had interhemispheric transfer for a time but lost it when they sustained a primary lesion. The later injury

TABLE 1 Mean Left, Right, and Total Ear Report Scores for Hemispherectomized, Callosal Agenesis, and Control Subjects

	Hemispherectomized	Agenesis	Control
Left	42.2	40.5	43.4
Right	29.5	46.0	45.6
Total	71.7	86.5	89.0

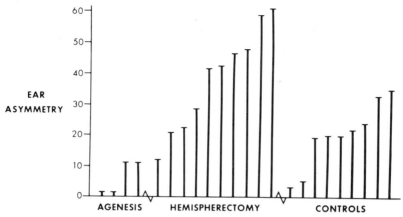

Figure 1. Ear asymmetry data for hemispherectomized, callosal agenesis, and control subjects.

cases, therefore, would have had the opportunity for some hemispheric specialization, which would suggest that the side of damage should be related to the degree of ear asymmetry. This is in fact was found since as in adult lesion cases (Oxbury & Oxbury, 1969), right-sided hemispherectomy produced larger asymmetries than did left hemispherectomy (Netley, 1972: Table 7).

STUDY 2: CASES OF SEX CHROMOSOME ANOMALY

The evidence implying a relationship between individual differences in hemispheric specialization and the sex chromosomes comes from a variety of sources. Some is inferred from the fact that the pattern of correlations between parents and children for spatial skills varies with the sex of both (Hartlage, 1970). That is, correlations are higher between differently sexed parent–child combinations and lower for same-sex combinations. This finding has been taken as evidence for the view that superior spatial ability is carried as a recessive gene on the X chromosome (Stafford, 1961). If it is assumed that hemispheric specialization is involved in individual differences in spatial ability, and this is a postulate underlying Buffery and Gray's (1972) theory, then it follows that sex chromosomes have some special relationship to hemispheric specialization. Indeed, some evidence has been found of actual anatomical differences between the sexes for those cortical areas subserving speech (Landsdell, 1964).

Further evidence comes from the study of the relationship between ability differences in normal men and women and their efficiency on laterally presented tasks. McGlone and Davidson (1973) examined this by administering tests of visuo-spatial ability, dichotic listening, and dot enumeration to young adults. Their findings indicate that females with a left-ear dichotic superiority (and assumed relatively greater right-hemispheric speech functioning) were particularly poor at spatial tasks. Left-handers, regardless of sex, showed the same tendency; but in the case of males, no relationship between spatial ability and ear superiority was found. McGlone and Davidson also reported that females tend to show greater right-field superiority on dot enumeration compared to males. It would seem, therefore, that females tend to process nonverbal tasks more frequently by the left hemisphere than do males, with this possibly being related to their generally poorer spatial functioning.

Additional evidence indicating the relationship of sex to hemispheric functioning is found in the literature dealing with the effects of localized cerebral lesions. Various studies have shown that the specific cognitive disorders associated with certain lesions may be commoner in one sex than the other. For example, Landsdell (1968) found the effect of right temporal lobectomy to be more disruptive of spatial abilities for men than for women. He also found that only for males could a correlation between the amount of right-hemispheric tissue removed and spatial impairment be established. McGlone and Kertesz (1973) report in contrast that only for females was it possible to demonstrate that spatial functioning was related to the verbal skills. The implication is that, for men, spatial skills are relatively more right-hemisphere dependent than they are for women, who seemingly employ more left-hemisphere based verbal strategies for these tasks. Additional evidence pointing to the significance of sex in determining the effect of brain lesions is found in the reports of Lansdell and Davie (1972) and Annett (1974). The significance of their findings is at present not clear, and the findings have not been incorporated into the few theories relating genetic processes to individual differences in ability which have been offered (e.g., Lehrke, 1974).

The evidence mentioned thus far has concerned the variable of sex differences at the phenotypic level, but some data exist pointing to the specific significance of the sex chromosomes in determining individual differences in cognitive functioning. Garvey and Mutton (1973), for example, report that individuals with an XXY sex chromosome complement are particularly handicapped on verbal tests. Developmental studies of children neonatally diagnosed as having similar disorders are in reasonable agreement with this report (Leonard, Landy, Ruddle, & Lubs, 1974).

The most well-established association between a sex chromosome abnormality and a specific cognitive impairment is that between Turner's syndrome and spatial impairments. Individuals with Turner's syndrome are phenotypically female but are without one X chromosome either completely or partially; they have been found to be essentially normal on verbal tests of various kinds but to perform relatively poorly on tasks described as nonverbal or spatial (Money, 1973; Garron, 1970). At present no explanation has been offered for this finding, but in planning our study it seemed reasonable on the basis of the evidence to hypothesize that some anomaly of hemispheric specialization might characterize Turner's syndrome patients. A more precise prediction than this for our study did not seem possible.

Our method consisted of testing a group of 14 Turner's syndrome patients being followed in the hospital's endocrine clinic. The assessment procedures consisted of a dichotic listening test given under free recall conditions, and the age-appropriate Wechsler test. The age range of the patients was 8 to 20 years, with a mean of 15.2 years. Verbal IQs were from 87 to 107, with a mean of 97; performance IQs ranged from 73 to 103, with a mean of 87.35. As a control group, 18 normal females of the same age range and ability were also tested.

The dichotic results are tabulated simply as the number of digits in the left and right channels which were correct and are presented in Figure 2. These data indicate that Turner's syndrome subjects show a definite tendency toward a bilateral distribution of ear scores in dichotic listening. Fifty seven percent of the Turner's syndrome patients are left-eared, while only 16 percent of controls show this phenomenon ($p < .02$ median test; Siegel, 1956, pp. 111–116). It seems, therefore, that the absence of one X chromosome in phenotypic females is associated with some tendency toward right hemisphere processing of verbal material. This is in contrast to the controls, who are predominantly right-eared and presumably left-hemisphere dominant for verbal functioning.

Explanations at this point are probably premature but speculations may not be, and the following is offered in this spirit. Assume with Stafford (1961) that superior spatial ability is mediated genetically by a recessive X-linked gene. Males would then be expected to show relatively good spatial skills, since only one X chromosome need be present for this ability to be manifested. Females on the other hand, will require two X-linked recessives in order to be spatially superior, and as a result their average level of spatial ability will be lower. Some further assumptions are required in order to translate these propositions about genetics and cognitive abilities into neural terms. Ounsted and Taylor (1972) have argued that the action of the Y chromosome is to slow the developmental rate so that more genomic

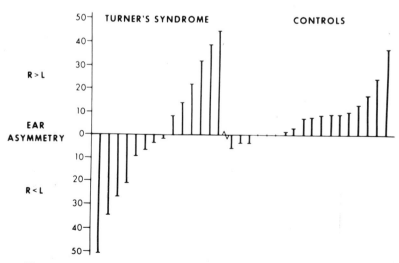

Figure 2. Ear asymmetry data for Turner's syndrome and control patients.

information may be expressed. Since it seems reasonable, on the basis of the data from agenesis patients, to accept Levy's (1969) hypothesis that hemispheric specialization follows a developmental course and arises from a competition for neural tissue, it may be that the Y chromosome acts in such a way that hemispheric specialization starts more slowly and terminates at a higher level for males. That is, the right hemisphere of a male would typically be more specialized for spatial tasks than the right hemisphere of a female. The X-linked recessive gene provides genomic information of a spatial nature which can be translated into available neural tissue. This may be best expressed in the presence of a Y chromosome, since this allows the right hemisphere to assume its spatial role. Thus, males fully express their spatial ability. Females are likely to possess high spatial skills rather rarely, with verbal ability being prepotent and resulting in less right-hemisphere specialization for spatial skills. Turner's syndrome patients would possess this high spatial latent ability but be unable, in the absence of a Y chromosome, to transcribe this into hemispheric specialization. A Turner's patient would, therefore, be more likely than a male to have verbal skill in the right and left hemisphere. This explanation, however, does not adequately account for why Turner's syndrome patients typically possess lower spatial ability than normal XX females. It appears necessary to invoke the additional concept implied by the Lyon hypothesis (Lyon, 1962). This concept, in the version offered by Russell (1964), states that sometime after conception there is a partial inactivation of one X chromosome in XX females. It has further been argued that the preserved and active portion shares some loci with certain loci on the Y chromosome (Ferguson-Smith, 1965). This suggests that the postulated braking effect of the Y chromosome would be, to a degree, also present in XX females. It would be absent, however, in XO Turner's syndrome cases and result in less expression of genomic spatial information in these individuals as compared to normal females. Figure 3 depicts the hypothesized development of hemispheric specialization in these three groups.

If a Turner's patient has verbal function mediated by the right hemisphere, spatial skills could be impaired by a kind of intrahemispheric occlusion. If this tendency were less pronounced and verbal skills were more left-hemisphere dependent, then some relative sparing of spatial impairment might be found. This possibility was examined by correlating the degree of dichotic ear asymmetry and

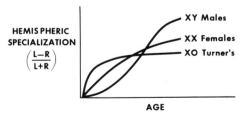

Figure 3. Hypothesized course of hemisphere specialization in XY male and XX female and XO Turner's syndrome subjects.

performance IQ within the group of Turner subjects with a right-ear superiority. The resulting correlation coefficient of .721 approaches significance at the $p = .10$ level and is consistent with the notion that the greater the degree of left-hemispheric involvement in language the less is the spatial impairment in Turner's syndrome. A similar correlation within the left-eared group resulted in an r of $-.220$. This of course is not significant, but it is in the direction expected if spatial skills were occluded by the verbal activities of the right hemisphere. The difference between these two correlations also approaches significance ($t = 2.084$, $p = .06$, 1-tail test).

CONCLUSIONS

To summarize the findings in the two studies: It appears that ear asymmetries are small in cases of agenesis of the corpus callosum. This suggests that if interhemispheric information transfer is absent or attenutated from birth, then the two hemispheres are less differentiated in terms of verbal processing. Evidence also was presented which suggests that the two hemispheres are not equally capable of assuming verbal and spatial functions, since genetic factors are at least correlated with indices of hemispheric specialization. It may be, therefore, that although an interactional interhemispheric information exchange underlies the development of neural specialization, the two brain halves are predisposed by a genetic program to development in certain directions and not others. This implies that hemispheric specialization has both a phylogenetic and an ontogenetic character.

REFERENCES

Annett, M. (1974) Laterality of childhood hemiplegia and the growth of speech and intelligence. *Cortex, 9,* 3–33.

Bryden, M.P. (1970) Laterality effects in dichotic listening: Relations with handedness and reading ability in children. *Neuropsychologia, 8,* 443–450.

Bryden, M.P. (1975) Speech lateralization in families: A preliminary study using dichotic listening. *Brain and Language, 2,* 201–211.

Bryden, M.P., & Zurif, E.B. (1970) Dichotic listening performance in a case of agenesis of the corpus callosum. *Neuropsychologia, 8,* 371–377.

Buffery, A.W.H., & Gray, J.A. (1972) Sex differences in the development of spatial and linguistic skills. In C. Ounsted & D.C. Taylor (Eds.), *Gender differences: Their ontogeny and significance.* London: Churchill.

Carlson, J., Netley, C., Hendrick, E.B., & Prichard, J.S. (1968) A re-examination of intellectual disabilities in hemispherectomized patients. *Transactions of American Neurological Association, 93,* 198–201.

Dennis, M., & Kohn, B. (1975) Comprehension of syntax in infantile hemiplegics after cerebral hemidecortication: Left hemisphere superiority. *Brain and Language, 2,* 475–486.

Ettlinger, G., Blakemore, C.B., Milner, A.D., & Wilson, J. (1972) Agenesis of the corpus callosum: A behavioural investigation. *Brain, 95,* 327–346.

Ettlinger, G., Blakemore, C.B., Milner, C.B., & Wilson, J. (1974) Agenesis of the corpus callosum: A further behavioural investigation. *Brain, 97,* 225–234.

Ferguson-Smith, M.A. (1965) Karyotype-phenotype correlations in gonadal dysgenesis and their bearing on the pathogenesis of malformations. *Journal of Medical Genetics, 2,* 142–155.

Garron, D.C. (1970) Sex-linked, recessive inheritance of spatial and numerical abilities, and Turner's syndrome. *Psychological Review, 77,* 147–152.

Garvey, M., & Mutton, D. (1973) Sex chromosome aberrations and speech development. *Archives of Disease in Childhood, 48,* 937–941.

Hartlage, L.C. (1970) Sex-linked inheritance of spatial ability. *Perceptual and Motor Skills, 31,* 610.

Kimura, D. (1961a) Some effects of temporal lobe damage on auditory perception. *Canadian Journal of Psychology, 15,* 156–165.

Kimura, D. (1961b) Cerebral dominance and the perception of verbal stimuli. *Canadian Journal of Psychology, 15,* 166–171.

Kimura, D. (1967) Functional asymmetry of the brain in dichotic listening. *Cortex, 3,* 163–178.

Kimura, D., & Durnford, M. (1974) Normal studies on the function of the right hemisphere in vision. In S. Dimond & G. Beaumont (Eds.), *Hemisphere function in the human brain.* New York: Halsted Press.

Kinsbourne, M. (1970) The cerebral basis of lateral asymmetries in attention. *Acta Psychologica, 33,* 193–201.

Kohn, B., & Dennis, M. (1974) Selective impairments of visuospatial abilities in infantile hemiplegics after right cerebral hemidecortication. *Neuropsychologia, 12,* 505–512.

Lansdell, H. (1964) Sex differences in hemispheric asymmetries of the human brain. *Nature, 203,* 550.

Lansdell, H. (1968) The use of factor scores from the Wechsler-Bellevue Scale of Intelligence in assessing patients with temporal lobe removals. *Cortex, 4,* 257–268.

Lansdell, H., & Davie, J.C. (1972) Massa intermedia: Possible relation to intelligence. *Neuropsychologia, 10,* 207–210.

Lehrke, R.G. (1974) X-linked mental retardation and verbal disability. *Birth Defects: Original Article Series, 10,* No. 1.

Leonard, M., Landy, G., Ruddle, F.H., & Lubs, H.A. (1974) Early development of children with abnormalities of the sex chromosomes: A prospective study. *Pediatrics, 54,* 208–212.

Levy, J. (1969) Possible basis for the evolution of lateral specialization of the human brain. *Nature, 224,* 614–615.

Lyon, M.F. (1962) Sex chromatin and gene action in the mammalian X-chromosome. *American Journal of Human Genetics, 14,* 135.

McGlone, J., & Davidson, W. (1973) The relationship between cerebral speech laterality and spatial ability with special reference to sex and hand preference. *Neuropsychologia, 11,* 105–113.

McGlone, J., & Kertesz, A. (1973) Sex differences in cerebral processing of visuospatial tasks. *Cortex, 9,* 313–320.

Milner, B., Taylor, L.B., & Sperry, R.W. (1968) Lateralized suppression of dichotically-presented digits after commissural section in man. *Science, 161,* 184–185.

Money, J. (1973) Turner's syndrome and parietal lobe functions. *Cortex, 9,* 385–393.

Netley, C. (1972) Dichotic listening performance of hemispherectomized patients. *Neuropsychologia, 10,* 233–240.

Oxbury, J.M., & Oxbury, S.M. (1969) Effects of temporal lobectomy on the report of dichotically presented digits. *Cortex, 5,* 1–14.

Ounsted, C., & Taylor, D.C. (1972) The Y chromosome message: A point of view. In C.

Ounsted & D.C. Taylor (Eds.), *Gender differences: Their ontogeny and significance.* London: Churchill Livingstone.

Russell, L.B. (1964) Another look at the single active X hypothesis. *Transactions of the New York Academy of Sciences, 26,* 726.

Siegel, S. (1956) *Nonparametric statistics for the behavioral sciences.* New York: McGraw-Hill.

Springer, S.P., & Gazzaniga, M.S. (1975) Dichotic testing of partial and complete split brain subjects. *Neuropsychologia, 13,* 341–346.

Stafford, R.E. (1961) Sex differences in spatial visualization as evidence of sex linked inheritance. *Perceptual and Motor Skills, 13,* 428.

Zurif, E.B., & Bryden, M.P. (1969) Familial handedness and left-right differences in auditory and visual perception. *Neuropsychologia, 7,* 179–187.

12

A Long-Term Study of Dichotic Speech Perception and Receptive Language Skills in a Child with Acquired Aphasia

GRACE H. YENI-KOMSHIAN

It is a well-known fact that when children and prepubertal adolescents incur localized brain injury, their recovery from aphasic symptoms is quite dramatic. The most striking clinical feature of children with acquired aphasia is the sharp reduction in the amount of voluntary speech output. When speech is produced, it is usually sparse and telegraphic in character. These children are reluctant to speak, and they have to be prodded into exchanging information verbally. In some cases, the patients go through a period in which they are described as mute, and then they show dramatic recovery (Alajouanine & Lhermite, 1965; Basser, 1962; Chase, 1972).

In a summary of published material and of his own experience Lenneberg states that two processes operate during the course of recovery from acquired aphasia in children between the ages of 2 and 10 years. First, there is interference with existing verbal abilities caused by the lesion, and second, there may be temporary interruption in active language acquisition normal to this age range. Cerebral trauma in 2- to 3-year-old children can cause all language accomplishments to disappear, and language is relearned by a repetition of all the stages seen in first language acquisition. Thus, in the very young, the primary recovery process is language acquisition. For a child between the ages of 3 and 4, the processes of language acquisition and language interference may be in competition for a few weeks. In patients older than 4 years, but younger than 10, the effects of language interference subside gradually, while at the same time the child is capable of expanding his vocabulary and learning new grammatical constructions. Lenneberg also states that it is generally agreed that recovery is complete in all cases of aphasia within the first 10 years of life; the course of recovery can be as short as a few weeks, and in most cases recovery is complete in less than 2 years. For children between the ages of 11 and 14, recovery might not be complete, and some aphasic symptoms become irreversible. Past the age of puberty, prognosis is the same as that for adult patients (Lenneberg, 1967).

Alajouanine and Lhermite (1965) describe the course of recovery in 32 patients between the ages of 6 and 15. They found no striking differences relating to age. In fact, they state that recovery was somewhat delayed in the group younger than 10 years of age. After 1 year of rehabilitation, most of the patients were able to go back to school; however, they had severe learning problems. The patients were able to regain their previous level of scholastic achievement but were unable to function satisfactorily at higher grade levels. The difficulties they encountered in school were in areas involving the use of language, such as history, geography, and foreign languages. Success in these school subjects would also require reading skills and the retention of newly learned material. The IQ of these children was either normal or lower than normal. Their performance on tests that measure retention of figures, retention of narration, arithmetic, and logic was not satisfactory.

More recently Hécaen (1976) described a series of 26 cases aged 3 years and 6 months (3:6) to 15:0 with left, right, or bilateral cortical lesions. His conclusions concerning the course of recovery were in general agreement with the previously published studies. Hécaen also stated that although recovery in childhood-acquired aphasia is very dramatic and more striking than in adult cases, certain aphasic symptoms, particularly deficits in writing, persist for a long time.

Many observers are probably overly impressed by the dramatic change that takes place in these patients. There is a great need to study the course of recovery more closely than has been done in the literature. Such an endeavor is difficult and time consuming. This report is one initial attempt at studying one patient over a period of 1 year and 10 months, following an episode of head trauma. The primary focus of investigation was whether recovery of language function in the patient would also be reflected in his dichotic listening performance.

THE CASE HISTORY

The patient is a male Caucasian born on 4 August 1964. At the age of 7:11, he sustained severe head trauma. Prior to his accident, he was a healthy normal child doing above average at school. He had successfully completed the second grade. He was left-handed; however, neither his parents nor his siblings are left-handed. On the day of the accident, he was riding his bicycle and was hit by a moving car. He was thrown 45 feet, landing on his head against the curb. He was unconscious, unresponsive, and in decerebrate posture (extended legs and flexed arms), with a skull fracture over the left temporal-occipital area. At surgery, 4 large bone fragments, which were depressed 2 cm into the brain, were removed. The area of lacerated brain was debrided and the dural defect closed. He remained comatose and decerebrate and suffered from seizures. One week later a craniotomy was performed on the right side because of evidence of increasing intracranial pressure thought to be due to cerebral edema. Frequent spinal taps were done to relieve the pressure. He remained comatose for 5 weeks. His records indicate that during the fifth week he would occasionally cry. Eight weeks after the accident he seemed to be more alert to his surroundings. Still he did not give any indication of communicative ability. It was evident that he had bilateral weakness, which was more pronounced on the right side. A pneumoencephalogram in the eleventh week indicated normal ventricular system with only slight enlargement of the left lateral ventricle. During this period he was receiving physical therapy with passive range of motion exercises. By the twelfth week he was able to sit in a wheelchair. His motor recovery was predominantly restricted to the left side. Three and a half months after the accident he began to show some attempts at communication by gesture. Within the next 2 weeks he started to vocalize *mama mama* and *go go go*, at first with no apparent communicative intent and later in a communicative and meaningful way. Following this his speech became echolalic, with frequent parroting of statements with no communicative function. He became adept at singing songs that he had known prior to the accident. No pronounced articulatory problems were noted; however, he had severe anomia. He was unable to name friends and familiar objects and places. He used gestures for communication. At this stage he was sent home, where he received physical therapy.

Five months after the accident he was admitted to another medical center for evaluation and rehabilitation. His EEG indicated an abnormal record in the left posterior-temporal-occipital region. His echoencephalogram indicated no lateral displacement of the midline structures; however, his lateral ventricles were enlarged bilaterally. He showed diminished strength bilaterally (quadriparesis), which was more pronounced on the right than on the left. In summary, the patient's cortical trauma was bilateral, with more extensive involvement of the left temporal-occipital area. His aphasic symptoms are best described as expressive with anomia.

HEARING, LANGUAGE, AND DICHOTIC LISTENING TESTS

In the course of the ensuing 17 months the patient was tested on several occasions. The following tests were administered: standard speech and pure tone audiometry, the Peabody Picture Vocabulary Test (PPVT), the Illinois Test of Psycholinguistic Abilities (ITPA), auditory memory for forward digits and sentences from the Binet, and a dichotic listening test.

The first testing session was 5 months posttrauma. The patient's hearing was within normal limits for pure tones and speech.[1] His lexical comprehension capa-

---

[1] The patient's hearing was within normal limits on all subsequent tests of hearing. These tests were performed prior to each dichotic test session.

bilities were tested by the PPVT, and he performed at 4:3 level. His score on the auditory reception test of the ITPA (*Do bananas telephone?*) was at the 3:8 level. The patient could not comprehend the nature of the task involved in the auditory association test of the ITPA (*grass is green : sugar is . . .*). His response on this test was echolalic, he imitated the examiner. On the Binet memory tests he scored at the 4:6 level for digits and at the 2:6 level for sentences. He could only repeat the first word of the sentences at the 4-year level. He was able to identify objects when defined by their function. However, he was unable to comprehend prepositions or point to parts of objects (*Show me the wheels of the car*). In the area of expressive language, he could produce a few automatic phrases and he would also say the names of his family members. He was unable to name simple objects that he knew receptively. He required extensive auditory clues (*shir for shirt*) before he could complete a naming task. Semantic clues (*bread and . . .*) did not help him produce the desired word. He was able to imitate words without difficulty. His articulation was intelligible but had a slow, labored quality.

He was enrolled in an extensive therapy program which provided him with general language stimulation and special emphasis on functional, everyday expressive vocabulary. The therapy sessions made use of a "triggering system," which provided him with auditory or semantic clues to elicit desired words. He was also taught how he could provide his own clues. This program, 30-min sessions, 5 times per week, was continued for 4 months.

At the age of 8:6, 7 months after his accident, he was given a dichotic listening test designed for normal 3- to 5-year-old children.[2] This test is composed of 12 monosyllabic names: *Ben, Bob, Bill, Pat, Dick, Doug, Tom, Tim, Ted, Ken, Jack, and Chuck.* Names that began with the same consonant, that had the same vowel and that exceeded more than 50 msec in duration were not paired. The test consisted of 50 single pairs of dichotic items. The initial portion of the test tape contained the 12 names binaurally. The patient was tested in a sound-treated booth. The stimuli were played on a Tandberg stereo tape recorder the output of which was connected to two attenuators and an amplifier. The stimuli were presented through Sharp earphones. He was first presented with the individual names binaurally and asked to repeat what he had heard. Then he was presented the dichotic stimuli, one pair at a time, and asked to tell the experimenter what he heard. This general procedure was followed on all dichotic testing sessions. The same dichotic test tape was used. However, sometimes the stimuli were presented at equal intensity to both ears and at other times the intensity was deliberately modified to favor the input of one ear.

The results of the first administration of the dichotic test at 60-dB SPL to both ears, indicated a complete extinction of the material presented to the left ear. His reporting of the right-ear stimuli was highly accurate (90%). After a short break he

[2] The results from 20 5-year-old children, the age group closest to the psycholinguistic age of the patient, showed a significant right-ear advantage on this test (Yeni-Komshian unpublished data). The results of an 8:1 male on the same test produced an REA of 22.58 as computed by R−L/R+L × 100.

was tested again, at 60 dB SPL to both ears, but this time he was given special instructions to attend to the left ear only. One experimenter continually reminded him, before each dichotic item, that he had to attend and report the material presented to the left ear. Again, all his responses were exclusively from the right-ear material. His performance on the binaural test and on monaural presentation to the left ear only was highly accurate.

One month later, at the age of 8:7 (8 months postaccident) he was given the same dichotic test at 60 dB SPL to both ears. His response pattern was essentially unchanged; that is, total extinction of the left-ear material and high accuracy for the right-ear material. At this and subsequent dichotic test sessions a new condition was added, the intensity of the stimuli was changed such that the left-ear channel was louder than the right-ear channel. One test was given at 60-dB SPL for the left ear and at 40-dB SPL for the right ear. Another test was given at 80-dB SPL for the left ear and 40-dB SPL for the right ear.[3] In both test conditions all correct responses were exclusively from the right-ear material.

At the age of 8:8, 9 months after the accident, he was discharged to go home and to attend a special school. His discharge note indicated that he had made considerable improvement in the quality and quantity of his expressive speech, although his scores on standard tests were not commensurate with his chronological age. On the PPVT he scored at the 5:2 level. On the ITPA, and this time he was given the whole scale, he scored an overall psycholinguistic age of 5:4. Auditory reception was at the 4:7 level and auditory association was at the 5:3 level. He was now able to ambulate with the help of a short brace on the right leg and the use of a cane.

One year after the accident, at the age of 8:11, he was called for follow-up testing. On the dichotic test no change in performance was observed when the channels were at the same level of intensity. When the intensity level between the ears was 35 dB SPL in favor of the left ear (left at 65 dB and right at 30 dB) he began to report some of the material presented to his left ear. His score for this condition was 50% correct for the right-ear material and 20% correct for the left-ear material. His error rate was 30%, and some of the errors were fusions. For example, he would report that he heard "Bog" when *Bob* and *Doug* were presented. Although he showed some signs of processing left-ear stimuli, he was still unable to report two responses even though he was told that the test consisted of two different speech signals. At that time his PPVT score was at the 6:4 level. On the ITPA, his score on the auditory reception test was at the 5:4 level and on auditory association it was at the 5:7 level. On the Binet he scored at the 7:0 level for digits and 5:0 level for sentences. The general quality of his speech production remained slow and labored.

At the age of 9:9, 22 months postaccident, he was tested again. For the first time after many dichotic test sessions he was aware of the fact that the stimuli were

---

[3] Discrepancies in channel intensity greater than 40 dB are hard to interpret because the ear with the weaker signal can receive input from the other ear through bone conduction.

dichotic, that is, he was able to report two responses on a dichotic item. When the stimuli were presented at equal intensity to both ears, 16% of the items were reported correctly for both ears. His performance showed a strong REA, with 54% correct for the right ear only, 19% correct for the left ear only, and 20% errors. Half of the errors were fusion. When the intensity level between the two channels was shifted in favor of the left ear, a difference of 5 dB produced a left-ear advantage. His performance on the standard language tests had also improved. He scored at the 7:10 level on the PPVT. On the ITPA auditory reception test he was at the 6:5 level, and on the auditory association test he scored at the 6:6 level. His score on the Binet memory tests remained at the 7:0 level for digits and the 5:0 level for sentences. In the area of expressive language, he was able to express his ideas in fairly complex sentences. His speech output was no longer slow and labored. His recovery was very impressive but not complete. Even his best skills were below age level. He was able to walk unassisted. This was, however, the last evaluation given to the patient.

The patient's performance over the period of 17 months of testing is summarized in Table 1. The table contains the patient's chronological age at the time of testing and the corresponding number of months posttrauma. His performance on the standard tests is listed in age equivalent scores. The dichotic test results listed in Table 1 only represent the scores obtained from the test condition of equal intensity to both ears. The results of the dichotic tests given to the patient during the seventh and eighth months posttrauma are combined, because there was no change in performance from one test session to another. The dichotic test scores

TABLE 1 Summary of Performance on Standard Tests and Dichotic Listening Tests at Equal Intensity in Both Channels

	$8:4^a$ $(5)^b$	$8:6-8:7^a$ $(7-8)^b$	$8:8^a$ $(9)^b$	$8:11^a$ $(12)^b$	$9:9^a$ $(22)^b$
Standard tests:					
PPVT	4:3		5:2	6:4	7:10
ITPA: Auditory reception	3:8		4:7	5:4	6:5
ITPA: Auditory association	$-^c$		5:3	5:7	6:6
Binet Digits	4:6			7:0	7:0
Binet Sentences	2:6			5:0	5:0
Dichotic listening tests:		$(N = 84)^d$		$(N = 50)^d$	$(N = 61)^d$
Both ears (%)		0		0	16
Right only (%)		89		88	54
Left only (%)		0		0	10
Error (%)		11		12	20

[a]Chronological age.
[b]Number of months posttrauma.
[c]Patient did not comprehend the task.
[d]Number of dichotic items.

were converted into percentages and the following response categories were used: the percentage of items when the two stimuli were reported correctly (both ears), the percentage of items when only the right-ear stimulus was reported correctly (right only), the percentage of items when only the left ear stimulus was reported correctly (left only), and the percentage of items when the response was either an error or a fusion (error).

It can be seen that over the period of 17 months of testing the patient showed the equivalent of a 43-month gain in comprehension of lexical items as measured by the PPVT. The language skills sampled on the two sub-tests of the ITPA include comprehension of sentences and verbal reasoning. His gain on the ITPA tests was equivalent to about a 36-month increment. His memory for digits and sentences shows an increment of about 30 months. The scores from the PPVT and ITPA indicate a sharply linear increment, whereas there is a plateau for the memory tests. In contrast, the dichotic test scores remained essentially stationary for a whole year posttrauma, but a change in performance was seen at the last testing period which was 22 months posttrauma.

DISCUSSION

This patient's recovery of language appears to agree with Lenneberg's (1967) description for the 5- to 10-year-old group. For this particular patient, the brain trauma resulted in severe disturbance of language skills, but his recovery did not mimic the pattern of stages seen in normal language acquisition. For example, throughout recovery his articulation was much more advanced than his naming capacity. His syntax appeared to have been unaffected, but unfortunately this was one of the many aspects of his language which was not studied systematically.

In considering those language skills which have been investigated in this patient it can be seen that his word and sentence comprehension was in the process of continuing improvement when the pattern of ear scores changed in the dichotic listening task. The data suggest that a substantial amount of language recovery took place when the patient was still incapable of processing competing speech signals. The fact that he had a very strong REA throughout the testing period would suggest that recovery of language function was taking place in the damaged left hemisphere. Furthermore, the fact that a relatively pronounced left-sided lesion caused his severe aphasic symptoms would support the assumption that language was represented in his left hemisphere prior to trauma.

Several possible interpretations are offered in discussing the results obtained from this patient. First, it is important to note that I have tested similar head trauma cases on the same dichotic listening test and the majority of these patients have shown a very strong REA with suppression of left ear input. Those patients who were followed showed a recovery of the left ear. In some patients recovery of the left ear response occurred within 3 months posttrauma.

During the first year posttrauma, this patient's dichotic listening performance was very similar to the dichotic results reported for patients with callosal disconnection (Milner, Taylor, & Sperry, 1968; Sparks & Geschwind, 1968). Only in this group of patients does one find such dramatic suppression of the left ear input in dichotic presentation of speech stimuli. This patient incurred bilateral damage with more acute involvement of the left hemisphere. It is conceivable that the bilateral damage resulted in a disconnection between the hemispheres in those areas relevant to auditory and language function. That is, the lesion does not have to be in the corpus callosum for a patient to demonstrate the behavioral manifestations of callosal disconnection (Geschwind, 1965). Informal testing of other head trauma patients suggests that if a hemispheric disconnection exists it is limited to language related functions. Results of these tests did not reveal left-sided apraxia, a syndrome associated with lesion of the corpus callosum. Assuming that a disconnection existed in this patient, then for the first year posttrauma this patient was simply performing in a manner predictable from models proposed by Sparks and Geschwind (1968), Kinsbourne (1975), and Cullen, Berlin, Hughes, Thompson, and Samson (1974).

In the case of this patient it can also be argued that, since he was just under 8 years of age at the time of the accident, mechanisms of neural plasticity were still operative to allow for some form of compensatory reconnection to take place. If this were the case, then the data reveal that it took more than 1 year posttrauma for the neural compensation to take place.

Another possible interpretation of the results is the phenomenon of extinction after simultaneous stimulation described by Bender (1970). Bender's work has focused on somatosensory stimulation. The phenomena he describes can be applied to dichotic listening. Like Bender's test, dichotic listening involves simultaneous stimulation. In Bender's test, for example, the face and the hand are simultaneously stimulated. Most neurologically involved patients would extinguish the hand and report the face. Bender has reported a hierarchy of dominance in the somatosensory system. In the case of simultaneous face and hand stimulation, the face stimulus is correctly perceived but the hand stimulus is either mislocalized or not perceived at all. Analogously, neurologically impaired patients might perceive the dominant stimulus (right ear or ear ipsilateral to the lesioned hemisphere) but might either misperceive or totally extinguish the less dominant stimulus (left ear or ear contralateral to the lesioned hemisphere). The analogy with somatosensory extinction as reported by Bender can explain dichotic results reported for normal listeners and neurologically damaged patients. In this context I would like to argue that the results of dichotic listening tests can be interpreted clinically in diagnosing central nervous system pathology. The greater the extinction of one ear—that is, the greater the left—right ear difference—the more severe the pathology. The pathology is diagnosed on the basis of the fact that the patient is incapable of processing two competing stimuli when presented simultaneously. Therefore, a sign of recovery would be seen when the patient begins to be able to process information from both ears in the dichotic listening test. Thus, in this particular patient only after some degree of central nervous system recovery was he able to process competing speech signals. It would then follow that the same recovery would be necessary for regaining language function.

It should be pointed out that this patient's dichotic test results do not match the pattern seen from adults with unilateral brain lesions (Cullen *et al.,* 1974; Goodglass, 1967; Kimura, 1967). In almost all of these studies the reported results indicate that the ear contralateral to the lesion does poorly on the dichotic listening test. This patient's brain injury was more acute in the left hemisphere, therefore, his right-ear score should have been worse than his left-ear score. The reverse was true. This reversal of results from what is seen generally in the adult patient population could be a major age difference between children and adults with brain injury. Or it could be that these results are obtained only for cases with bilateral head injury due to trauma. The most common source for adult studies of dichotic listening in neurologically impaired patients is epileptics who have undergone lobectomies, and stroke patients. This patient suffered a general and severe head trauma.

One final interpretation is proposed. When the central nervous system is severely traumatized, as in the case of traumatic head injury, and if some sensory function is still in operation, then those sensory pathways that are most prominent are the ones that will be able to function after the trauma. Then, with recovery, the secondary sensory pathways will come back into function. In the auditory system, the crossed pathways—the right ear to the left hemisphere and the left ear to the right hemisphere—are the prominent pathways. After injury the crossed pathways might be the only ones that can transmit impulses; only later, with recovery, can the secondary pathways, the ipsilateral and callosal, come into play. Since the dichotic listening task used in this investigation was language based, the right ear to left hemisphere pathway would be the only channel of information the patient was capable of processing. With recovery, the secondary auditory pathways become functional and then the patient was able to process the left- and right-ear stimuli. Only long-term studies of dichotic listening with brain trauma cases can test the suggestion put forward here.

ACKNOWLEDGMENTS

The author wishes to thank the staff members of the Hearing and Speech Clinic at the Kennedy Institute for the Physically and Mentally Handicapped Child for their cooperation and help throughout the testing period. Special thanks are due to Mr. Stephen Shevitz, Dr. Robert Johnson, and Dr. Joan Sinnott for their help.

REFERENCES

Alajouanine, T., & Lhermite, F. (1965) Acquired aphasia in children. *Brain, 88,* 653–662.
Basser, L.S. (1962) Hemiplegia of early onset and the faculty of speech with special reference to the effects of hemispherectomy. *Brain, 85,* 427–460.

Bender, M.B. (1970) Perceptual interactions. *Modern Trends in Neurology, 5,* 1–28.

Chase, R.A. (1972) Neurological aspects of language disorders in children. In J.V. Irwin & M. Marge (Eds.), *Principles of childhood disabilities.* New York: Appleton. Pp. 99–135.

Cullen, J.F., Jr., Berlin, C.I., Hughes, L.F., Thompson, C.L., & Samson, D.S. (1974) Speech information flow: A model. In *Proceedings of a symposium on central auditory processing disorders,* Univ. of Nebraska Medical Center, Omaha, 108–127.

Geschwind, N. (1965) Disconnection syndromes in animals and man, Part I. *Brain, 88,* 237–294.

Goodglass, H. (1967) Binaural digit representation and early lateral brain damage. *Cortex, 3,* 295–306.

Hécaen, H. (1976) Acquired aphasia in children and the ontogenesis of hemispheric functional specialization. *Brain and Language, 3,* 114–134.

Kimura, D. (1967) Functional asymmetry of the brain in dichotic listening. *Cortex, 3,* 163–178.

Kinsbourne, M. (1975) Mechanisms of hemispheric interaction in man. In M. Kinsbourne & W. Smith (Eds.), *Hemisphere, disconnection and cerebral function.* Springfield, Illinois: Thomas. Pp. 260–285.

Lenneberg, E.H. (1967) *Biological foundations of language.* New York: Wiley.

Milner, B., Taylor, L., & Sperry, R.W. (1968) Lateralized suppression of dichotically presented digits after commissural section in man. *Science, 161,* 184–186.

Sparks, R., & Geschwind, N. (1968) Dichotic listening in man after section of neocortical commissures, *Cortex, 4,* 3–16.

13

An External View of Neuropsychology and Its Working Milieu

J. JACOBS

From error to error one discovers the truth.

—Sigmund Freud

In the scientific context, the clinical neuropsychologist can be seen as an intermediary between two groups: the clinical neurologists, who provide him with his case material and criterion information, and the experimental physiological psychologists, who provide findings and theories about brain–behavior relationships and thus establish a conceptual basis for his clinical practice. The objective is that of predicting diagnoses from a class of data that are relatively independent of, and different from, the conventional neurological procedures. The clinical neuropsychologist concerns himself with neurological structures and functions insofar as they are relevant to the understanding of some dimension of behavior. He holds the belief that since the cerebral hemispheres are the organs of behavior, analyses of psychological functioning is a highly effective means of reaching an understanding of brain functioning. Thus the integrity of the conceptual constructs must be real, and each and every step clear and based on substantial data.

Assessment of brain–behavior relationships requires continued complementation between experimental and clinical psychology. There continues to exist an experimentally (and physiologically) orientated approach, as contrasted with the clinical approach. The experimental approach often emphasizes the research model derived from animal work and focuses on abstract problems of content rather than upon prediction or conclusions regarding the individual subject. The clinical approach emphasizes the psychometric model of assessment and focuses on classification (or diagnosis) of the individual subject, sometimes to the neglect of more basic conceptualization (Meier, 1974).

A number of testing techniques and procedures have become well accepted in neuropsychological research. However, the clinical worker often perceives sources of error not only in the measurement but also in the interpretation of these measurements, which, although not necessarily invalidating the research, should certainly be recognized and the necessary allowances made by research scientists. In this paper, a number of sources of error will be discussed as they are seen to arise in neuropsychological research allied to the medical sphere in general, with special mention of some relating to research on the lateralization of brain function.

THE INFANT AND EXPERIMENTAL OBSERVATION

Often, neonatal animal research is compared directly with human neonatal research. Some basic differences occur regularly. Usually, in an animal study, all the replication members of the litter are treated equally, that is, individual differences are probably minimal and, in any event, are not taken into account. However, there are difficulties in extrapolating from the animal model to a human model, where each and every infant is unique. For example, all 10-day-old infants may be tested for their visual and other responses and, while chronologically 10 days old, are really 10 to 40 days old, with all that this entails neurologically (since the gestational age is the important factor, rather than the birth day as such) (Dubowitz, Dubowitz, & Goldberg, 1970). Thus, in order to control for idiosyncratic factors related to infant risk factors and maternal age; socioeconomic status; obstetric, anesthetic and analgesic medication; and infant neurological and physical status, Brown (1975) used the following criteria: (1) the mother planned to bottle feed her infant; (2) the mother's age was between 18 and 38 years; (3) the mother had no history of previous abortions, miscarriages, or premature deliveries; (4) maternal analgesics and tranquilizer drugs did not exceed 150 mgm 1 to 6 hr prior to delivery; (5) there were no signs of fetal or postnatal anoxia; (6) infant was presented in the vertex position; (7) Apgar rating was between 8 and 10 at 1 to 5 min after delivery; (8) the infant was Rhesus positive; (9) the estimations by the obstetrician and the pediatrician of the infant's gestational age did not differ by more than 2 weeks; (10) the infant was between 55 and 80 hr of age at 7 A.M. on the day on which he was examined and observed.

The clinician is immediately aware that each infant is a highly variable organism, making the measurement of an ability a gross problem of potential versus actual behavior. Consequently, laboratory controls must be made. But it is also possible that many of the ways in which infant behavior is studied in the laboratory impose artificial conditions, so that some of the more naturally flowing patterns of behavior are seriously interrupted or disturbed. The controlled laboratory atmosphere is certainly justifiable. If science is a process of identifying variables and describing the ways in which they interact to control simple and complex phenomena, then, by being able to determine the turn of events, by the use of a variety of sophisticated recording devices, and by the ability to control the presentation of stimulations, interfering variables can be reduced to a minimum, precision in recording behavior can be maximized, and highly controlled manipulation can be undertaken. However, the price of such external control in laboratory research on infant behavior can be very high. The complexity of cooccurring natural events of the normal environment are reduced to a minimum, responses to be observed are often made to occur in immature densities, and normally occurring interspersed environmental events that possibly maintain attending behavior (such as caretaker soothing, position changes, and shifts in tactile stimulation) must be eliminated from many experimental procedures.

As with any other infant research laboratory, all of the procedures with regard to health, hygiene, risk levels, and equipment apply equally to a newborn research laboratory. It must be remembered that the newborn infant is making many adjustments to extrauterine life. These adjustments sometimes involve unstable functioning or functioning that changes radically and suddenly.

Not to be forgotten in research with the newborn, is the requirement of a careful development of relationships with physicians, nurses, and hospital administrators. In overcrowded and understaffed settings, a researcher can be annoyingly intrusive and disruptive.

INDIVIDUAL DIFFERENCES IN BRAIN ORGANIZATION

Although researchers like to consider, for the sake of theory, all brains as similar, clearly this is not so. First of all, lesions in a given region may produce different effects in different individuals (Butler, 1971). Moreover, very small lesions often produce no symptoms, and when the damage is more extensive, it seldom affects abilities singly. One well-accepted dimension of individual difference is the individual variation in cerebral dominance that may account for some of the unexpected clinical anatomical variations found (e.g., Geshwind & Levitsky, 1968; Wada & Rasmussen, 1960).

Reitan (1974) emphasizes that it is important to remember that neuropsychological assessment is based on behavior data related to brain functions, as contrasted with physical sources of evidence, such as X-rays, EEG tracings, tissue secretions, and similar neurological diagnostic evidence. Neuropsychological evidence, therefore, is relevant not only for brain inferences but also for assessment of the behavioral consequences of brain lesions. These consequences vary from one individual to another and raise many clinical questions regarding the interface between the patient's psychological deficits and his environment.

TEST–RETEST RELIABILITY WITH NORMALS VERSUS
BRAIN-DAMAGED PATIENTS

Whereas, in the medical world, there are well-established percentile charts for height, weight, and head circumference, with confidence limits, this is not yet present to any major degree in psychological tests, and one has to select those with the greatest reliability coefficients. It might be supposed that tests of crystallized intelligence (those involved in such skills as information processing, vocabulary, spelling, etc.) are likely to have high test–retest reliability when compared to measures of fluid intelligence (the capacity to adapt to solve problems) if crystallized intelligence is a stable characteristic despite brain damage. When test–retest coefficients are considered for instruments such as the WAIS or WRAT this appears to be a reasonable hypothesis. Even in the WAIS, tests thought to be sensitive to cerebral dysfunction had lower coefficients than those subtests that might be labeled as belonging to the crystallized intelligence groups as described in a similar way by Wechsler (1958).

Another example of this type of problem involves the dichotic listening task as a testing technique. Many subject and stimulus variables must be controlled for a valid interpretation (see Chapter 7). It is often assumed that, in a statistical analysis, the differences within the sample will be evened out provided a large enough sample is taken. This has some validity, but unless one is aware of the individual members of the sample in terms of hearing capacity, presence of wax, presence of the "allergic diathesis" (with middle ear compliance problems, eustachian tube difficulties, mucous membrane reaction difficulties, perennial allergic rhinitis, "pollenosis"), possible incipient viral infections, and so forth, results of testing can be invalidated. It is essential, therefore, to have an adequate individual and family medical history for each subject, to include the possibility of such interfering situations and adequate reassessment prior to each test (although such reassessment need not be entirely complete each time) and for an appropriate physical examination of upper airways and ears to be carried out.

INTERPRETING RESULTS OF SURGERY

In life, the "surgical" areas involved in hemisphere studies include hemispherectomy—surgical removal of a total cerebral hemisphere as treatment for a variety of disease processes (Dennis & Whitaker, 1975; Kempe, 1968; Neilson & Raney, 1939) Unfortunately, the operation concerned is described variously as "hemidecortication," "surgical removal of the diseased cortical tissue," or "resection" of one or other hemisphere. There are really enormous differences in the possible extent of these procedures and hence the amount of brain tissue removed. A complete hemispherectomy may be indicated for persistent focal seizures, hemiplegia, and mental deterioration in an infant or child with unilateral cerebral atrophy (Campbell, 1976). In a coronal section of the brain, the line of excision at the side of the hemisphere leads through the corpus callosum and goes lateral to the striation (caudate nucleus and putamen). Arteries like the middle cerebral artery will be clipped—perforating vessels are dealt with and draining veins coagulated. Anteriorly the incision leads to the limen insulae, and posteriorly the incision transects the internal capsule (including its posterior limb consisting of the lenticulothalamic, retrolenticular, and sublenticular portions, see Figure 1).

This is the classical description of a hemispherectomy; but it is by no means performed consistently in exactly the same way, either by the same surgeon in successive operations or by different surgeons. The depth of the incision will vary and so will the amount of residual tissue. Sometimes the basal ganglia are removed, sometimes the hippocampus. The thalamus may remain, but since there is nearly complete degeneration of this area following such an operation, except in the midline and intraluminar nuclei, the end result is difficult to assess.

In cases of diffuse calcification and meningealangiomatosis of one hemisphere (Sturge–Kalisher–Dimitri–Weber syndrome), discussed by Dennis and Whitaker (Chapter 8) as "hemicortectomy" or "hemi-decortication," the surgeon tends to remove the naevoid lesions (which differ in extent from case to case), removing the pararterial areas of calcification, and coagulating a varying number of vessels. The blood supplies remaining will vary, and the tissue removed will vary in quantity, size, and depth. How can we then compare one case with another, whether a right-

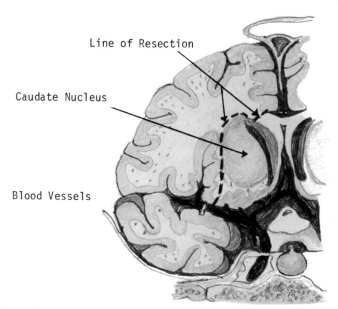

Figure 1. Coronal view of left hemisphere. Line of excision for complete hemispherectomy.

or left-sided removal is considered, unless we have a photograph of start and finish in three dimensions? It is difficult to equate the clarity and expertise of sensitive testing to the anatomical situations that may seem to present predictable consequences, yet may be wide of the mark. For example, Neilson and Raney (1939) indicate that a localized lesion in the left temporal lobe will cause a greater degree of aphasia than surgical removal of the entire lobe.

Similar problems of extent and depth of removal occur when temporal lobe resection is described. This operation includes the removal of the anterior 5.5 to 6.5 cm performed in one block, including the major portion of the hippocampus, the dorsolateral part of the amygdala and the parahippocampal gyrus and uncus, together with the more superficial temporal gyri (Falconer, 1973; Milner, 1971).

INTERPRETING EEGS

The electroencephalograph records the continuous changes in electrical potential within the brain itself. With the development of computers and advanced electronic equipment, a new dimension has been added to the study of the brain's electrical activity. These nonrandom changes of electrical activity in response to sensory stimulation are called *evoked potentials* and are the electrical signs of information processing in the brain.

Interpretation of the EEG (at times regarded by the nonexpert as limitless in its diagnostic possibilities) has many difficulties. It must be appreciated that the initial focus may be quite small even though, in its EEG spread, apparently a larger area may be involved. Given a primary lesion, a transsynaptic mirror lesion may be produced in the opposite hemisphere, with resultant difficulty in isolating primary from secondary lesions.

A great deal of knowledge is needed to check on the use of the apparatus (Kiloh, McComas, & Osselton, 1972). Artifacts in terms of tongue movements, sweat, microreflexes, intravenous infusions, respirators, people walking around in the room, paging systems, and various monitors (needed for other systems such as the heart, etc.) all may appear on the tracing and be misread. Even asymmetries in skull thickness (Leissner, Lindholm, & Petersen, 1970) may correlate with EEG asymmetry.

EXAMPLES OF FALSE DIAGNOSES

Although neuropsychological theorizing is necessary for the field to progress, the clinician must always look very critically at false diagnoses based on dependence on neuropsychological clues wrongly particularized from theoretical generalizations. The following are some typical examples, taken from personal case studies where clearly neuropsychological findings alone proved to be inadequate.

Known Brain Trauma to a Young Child with Apparent
Neuropsychological Test Confirmation of Damage, Disproven by
Twin Study

A patient, age 6, was kicked by a horse on the left occipitoparietal region, resulting in a compound fracture, coma, and removal of some damaged areas of the brain. The child recovered, and the neurological status and the EEG became normal. The mother then indicated that the child had changed in terms of personality; she was now much more subservient than before and her speech abilities were diminished. A neuropsychological profile was undertaken which suggested visual motor and visual spatial integration difficulties compatible with brain damage.

However, when a twin sister was evaluated, her neuropsychological profile proved to be exactly the same as her sister's, at a slightly higher level. The mother acknowledged that there had always been some difference between the two children; her anxiety and feelings of guilt had exaggerated her fears.

Apparent Organic Brain Abnormality with Apparent Positive Test
but Behavioral Therapy Removes "Non-organic" Symptom Basis

A boy, age 12, had a 5-year history of headaches, with objects appearing smaller and larger at intervals. The frequency had increased of recent months and school performance diminished. Neurological examination was normal but the eyegrounds were regarded as showing papilloedema (oedema of the optic discs indicating increased intracranial pressure). The EEG was normal.

A psychologist (with neuropsychologist supervision) did a battery of tests and the results were "more than suggestive of organic brain disease." The eyegrounds were then more expertly shown to reflect "pseudopapilloedema," rather than true papilloedema. Family therapy applied to a grossly dysfunctional family improved the interrelationships of the group and improved the boy's headaches and subsequently his school work. A 2-year follow-up has confirmed the nonorganic nature of the problem.

Confirmation of Epilepsy, Drug Therapy, and Family
Malfunction Highlight Difficulty of Neuropsychological
Test Specificity

A 2-year-old boy commenced epilepsy—the epilepsy was difficult to control especially since multiple drugs were used; the family reaction and communication was poor; paternal expectations were not realized; behavior became more difficult and the boy at age 12 was removed from the home and placed in various foster homes. A variety of psychological testings gave global results varying from 60 IQ to 83 IQ with one common finding of "organic brain syndrome." In fact, the tests could have been done in varying stages of pre- or post-epileptic aura, with under- or overmedication, and in varying states of emotional stress. The need to give findings "uncontaminated" by value judgment in the context of the medical interpretations was very real. Provision of more realistic single-drug, anticonvulsant therapy and family therapy to the total group, with adequate behavioral control, helped remove the "organicity."

"Hyperactivity," Minimal Brain Dysfunction, and Professional Biases

The presentation to professionals of any child with problems of increased activity, short attention span, school and/or home difficulties involves the problem of "minimal brain dysfunction [Walker, 1974]." The ability of psychologists, neurologists, pediatricians, teachers, and others to diagnose hyperactive cases in the presence of hyper- or hypoactivity, family dysfunction, lack of appreciation of normality in an overcrowded class, conditioning situations reflect on the need for objective "noncontaminated" evaluation.

It must be realized that not only neuropsychological testing but an individual psychiatric assessment of the child, a physical (including neurological) assessment, a family evaluation, as well as a full school evaluation is mandatory in each case. This may then allow for a residue of "true" cases.

The fallibility of research tools underscores the importance of the following strictures for research.

1. Tests should be used whose repeatability reflects techniques that are above reproach; tests should be performed with clearly defined populations; and selection of criteria should be such as to make parallel studies possible.

2. When techniques entail instrumentation belonging to other disciplines (EEG, audiology, etc.), professionals in those disciplines should be involved and consulted throughout.

3. In dealing with human subjects, professionals in allied disciplines (ophthalmologists, audiologists, physicians, pediatricians, obstetricians, anatomists, etc.) should be involved in setting out the parameters of the experiment, so that available knowledge will be taken into account.

4. When human beings are the experimental subjects, the influence of health changes on the investigation must be considered (e.g., the influence of allergic mucosal reaction on hearing test results).

5. When a hypothesis is expounded and "validated" the possibility of other hypotheses answering the same questions has to be recognized. The apparent validation must not be taken to invalidate all other parallel hypotheses.

6. When working with other professionals, their knowledge and expertise should be used to gain a more precise picture. For example, if specific areas of the brain are to be considered, then the neurosurgeon will be competent to supply exact details of surgical excision and all the implications thereof.

7. When making use of sophisticated equipment the researcher should not be misled into believing that he has developed sophisticated answers. More elegant mythologies are no more useful or truthful than simpler mythologies.

8. It must always be remembered that things easy to measure are not necessarily important and those not measurable may be very important.

REFERENCES

Brown, J.V., Bakeman, R., Snyder, P.A., Frederickson, W. Timm, Morgan, S.T., and Hepler, R. (1975) Interaction of black inner-city mothers with their newborn infants. *Child Development, 46,* 677–686.

Butler, S.R. (1971) Organization of cerebral cortex for perception. *British Medical Journal, 27,* 544–547.

Campbell, E.J.M. (1976) Basic science, science and medical education. *Lancet* (1), January 17, 134–136.

Dennis, M., & Whitaker, H.A. (1975) Language acquisition in the right and in the left hemisphere. *Conference Proceedings:* A Conference in Language Development and Neurological Theory, St. Catharines.

Dubowitz, L.M.S., Dubowitz, V., & Goldberg, C. (1970) Clinical assessment of gestational age in the newborn infant. *Journal of Pediatrics, 77,* 1–10.

Falconer, M.A. (1973) Reversibility of temporal lobe resection of the behavioural abnormalities of temporal-lobe epilepsy. *New England Journal of Medicine, 289*(9), 451–455.

Geschwind, N., & Levitsky, W. (1968) Human brain: Left-right asymmetries in temporal speech region. *Science, 161* (July 12, 1968), 186–187.

Kempe, L.G. (1968) *Operative neurosurgery,* Vol. 1. Springer-Verlag. Chap. xvii, p. 180.

Kiloh, L.G., McComas, A.J., & Osselton, J.W. (1972) *Clinical Electroencephalography.* London: Butterworth.

Leissner, P., Lindholm, L.E., & Petersen, E. (1970) Alpha amplitude dependence on skull thickness as measured by ultra sound technique. *Electroencephalic Clinical Neurophysiology, 29,* 392–399.

Meier, M.J. (1974) *Some challenges for clinical neuropsychology. Clinical neuropsychology. Current status and applications.* Washington, D.C.: Winston.

Milner, B. (1971) Interhemispheric differences in the localization of psychological processes in man. *British Medical Bulletin, 27*(3), 272–277.

Neilson, J.M., & Raney, R.B. (1939) Recovery from aphasia studied in cases of lobectomy. *Archives of Neurology and Psychiatry, 42,* 189.

Reitan, R.M. (1974) *Assessment of brain-behaviour relationships.* In P. McReynolds (Ed.), *Advances in psychological assessment,* Vol. iii. San Francisco: Josey-Bass.

Wada, J., & Rasmussen, T. (1960) Intracarotid injection of sodium amytal for the lateralization of cerebral speech dominance. Experimental and clinical observations. *Journal of Neurosurgery, 17* (March '60), 266–282.

Walker, S., III (1974) We're too careless about hyperactivity. *Psychology Today, 8* (No. 7), December, 43–44.

Wechsler, D. (1958) The measurement and appraisal of adult intelligence. (4th ed.) Baltimore: Williams and Wilkins.

Part III

The Development of Cerebral Dominance

WHY IS LANGUAGE LATERALIZED TO THE LEFT?

There is now overwhelming evidence that lateral cerebral asymmetries exist for psychological as well as physiological functions (Corballis & Beale, 1976). A question immediately arises: Why are language functions lateralized primarily to the left? Four alternatives have been suggested.

Acoustic Specialization

Newborn infants can distinguish speech sounds from nonspeech sounds such as muscial chords, and show cerebral asymmetries in the processing of them (Molfese, 1972). What acoustic features could be responsible for such asymmetric cerebral responses (see Chapter 2)? Speech sounds and piano chords differ with respect to a number of features: the bandwidth of the signal, the concurrence of harmonic and nonharmonic formants, the signal transitions, and so forth. It is possible that the human auditory system has specialized to the point of producing asymmetric cerebral responses with respect to such features, separating speechlike from nonspeechlike sounds. Since the principal channel for language is speech, it would not be surprising if the left hemisphere, which from birth shows a prepotency for speech sounds, were to take on the psychological function for language processing as a whole.

If this were the sole reason for left-hemisphere specialization for language, then nonspeech, language-related abilities should only gradually become left lateralized as the child matures, while the representation of speech-related tasks should not increase in asymmetry. What is needed are developmental data on the relative asymmetry of the representations of psychological abilities, such as nonverbal communication or the nonverbal analytic and serial processing of information. Relevant to this issue is Neville's study (Chapter 10) on lateralization of responses to visual stimuli. Whereas recognition of household objects usually is associated with right-hemisphere activity (being visual, nonlinguistic), she found the opposite in congenitally deaf children who communicate with sign language. Perhaps linguistic functions in deaf signers as well as in hearing individuals are left lateralized. However, the spatial nature of sign language may also result in the left lateralization of other, nonlinguistic spatial abilities in signers. It would be interesting to find more direct evidence of left-hemisphere representation of sign language in the congenitally deaf.

Lateralization of Speech Mechanisms

A second, similar hypothesis relating to output processes can be offered. Sussman (1971) and Sussman and MacNeilage (1975) had subjects track a stimulus tone. The stimulus tone was presented in one ear, the subject-controlled tone in the other. In one condition, the subject controlled the tone by movements of the tongue; in the other condition the subject controlled the tone with the right hand. Sussman found that the tongue-to-right-ear condition provided significantly better control than the tongue-to-left-ear condition. The hand-controlled condition did not produce a significant difference favoring either ear. The tongue-to-right-ear advantage is interesting in light of the fact that there was no advantage in either hand-to-ear condition and that the stimulus was nonverbal. Why should the right ear (left hemisphere) be better at coordinating the tongue in a nonlanguage auditory task? Sussman (1971) concludes that "the left hemisphere is especially adept at integrating the afferent discharges from the speech musculature with the resultant self-generated auditory input [p. 1878]." Perhaps some special relationship exists between the speech musculature and the left hemisphere independent of language use. Seen in this light, the physical proximity of Broca's area to the cortical motor control area for the tongue in the left hemisphere is suggestive of a previously unexplored hypothesis for the location of Broca's area.[1]

Returning to our original question, What does the above information suggest about left lateralization for language? Consider this hypothesis: Is it possible that because of a quirk in the organization of the central nervous system, the left hemisphere has from birth more efficient motor and sensory control over the speech musculature, especially the tongue? As was argued in the preceding section, since human language is generally closely linked to speech mechanisms, the left hemisphere would come to have more efficient control over language and language-related activities.

---

[1] We are indebted to Dr. Charles Berlin for pointing this out.

Once again, developmental data on speech and nonspeech language-related tasks are needed; a gradual increase in the asymmetry of the representation of the latter alone would lend credence to this kind of hypothesis. Lateralization data from congenitally deaf children using sign language would also be relevant.

Cognitive Style and Hemispheric Development

The previous two hypotheses have been based on a relationship between language and its usual interpersonal channel, that is, speech. Another approach deals with the cognitive aspects of language processing, that is, the analytic versus the holistic mode. This approach has been presented in detail elsewhere. Bever (1975, pp. 252–254), for example, makes four statements concerning mental activity and neurological structure:

Statement 1: The mind is self-organizing. Different modes of processing that are incompatible with one another are organized separately in "mental space," and ultimately in separate parts of the brain. Holistic and analytic modes are examples of incompatible, and therefore spatially separated, processes.

Statement 2: Analytic processing requires more mental activity than holistic processing. The logical support for this is that in order to analyze a signal, the whole must be processed anyway; therefore analytic processing includes holistic processing. Savin and Bever (1970) found, for example, that subjects can respond faster to a whole syllable than to the initial phoneme in the syllable.

Statement 3: The dynamic mapping of mental processes onto functional brain structures is maximally simple. By this, Bever means that similar mental activities are represented anatomically in similar parts of the brain.

Statement 4: The left hemisphere is more "adaptable" at birth. There is some evidence that certain areas of the left hemisphere are larger at birth than their counterparts in the right hemisphere (Wada, Clarke, & Hamm, 1975; Witelson & Pallie, 1973). Statement 4 only claims, however, that the left hemisphere is more able to deal with mental activity at birth; it is more flexible.

Bever concludes that the mentally more demanding kind of activity (analytic) will become localized in the more adapatable hemisphere (the left hemisphere). In this way, language, an analytic process, becomes left lateralized.

These statements need clarification, as well as empirical support. Statement 1, for example, could be criticized on the grounds that different areas of the brain must be able to communicate with one another, that is, incompatibility of processing modes cannot exist (Klein, 1976). Similar problems of definition exist in the other statements as well. However, the hypothesis is interesting because of its potential for a general cognitive theory of brain functioning.

An argument similar to Bever's has been offered by Carmon, Harishanu, Lowinger, and Lavy (1972), but with two premises conflicting with his. They provide evidence that the right hemisphere matures physiologically earlier than the left, because, in part at least, the blood flow to the right side of the brain is greater. They reason that since visuo-spatial processing is required of the infant long before speech and dexterity are required, it should not be surprising that the more advanced hemisphere, the right hemisphere, takes on this function.

Nonequipotentiality for Language

This hypothesis states that the hemispheres do not have equal prepotency for language functions; some facet of the structure of the left hemisphere predisposes it to whatever abilities are needed for linguistic behavior. Dennis and Whitaker (Chapter 8) review some remarkable cases of patients with very early hemispherectomies and follow their development through childhood. The two patients with only a right hemisphere showed poorer performance on tests of syntactic abilities (perhaps an analytic ability) than the patient with only a left hemisphere.

This hypothesis is similar to Bever's but is not really compatible with it. According to Bever, the analytic mode is more complex than the holistic mode, and the left hemisphere comes to take on the more complex activity because it is more flexible. In this way, the relative abilities in language (analytic) tasks and nonlanguage (holistic) tasks should not be different for left versus right hemispherectomies, although the less flexible right hemisphere should show lower overall ability. This does not appear to be the case (see Chapter 8).

Although the nonequipotentiality hypothesis has good supporting data and is intuitively pleasing, it is the least explanatory at this time of the four hypotheses discussed. We need to specify what general functions are included in the nonequipotentiality scheme and eventually must explain by what mechanism or structure this differential prepotency is determined.

These four hypotheses are speculative, and there is no reason to consider them exclusive of one another. For example, the first two deal with input and output systems and are not incompatible with either the "nonequipotentiality" or the "cognitive style" approaches. All of the hypotheses agree on one main point, however. Asymmetries in brain function are present at birth (perhaps as an accident of evolution?) and the asymmetries found in adulthood have probably evolved from them. The following four chapters discuss the asymmetry-at-birth proposal.

REFERENCES

Bever, T. (1975) Cerebral asymmetries in humans are due to the differentiation of two incompatible processes: Holistic and analytic. In D. Aaronson and R.W. Rieber (Eds.), *Developmental psycholinguistics and communication disorders.* New York: New York Academy of Sciences.

Carmon, A., Harishanu, E., Lowinger, E., & Lavy, S. (1972) Asymmetries in hemispheric blood volume and cerebral dominance. *Behavioural Biology, 7,* 853–859.

Corballis, M.C., & Beale, I.L. (1976) *The psychology of left and right.* New York: Lawrence Erlbaum.

Klein, D. (1976) Visual perceptual asymmetries and hemispheric specialization. Mimeo, Univ. of Toronto.

Molfese, D.L. (1972) Cerebral asymmetry in infants, children and adults: Auditory evoked responses to speech and music stimuli, Unpublished doctoral dissertation, Pennsylvania State Univ.

Savin, H., & Bever, T.G. (1970) The nonperceptual reality of the phoneme. *Journal of Verbal Learning and Verbal Behaviour 9,* 295–302.

Sussman, H.M. (1971) The laterality effect in lingual–auditory tracking. *Journal of the Accoustical Society of America, 49,* 1874–1880.

Sussman, H.M., & MacNeilage, P.F. (1975) Studies of hemispheric specialization for speech production. *Brain & Language, 2,* 131–151.

Wada, J.A., Clarke, R., & Hamm, A. (1975) Cerebral hemispheric asymmetry in humans. *Archives of Neurology, 32,* 239–246.

Witelson, S.F., & Pallie, W. (1973) Left hemisphere specialization for language in the newborn: Neuroanatomical evidence of asymmetry. *Brain, 96,* 641–646.

14

Does Cerebral Dominance Develop?

MARCEL KINSBOURNE
MERRILL HISCOCK

The development of cerebral dominance has attracted both academic and clinical attention. The popular line of argument may be caricatured as follows:

1. Most adults have language lateralized to the left side of the brain; therefore, it is good to have it lateralized to the left; therefore, the more lateralized to the left a person is, the better he speaks; and the better he speaks, the more lateralized to the left he must be.

2. Left-handers often do not have left lateralization of language; therefore, they must be less intelligent than right-handers.

3. Infants do not have language at all, so it cannot be lateralized in them.

4. As language skill develops and gains in richness and flexibility, its lateralization must be developing. Therefore, language lateralizes over time to the left hemisphere from a bilateral base state.

5. Those children who are quick to learn to speak are so because they lateralize faster, and those who lateralize faster supposedly learn to speak more quickly.

6. Now, here comes the therapeutic twist: If it is good to possess language skills, then the sooner, the better. So let us get language over to the left right away. How? By whatever peripheral manipulations we can dream up (tying the infant's left hand behind his back and turning him onto the left side?)

Here is a line of argument that not only lacks validity in its every step but also sets the scene for a variety of bizarre managements that, in fact, are being practiced up and down this continent. So, there is practical as well as theoretical relevance in addressing oneself to the questions raised by these various assumptions. We will do so admittedly on the basis of circumstantial rather than definitive evidence. But, as

171

Sherlock Holmes has shown us, one can derive a lot of mileage out of circumstantial evidence.

In this chapter we will argue (1) that, in adults, anomalous language lateralization per se does *not* entail cognitive deficit; (2) that, in children, there is neither neuropsychological evidence nor evidence from the ontogency of asymmetry in normal behavior that validates the concept of developing lateralization; and (3) that certain asymmetries in newborn behavior can plausibly be regarded as precursors of cerebral dominance and as indicators of its very early reign in ontogeny.

LEFT-HANDEDNESS

Left-handers provide a convenient starting point for sorting out the implications of anomalous lateralization. From studies of patients with brain damage (Milner, Branch, & Rasmussen, 1964; Roberts, 1969; Zangwill, 1967) and from clinical use of the sodium amytal technique (Wada & Rasmussen, 1960), we can be quite sure that virtually all right-handers are left lateralized for language. In contrast, left-handers form a mixed group (Ettlinger, Jackson, & Zangwill, 1956; Goodglass & Quadfasal, 1954; Hécaen & Piercy, 1956; Hécaen & Sauget, 1971; Humphrey & Zangwill, 1952; Milner *et al.,* 1964, Zangwill, 1960); between one-half and two-thirds of sinistrals do seem to have left-lateralized language, but almost one-third are right lateralized for language, and an appreciable number seem to use both hemispheres for language purposes (Rasmussen & Milner, 1976). Even this latter group is divisible into two subgroups: those who appear to use both hemispheres for similar language purposes and those who allocate different roles in language processing to each hemisphere (e.g., naming to one, sequential verbal production to the other) (Rasmussen & Milner, 1976).

At this time, specialized techniques are required to allocate left-handers to each of these differently lateralized subgroups, and this is not practical with large-scale normal samples. But it is clear that any representative sample of left-handers will include a substantial number of individuals with deviant language lateralization. It follows that if there is some measurable behavioral advantage associated with the left lateralization norm, then, on the appropriate dependent variable, a group of left-handers should show both more variability and lower mean performances than an appropriately matched group of right-handers.

Are left-handers really less intelligent than right handers? There is much evidence that among certain damaged populations and institutionalized populations there are proportionately more left-handers than in the normal population (Bakwin 1950; Doll, 1933; Hicks & Kinsbourne, 1977), but no one really has sampled across all human beings. Even Wechsler did not sample inside institutions (Wechsler, 1944). For purposes of the present discussion, we are even more restricted; we refer to a subset of the general population, undergraduates. Among undergraduates, are there intellectual differences between right-handers and non-right-handers? If so, do they relate to language lateralization or do they not? Levy (1969) has argued that, in left-handers, language is less lateralized than in right-handers. Therefore, there is some language representation in both hemispheres of left-handers, and this in some way interferes with spatial functions. It follows that left-handers should be as good verbally as right-handers, but less good spatially. She found 15 right-handed and 10 left-handed Cal Tech graduate students to be matched on Wechsler verbal IQ (with if anything, advantage to the left-handers). The left-handers were less good on performance IQ; however, the group had an average IQ in the mid-130s, which makes it a quite unrepresentative sample, and the sample size is so small as to leave it open to incalculable fortuitous effects.

As a corrective, let us consider the outcome of a very large-scale analysis performed by a group from the National Institutes of Health (Robert & Engle, as reported in Hicks & Kinsbourne, 1977). In a sample of 6350 right-handers and 762 left-handers with an age range of 6 to 11 years, no trace of a difference in Wechsler IQ emerged between the groups.

Where does this leave the data on the prevalence of left-handers in subnormal groups, and the concept of pathological left-handedness (Gordon, 1920; Satz, 1972)? The explanation is that some left-handers were potential right-handers but they sustained brain damage that shifted their handedness to the left; the ranks of left-handers are thus swelled with individuals who may have lowered cognitive capabilities on account of the brain damage. In other words, the left-handed population has more of a sprinkling of brain-damaged people than does the right-handed. That sprinkling should be attributable largely to the "sporadic" left-handers, those who do not have family history of sinistrality. They would be the ones at risk, whereas the ones with a family history of sinistrality are considered to be left-handed for biological reasons, as an expression of normal variation.

Sporadic non-right-handers constitute a substantial segment of the total non-right-handed population. If the hypothesized brain damage occurred in this group, surely its effect should reflect on the cognitive performance of non-right-handers. Yet, in fact, in normal samples, that performance is not impaired (Hicks & Kinsbourne, 1977). It follows that the concept of pathological left-handedness should be restricted in its use to populations that can otherwise be documented as brain damaged (as, for example, subsets of the mentally retarded population). Among the general population this concept has little validity. Correspondingly, the claims of Bakan (1971) and of Bakan, Dibb and Reed (1973) that non-right-handers experience more adverse circumstances of birth can be dismissed, both on the grounds already mentioned and on grounds of directly contradictory evidence (Hubbard, 1971; Schwartz, 1976).

When there is a difference between right-handers and certain subgroups among left-handers on various cognitive measures, that difference need not be related to language lateralization. If a group of non-right-handers scores poorly on some measure, it need not be because these people are differently lateralized for language. It more likely is because there is an insufficiency in brain organization concomitant with the left-handedness but independent of language lateralization.

ONTOGENETIC CHANGES IN LATERALIZATION

In this section we shall consider two sets of data that have been much propagandized as evidence for cerebral dominance as a developing characteristic of cerebral organization (Gazzaniga, 1970; Hécaen & Sauget 1971; Zangwill, 1960). One is neuropsychological, the other derives from perceptual asymmetries.

Neuropsychological Evidence

The neuropsychological data are summarized by Lenneberg (1967), who in the main derived them from a review by Basser (1962). Lenneberg makes two claims. One claim is that when children experience unilateral brain damage and that brain damage causes aphasia, the aphasia that it causes is less severe and more transitory than it would have been in an adult who sustained comparable brain damage. This is attributed to a concurrent right-hemisphere role in language function. There are problems with this claim. It is virtually impossible to compare the extent of brain damage incurred by small children with that incurred by adults, both because the brain is a different size and because the common causes of such damage are quite different at different ages. But even if children really do recover more quickly from aphasia, this does not necessarily indicate that in children the right hemisphere is more involved in ongoing language control than it is in adults. It merely illustrates the greater plasticity of the less mature organism as it compensates for functional loss due to damage (Isaacson, 1968). Except in the rare type of case in which the whole left hemisphere is abruptly inactivated, it is not clear whether this compensation is based on the right hemisphere, or residual left hemisphere, or both. So, instead of resorting to the concept of a shrinking neuroanatomical base for a particular function (language), we can use the ancient and well-established neurological concept that plasticity of the nervous system diminishes with increasing age.

Whereas a *shifting* brain base for specific behavior (to higher levels of organization) is familiar in phylogeny as "encephalization" of function (Sarnat & Netsky, 1974) and even appears to occur in ontogeny (Miller, Goldman, & Rosvold, 1973), we know of no animal model and of no human analogue to the idea that, for a given behavior, the brain base *shrinks* with increasing functional sophistication. It is a totally new creation, and until its explanatory value is clearly demonstrated, it should be treated with skepticism.

The second, apparently more powerful claim put forward by Lenneberg (1967) and refined by Krashen (1972) is that, for children between ages 2 and 5, damage to either side of the brain is likely to cause aphasia. Therefore, the younger the child, the greater the extent to which both hemispheres are involved in language. Now, there are five criteria on which one can judge this statement. They are (1) the adequacy of the sampling of cases, (2) the representative character of the case material, (3) the evidence for lateralized lesion, (4) the evidence for aphasia, and (5) the logic of the inferences made. The proposition fails on every one of these criteria.

First, sampling: Basser (1962) mostly derived his cases from sporadic reports in the literature. Now, what inferences can we make about data so gathered? If someone comes across a case of aphasia after right-sided damage, he might report it, as a way of getting his name into the literature. No such purpose would be served by reporting childhood aphasia after left-hemisphere damage. Even among adults, some 3% of people would indeed become aphasic through right-sided lesions (Zangwill, 1960). Why should not occasional children also behave in this way? They might then selectively be reported. (A more representative sample, taken not from the published literature, but from the records of a large hospital, is discussed later.)

Second, how representative of the general population are children who suffer severe brain damage? Many of the causes are potentially recurrent or more apt to occur to children who have already previously suffered brain damage. Some of the children with right-sided aphasia might have switched language lateralization from left to right on account of earlier damage implicating the left.

Third, the adequacy of anatomical definition: Neurologists can tell which part of the brain is affected, but they cannot tell the limits of involvement. Referring to primary sources, one finds that in virtually none of the reported cases is it certain that the other hemisphere was spared. In the presence of left hemiplegia one can be sure that the right brain was involved, but for all one knows, the left side might have been, too. The type of disorder these children had often does implicate the brain bilaterally; a recent report by Hécaen (1976) illustrates this problem. Hécaen observed aphasic symptoms in 15 of 17 children with damage classified as left-hemispheric and in 2 of 6 children with lesions classified as right-sided. Although the frequency of language impairment with right-sided lesions was high (33%), it clearly is a dubious statistic. One of the right-hemisphere cases with language disorder was left-handed and the other one had an etiology of cranial trauma. Hécaen concedes the inability to rule out bilateral involvement in his cases of traumatic etiology. Once again, we find that we must look elsewhere if we are to find compelling evidence of bilateral representation of language.

Fourth, the adequacy of behavioral definition: In the absence of strict and consistent criteria for defining aphasia, it is impossible to know how many cases actually involved impairment of language. We obtained the case reports of all children at the Hospital for Sick Children, Toronto, recorded as having aphasia due to early brain damage. These are the figures: above age 5, 24 left-brain lesions, and 4 right; age 5 and below, 26 left-brain lesions and 4 right. So only some 13% of the children aged 5 or less who were reported to be aphasic had right-sided lesions. Now, this is by far the largest of such series, and the percentages are a far cry from equiprobability. This makes the sampling problem a little bit less serious. Still, the data are equivocal, because the evidence for aphasia in clinical charts often is no better founded than "the child would not talk to the doctor." There are many reasons why that might happen. So, the figure of 13% could be an overestimate. When strict criteria were used for conceding that a speechless child is aphasic, the number of our cases below age 6 was reduced to eight; all of them had left-sided damage.

Finally, what of the logic of the whole enterprise? Suppose it had been true that many children become aphasic when the damage is on the right side of the brain. Would that prove that language is bilaterally represented? Surely not. It would merely show that in those children language was represented on the right side. What would it take to prove language bilaterality?

First of all, one would have to define operationally what this means. Is it that the two hemispheres are redundant for language? Then it would be bilateral damage to generate language symptoms. Or, is it that both are necessary for language, and neither one is sufficient? Such a patient would risk becoming aphasic with insult to either side. Or, maybe, one hemisphere performs some language functions, the other hemisphere, the rest. Then, which does what? No one seems to know. One cannot logically make any inference about bilaterality of language representation unless one studies both hemispheres of a given individual. So, if one were able to arrange abrupt damage first to one hemisphere and very soon afterward to the other, and one observed partial aphasia after the first injury and total aphasia after the second, then one might begin to build up a case. Pending such an unlikely event, the neuropsychological evidence for the emergence of cerebral dominance out of initial equal participation of the two hemispheres in language behavior is lacking.

Perceptual Asymmetries

Let us now turn to the evidence from perceptual asymmetries (White, 1969). When people process input, they perform more effectively when the stimuli come from the side of space opposite to the hemisphere which is going to analyze them. A right-ear advantage in dichotic listening for verbal input, for instance, indicates left lateralization of language (Kimura, 1961, 1967). It has further been argued that by comparing different groups with respect to the extent of the mean right-ear effect, one can directly compare the extent of language lateralization in those people. (In fact, attentional, motivational, cognitive, and situational variables intervene.) Disregarding the dubious nature of that assumption, people have looked for changes in dichotic ear effect across the years of childhood. And in fact, there really is not any reliable demonstrable difference in degree of ear effect with age, even down to age 2 or 3.

The original study of dichotic listening in children (Kimura, 1963) reported a significant REA for digits in children as young as 4 years. Although Kimura failed to test age differences in an analysis of variance, her data suggest no increase in asymmetry with increasing age. Subsequent studies yielded similar results (Kimura, 1967; Knox & Kimura 1970). A more recent study by Berlin, Hughes, Lowe-Bell, and Berlin (1973) bolstered the tentative conclusion that listening asymmetry is established by 5 years and undergoes no developmental increase from that point. The Berlin et al. study is notable because precisely matched pairs of consonant–vowel nonsense syllables replaced the usual digit strings; yet a consistent REA between the ages of 5 and 13 years was found. Thus, the REA in children is not limited to digit lists, nor would it seem totally dependent on memory or response set factors.

In addition to the studies demonstrating a constant degree of asymmetry over a wide age span, other dichotic experiments have yielded a REA advantage for verbal material in children as young as 2- and 3-year olds (Bever, 1971; Gilbert & Climan, 1974; Ingram, 1975; Nagafuchi, 1970).

What appears to be strong evidence for the absence of a developmental increase in listening asymmetry, especially after 5 years of age, is mitigated by a smaller number of other studies that do show a developmental increase (Bryden, 1970; Bryden & Allard, 1976; Satz, Bakker, Teunissen, Goebel, & Van der Vlugt, 1975). The issue is further complicated by the Satz group's use of long digit strings (four pairs of digits) and by Bryden's (1970) preference for using as his datum the proportion of subjects at each age level showing a REA. Satz *et al.* suggest that previous failures to find an age by ear interaction can be attributed to ceiling effects; but their use of longer digit lists may have introduced an equally distorting floor effect (the mean score at age 5 was less than 25% for each ear in the Satz *et al.* study). Similarly, Bryden's method of analyzing his data avoids certain scaling difficulties (cf., Richardson, 1976) but probably capitalizes on the decreasing noisiness of the data with increasing age. In any event, a great deal of information is lost when only a single percentage is used to describe performance at each grade level.

Studies of Ontogenetic Trends in Perceptual Asymmetries

Study 1: Children's Free Recall of Dichotic Digits. Although our first dichotic study demonstrates the invariance of the REA for verbal material over the age range of 3 to 12 years, the results also exhibit some of the vagaries characteristic of the free-recall procedure for strings of digits.

Subjects were 150 right-handed children attending a laboratory school. The source of stimuli was a tape made at Haskins Laboratories that was composed of synthesized dichotic digit pairs arranged in groups of three. Presentation rate within the triads was two pairs per second. We instructed our subjects to report as many digits as possible, and we placed no constraints on the order of report. There were 2 practice trials and 16 test trials (i.e., a total of 48 digit pairs was scored).

The mean number of digits recalled from each ear and at each grade level is shown in Figure 1. It is evident from the figure that the mean right-ear score at each grade level exceeds the left-ear mean; the overall REA—mean recall of 32.8 digits in the right ear versus 28.7 in the left—was statistically significant, $F(1,132) = 28.91$; $p < .001$. As there was no sex difference ($F < 1$), scores of males and females were pooled. Then, scores were transformed using Kuhn's (1973) formula for the ϕ coefficient. This index was chosen instead of the Fechnerian ratio, $(R - L)/(R + L)$, because the latter ratio restricts the maximum value of the asymmetry when total performance exceeds 50%. Since total performance increases with grade level, the

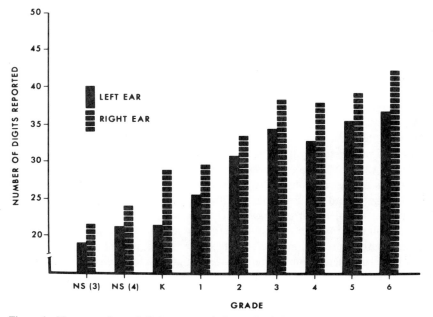

Figure 1. Mean number of digits reported from the left and right ears in a free-recall dichotic listening task. NS (3) and NS (4) denote 3-year-old and 4-year-old nursery school classes, respectively, and K denotes kindergarten.

use of phi favors finding an increasing degree of asymmetry with increasing age. Nonetheless, analysis of variance yielded no significant grade-level effect ($F < 1$), and the grade-level linear trend also was nonsignificant, $F(1,132) = 1.62; p > .10$.

Thus, the data seem to support those studies finding no developmental differences in REA for verbal material (Berlin *et al.,* 1973; Kimura, 1963, 1967; Knox & Kimura, 1970). However, when the results were examined on a grade-by-grade basis it was discovered that, even though the four oldest groups all showed significant REA, only one of the five youngest groups—the kindergarten group—displayed an ear effect that reached statistical significance. Since the right-minus-left scores differed little between old and young children (4.46 digits for Grades 3–6 versus 3.85 digits for preschool–Grade 2), the statistical weakness of the REA among the young children must be attributable largely to their high degree of variability. This increased amount of noise in the data could account for findings that young children are less likely to show a REA than are older children (Bryden, 1970). In fact, 63% of our younger children and 70% of our older children showed a REA. This pattern is consistent with Bryden's (1970) results, but the difference is nonsignificant ($\chi^2 = .63$, n.x.).

Studies 2, 3, and 4: Listening Asymmetries in Preschool Children. The shortcomings of the free-recall procedure for digit lists are well known (Bryden, 1972; Bryden & Allard, 1976). Measured performance presumably comprises an unknown mixture of perceptual, attentional, memory, response set, and perhaps other factors. The results of our first study suggest that the ambiguities of this method are especially marked in young subjects, and it is precisely these subjects in whom we are most interested. Consequently, we chose other procedures to ascertain the existence of listening asymmetries in preschool children. In addition, we adjusted the difficulty of our tasks so that total performance would be as close as possible to the 50% level. Not only does this precaution minimize the likelihood of floor effects; it also makes the task more interesting and engaging for the young child. We expected that the child might repay us for this extra consideration by trying harder and perhaps applying a more consistent and adaptive strategy than if he were overwhelmed by an excessively difficult task.

The first study with preschool children (Kinsbourne, Hotch, & Sessions, 1976, Experiment 1) used an auditory search paradigm, in which the child listened for a target presented to one or the other ear and indicated the presence or absence of that target. This paradigm deconfounds input (i.e., perceptual and attentional) from output (i.e., response set and memory) asymmetries. Twenty children between 3 and 5 years of age completed 24 trials each using this technique. Single dichotic pairs of digits were presented, and the child reported whether or not he or she heard the target digit, either an "8" or a "5." The target was present on half the trials and it occurred equally often in the right and left ears.

The mean number of errors (i.e., "misses") for trials with the target at the left ear was 3.2 out of a possible 6 but the mean number of right-ear errors was only 2.2. This ear asymmetry was statistically significant, $F(1,18) = 9.80$; $p < .01$.

A subsequent dichotic study (Kinsbourne et al., 1976, Experiment 2) used selective report instructions to demonstrate a very strong asymmetry in 3-year-old children. Sixteen children from 3:6 to 3:11 years of age completed the experiment. Each of them showed a right-hand preference for at least five of six standard handedness-assessment tasks.

The children heard 24 dichotic trials of randomly paired digits. Prior to each set of 12 trials, the experimenter pointed at the ear to which the child was to attend. Half the children began with the left ear and half began with the right; they switched attention to the opposite ear after the first 12 trials. The experimenter periodically questioned the child between trials to ensure that the child was trying to attend to the designated ear.

Again a striking asymmetry was found; these 3-year olds had much less difficulty attending to the right ear than to the left. Correct right-ear identifications were made 67% of the time, but correct left-ear identifications were made on only 26% of the trials. Analysis of variance confirmed that the effect was statistically significant, $F(1,12) = 12.61$; $p < .005$. Moreover, incorrect responses showed a corresponding asymmetry. Nearly all errors were intrusions from the opposite ear; and the majority of these intrusions were digits arriving at the right ear that were reported instead of the requested left-ear digits.

Thus far our results demonstrate that dichotic digit tasks of age-appropriate difficulty will yield a marked REA in children as young as 3 years. Moreover, the asymmetry appears to be either perceptual or attentional in origin, since the auditory search and selective listening techniques presumably obviate any asymmetries introduced by memory or response set factors.

The next step taken was to replicate the selective listening asymmetry in a larger study and to further examine the attentional component. This final dichotic study (Hiscock & Kinsbourne, 1977a) differed in several ways from the earlier selective listening experiment. First, the attended ear was randomly selected. The experimenter designated the attended ear on each trial by touching the child near the ear with a hand puppet mounted on a stick. This cuing occurred 3 sec prior to the dichotic stimuli for one set of 30 trials and immediately after the stimuli for another set of 30 trials. The precuing and postcuing conditions were administered on different days and the order was counterbalanced across subjects. The stimulus source was the same synthesized digit tape used in the free recall study reported above, but the tape was edited so that only single pairs of the digits 1 through 6 were heard.

Subjects were 12 3-year-olds, 14 4-year-olds, and 16 5-year-olds. Mean ages were 3.6, 4.5, and 5.4 years, respectively. All the children were judged to be right-handed on the basis of their observed hand preference for at least six of seven tasks selected from the Edinburgh Handedness Inventory (Oldfield, 1971).

Three dependent variables were considered: (1) the number of correct responses from the left and right ears, respectively; (2) the number of intrusions from the unattended ear; and (3) the total number of digits reported from each ear, regardless of whether that ear was the attended or unattended ear. The third variable, in other words, is the number of correct responses for an ear plus intrusions from that ear reported when the opposite ear was the designated ear. The pattern of results for all three dependent variables is shown in Figure 2. Several observations can be made: (1) there is a marked overall REA, especially for 3- and 4-year-olds; (2) the asymmetry occurs in both the pre- and postcuing conditions; (3) the asymmetry occurs for total responses and intrusions as well as for correct responses; and (4) regardless of ear, the number of correct identifications was only about half the number of total responses.

Since there were no sex differences in degree of asymmetry ($F < 1$), scores of males and females were pooled. Analysis of correct responses yielded a significant ear effect, $F(1,30) = 10.38, p < .005$, reflecting an overall performance level of 51% for right-ear digits versus 38% for digits entering the left ear. Scores were transformed to phi coefficients prior to examination of grade-level effects. Analysis of variance failed to reveal any developmental change in degree of asymmetry, $F(2,30) = 1.34, p > .25$, although separate analyses of variance for each age level indicated that the asymmetry if more marked in 3-year-olds, $F(1,8) = 3.49, p < .10$, and 4-year-olds, $F(1,10) = 5.41, p < .05$, than in 5-year-olds, $F < 1$.

Time of cuing had no effect on overall asymmetry; the REA was as great when children knew in advance which ear to monitor as when they had no advance information. Cuing condition, however, did interact with age level, $F(2,30) = 6.70, p < .005$. Postcuing decreased the asymmetry of 3-year-olds, tended to enhance the

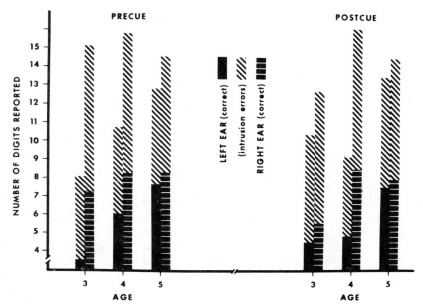

Figure 2. Mean number of digits recalled by young children in a selective listening task (from Hiscock & Kinsbourne, 1977a).

asymmetry of 4-year-olds, and had little effect on the 5-year-olds. Although this specific pattern is not readily interpretable, it appears that output factors (i.e., in the postcuing condition) combine with input asymmetries to produce a different, and less ordered, developmental pattern than that seen in the precuing condition. The most interesting finding is that the addition of these various output factors did not change the strength of the overall REA.

Two additional findings are noteworthy. First, there were almost as many intrusions from the opposite channel as there were correct responses from the designated channel. The children simply were poor at assigning an input to the correct ear. Moreover, the intrusions showed the same asymmetric bias as the correct responses. In other words, incorrect responses tended to be digits at the right ear that were reported when the left ear was the designated ear. Consequently, the second and third dependent variables—intrusion errors and total digits reported—yielded results very similar to those obtained from analysis of correct responses.

Implications and Limitations of Perceptual Data

All in all, our listening studies provide no reason to believe that the REA develops. On the contrary, we have found repeatedly a large mean REA in preschool children. In both of our selective attention studies, preschool children tended to report the right-ear digit, regardless of which one they were asked for. This suggests an attentional bias to the right when children adopt a verbal set. When people think in words, they tend to attend to the right; this effect seems actually to be more marked in children than in adults. In a sense this is not surprising, because perceptual asymmetries, which we believe to be primitive and adaptively irrelevant aspects of cerebral organization, might well *decrease* as control over behavior increases in sophistication during cerebral maturation. We would expect these archaic arrangements to become more fleeting and vanish with increasing age rather than become greater.

However, there also are serious general problems associated with the interpretation of perceptual asymmetries. It is one thing to say that, since this group has an overall right-ear effect, or a right half-field effect, therefore within this group left-sided language specialization predominates. It is quite another thing to assume that the degree of ear effect provides a direct metric for individual differenes in brain organization (cf. Shankweiler & Studdert-Kennedy, 1975). The very notion that the degree of asymmetry in performance directly measures a structural characteristic depends on a particular model of asymmetries (Kimura, 1961; 1966). That model does not offer the only way to explain the data. An alternative concept is the following: The left hemisphere, when engaged in its specialized (i.e., verbal) activity, whether acticipatory or ongoing, generates a right-sided selective orientation by virtue of the functional proximity of the left frontal rightward turning center, which becomes synergically activated. As verification, the lateral gaze studies show just such an effect (Kinsbourne, 1972; 1974). If a person is verbally active, he tends more naturally to listen to the right side of space than to the left side of space. In fact, Treisman and Geffen (1968) inadvertently demonstrated this to be true with a selective shadowing experiment. Once one accepts the possibility of a relationship between degree of asymmetry in performance and attention variables, it becomes obvious that there are other dimensions that might control the degree of asymmetry in performance in addition to brain specialization. The amount of effort a subject makes and the extent to which his strategy is specifically verbal, will determine how much the left hemisphere is activated, as compared to the right, and thus the degree of any asymmetry in processing ability. The relative activation of the two hemispheres will vary with task difficulty, motivation, cognitive strategy, and more conscious attentional shift to compensate for known or inferred shortcomings in processing one of the inputs.

When comparing males and females (Kimura, 1967; Buffery, 1971), rich and poor (Geffner & Hochberg, 1971), young and old (Satz *et al.,* 1975), before one arrives at statements about how these groups' brains differ, based on a few more mistakes committed on one side than on the other, one should take pains to hold these potentially biasing variables constant. For instance, a child of low socioeconomic status might not be adopting a verbal strategy or any strategy at all when the experimenter shoves earphones over his head. Failure to demonstrate asymmetry under such circumstances (Geffner & Hochberg, 1971) need imply nothing about brain or organization. Males and females may use different strategies even though the brains which generate them may be identically organized (Maccoby & Jacklin, 1974). There is much work to be done before we can translate these data into something revealing about the brain. After all, in any sample of verbal dichotic data, at best about 80% of people show even a minimal (insignificant) REA. Now, what happened to the remaining 20%, who presumably are also left lateralized for language? Does their language area migrate to the other side for the duration of the experiment? Clearly a method that so grossly misclassifies a substantial minority of the normal population cannot be a valid index of lateralization with individuals when used in the usual manner. Unless one can show within one subject that his performance is significantly asymmetrical, that the degree of asymmetry is reliable on retest, and that the asymmetry is not based on attentional factors, one has not elucidated the language lateralization of that subject. Once a method has been developed which can do this, it still is unlikely that subjects can be arranged on a continuum of "degree of lateralization" of language or any other functions that are represented asymmetrically in the brain (cf., Shankweiler & Studdert-Kennedy, 1975).

For all these reasons, it is desirable to support arguments about the structural asymmetry of cognitive processes in the brain with measures less susceptible to situational bias. To achieve this, we leave the realm of perceptual phenomena and turn to the observation of motor concomitants of lateralized cerebral processes, and to capacity measures of laterally controlled performance. We now describe attempts to design techniques to enable this to be done.

New Techniques for Assessing Lateralization

We have used two novel tasks to examine the ontogeny of lateralization. In one study we used the lateral gaze effect reported elsewhere for adults (Kinsbourne, 1972). When thinking about the solution to problems, subjects look to the side opposite the hemisphere specialized for the required mode of thinking: They look rightward for verbal and leftward for spatial thought. We asked 5-year-olds verbal questions and spatial questions and, as expected, they looked to the right immediately after the verbal questions and to the left after the spatial questions (Kinsbourne & Jardno, 1974, unpublished). This indicates the customary specialization as early as age 5.

We also used a finger-tapping task with verbal interference (Kinsbourne & McMurray, 1975). This is an instance of a type of experiment that contrasts subjects' ability to perform concurrent activities when they are programmed in the same hemisphere (e.g., speaking and right manual activities) and when they are programmed in separate hemispheres (e.g., speaking and left manual activities) (Kinsbourne & Cook, 1971; Hicks, 1975). "Sharing" of the same hemisphere for two independent activities results in more marked impairment of performance. We had children tap as fast as they could with the one index finger and then with the other. In this control condition we found the right-sided superiority one might expect. We also, in counterbalanced order, had them do the same thing over, while talking. Now they were tapping faster with the left than with the right index finger. In other words, we found the expected greater interference between two activities programmed by the same hemisphere, the speaking and the right-hand tapping, as compared to two activities programmed in opposite hemispheres, speaking (programmed in the left hemisphere) and left-hand tapping (programmed in the right hemisphere). So, again there is evidence for lateral specialization by age 5.

We speculated that the finger-tapping task would be appropriate for use with children of various ages (Hiscock & Kinsbourne, 1977b). In fact, we reasoned that this technique might be superior in many respects to traditional perceptual tasks for evaluating the pattern of asymmetries in children. As we have seen, floor and ceiling effects constitute a serious problem in dichotic listening. The use of a rate measure enables us to handle a wide range of performance levels without encountering either floor or ceiling effects. The tapping task seems easy enough for 3-year-olds but challenging enough for adolescents. It is an interesting task and it takes little time to administer. Probably the most important advantage of the technique is its control over the allocation of attention. When two channels of input information compete for attentional resources over a long series of trials, as in dichotic listening, there is a great temptation for the subject to indulge his curiosity and relieve his boredom by distributing attention between the two channels in various ways. Any such variability in strategy, of course, contributes to experimental error. In the tapping task, only one hand is engaged at a time, and a certain minimal level of attention is required to maintain the tapping. Thus, there is much less opportunity for attentional shifts, and those variations that do occur involve redistribution of attention between the two concurrent tasks and not between right and left hands. In other words, an attentional shift in dichotic listening away from one channel implies a shift toward the other channel, and this magnifies the effect of the shift; however, this is not the case for the tapping task, in which an attentional shift from tapping only implies more attention to speaking.

We applied the Kinsbourne and McMurray (1975) procedure to the group of preschool and grade-school children described previously. This time we had 151 right-handed subjects aged from 3 to 11 years. Each child was instructed to tap as fast as possible in six counterbalanced conditions: (1) right-hand tapping without concurrent activity, (2) left-hand tapping without concurrent activity, (3) right-hand tapping and recitation of a nursery rhyme, (4) left-hand tapping and recitation of the rhyme, (5) right-hand tapping and recitation of a list of four animal names, and (6) left-hand tapping and recitation of the animal names. The only significant deviation from the Kinsbourne and McMurray technique was our requirement that subjects tap a telegraph key rather than simply tap on the table top. The key controlled an audio oscillator, which was connected to the input of a stereo tape recorder. Thus, the tapping data could be scored blindly and at the scorers' convenience.

We looked first at tapping rates in the control conditions, that is, without interference, and found a very strong overall right-hand superiority that manifests itself at all grade levels. Furthermore, tapping rate for both hands increases with age. The primary object of the technique is to determine the degree to which the concurrent task depresses tapping rate for either hand. Especially since there were hand and grade level effects for the control conditions, it was necessary to use a

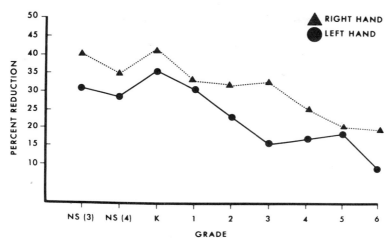

Figure 3. Mean reduction in right-hand and left-hand tapping rate, relative to the control condition, when the concurrent task was recitation of a nursery rhyme (from Hiscock & Kinsbourne, 1977b).

measure of rate depression that would be independent of overall performance. We simply converted our scores to ratios representing the proportion of decrease in tapping rate from control condition to concurrent task condition. Our dependent measure can be expressed as

$$x_i = \frac{r_c - r_v}{r_c}$$

where r_c is tapping rate for either hand in the control condition and r_v is the tapping rate for the same hand in one of the concurrent task conditions.

Figure 3 shows our findings for the nursery rhyme task. Values in the figure represent the percentage decrease in tapping rate for either hand. There is a decreasing interference effect with age for both hands, $F(8,115) = 6.02, p < .001$, and a strong asymmetry such that the right hand is affected more than the left hand, $F(1,115) = 34.14, p < .001$. The Hand × Grade-Level interaction is nonsignificant, $F(8,115) = 1.38, p > .20$, as is the Hand × Grade-level linear trend interaction, $F < 1$.

The analogous data for the animal-naming task are illustrated in Figure 4. Again, there are significant effects for both grade level, $F(8,115) = 5.36, p < .001$, and hand, $F(1,115) = 21.56, p < .001$. Again there is neither a Hand × Grade-Level interaction, $F < 1$, nor a Hand × Grade-Level linear trend interaction, $F < 1$.

We are continuing to examine the finger-tapping task in order to achieve a better understanding of the underlying mechanisms. We are looking at the task's reliability over time, the variability of tapping rate within each condition, and the temporal nature of the verbal–manual time sharing. At our present level of understanding, it

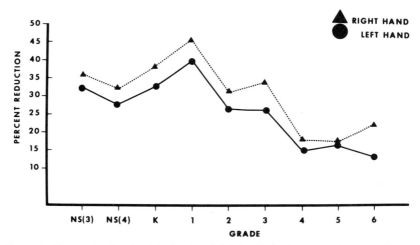

Figure 4. Mean reduction in right-hand and left-hand tapping rate, relative to the control condition, when the concurrent task was recitation of animal names (from Hiscock & Kinsbourne, 1977b).

seems clear that the results complement our dichotic listening findings: Asymmetries are seen in children as young as 3 years, and the asymmetries remain relatively constant until age 13.

The Concept of Developing Lateralization

As has been discussed, the concept of varying degrees of lateralization of language, viewed ontogenetically, is based on hopelessly inadequate evidence. In addition, the concept is vague. If it implies varying degrees of ongoing participation of the minor hemisphere in verbal activity, then the manner and mechanism of this hypothetical contribution remains virtually undiscussed, not to mention unexplained. If all that is implied is varying degrees of contralateral compensatory capacity after insult to the language-dominant hemisphere, then the concept is misleadingly named. It certainly is possible that males and females differ in this respect, and it is likely that age is a correlated variable. But only the neuropsychological data can speak to this point. The normal perceptual asymmetry literature is not pertinent.

Applying these considerations to the ontogenetic data, we remain with one reliable conclusion: It has repeatedly been found possible to demonstrate performance asymmetries down to the preschool years, and even as low as 3 years of age. The data about relationship of degree of that asymmetry to age is equivocal, but, as we have seen, it would be hard to interpret even if a consistent age-related function could be supported. Floor and ceiling effects, different degrees of motivation, differences in task difficulty, asymmetries and extraneous focal points of interest in the experimental situation, and the varying use of cognitive and attentional strategies all could account for any age-related systematic variation (cf. Kinsbourne,

1975). Let us concede only that lateralized individuals occur with substantial frequency at those young ages.

ASYMMETRIES IN INFANTS

Striking findings were reported by two separate groups some years ago. Newborn babies turn their heads spontaneously to the right four times as often as to the left (Turkewitz, Gordon, & Birch, 1968). When operant conditioners used rightward turning as an instrumental response, their data were so contaminated by spontaneous rightward turning that they systematically had to use leftward turning only (Siqueland & Lipsitt, 1966). These are sizable asymmetries. Second, although hand preference for reaching cannot be demonstrated until the last few months of the first year of life (Gesell & Ames, 1947), that is merely because young infants are not very good at reaching, and if you ask babies a silly question, you get a silly answer. The notion that infants do not have manual asymmetry comes from the choice of an inappropriate dependent variable, reaching. In the first place, infants tend to reach bimanually, and they are notorious for not crossing the midline. If they are exactly lined up, they are likely to reach with both hands; if not, they are likely to reach with the ipsilateral hand. So Caplan and Kinsbourne (1976) decided to study the duration of reflex grasping instead. An experimental rattle was placed into the right hand and the left hand of 3-month-old babies. There was a significant manual asymmetry in terms of longer duration of clutching of the rattle by the right hand. Again, then, we find an early asymmetry.

We now refer to two experiments described in this volume—Molfese's in Chapter 2 (also cf. Gardiner & Walter, 1976; Molfese, 1973; Molfese, Freeman, & Palermo, 1975) and Entus's in Chapter 6. What do we learn from the higher amplitude of electrophysiological response over the infant's left hemisphere in the presence of verbal information—an asymmetry even greater in infants than in adults (Molfese *et al.*, 1975)? What do we conclude that the infant's greater propensity to respond to a phoneme transition on the right-ear channel during dichotic presentation of speech sounds? Here we have an asymmetry for language-related processes long before language behavior as such is detectable. In other words, instead of lateralization accompanying the development of this ability, it is there long before. Now, can one's brain be specialized for something before it can be performed? We would suggest that it can. What is more, this is quite characteristic of infant development. Infants typically manifest the pattern of an activity before they can perform that activity in any goal-directed manner. The vehicle, the manner of performing, precedes the content, the capability. For instance, toddlers toddle from point to point and back again for no demonstrable reason. Infants put things into other things without there being any reason to put the one thing into the other or take it out from there. They make all sorts of speech sounds before they are using them to communicate, and they show interactional synchrony; in other words, much patterning of behavior precedes the adaptive use of that behavior. Language development seems to be a case in point. The left half of the brain is programmed to subserve language, and that is why under normal circumstances it usually does so. But the preprogramming need not be explained by invoking a radical difference between the two hemispheres in neuronal organization (Semmes, 1968). The neuronal substrate cannot be much different in the two sides, though there may be minor differences; we learn this, for instance, from the early hemispherectomy data, which show the nondominant hemisphere to be largely, though not completely, capable of subserving the unaccustomed function (Chapter 8, this volume; Kohn & Dennis, 1974). We need assume no more than that there is a preprogrammed arrangement for one side of the brain to be more activated than the other by a particular stimulus type. That side of the brain which will later deal with language shows its material-specific activation pattern long before its neuronal equipment is sufficiently developed for the actual behavior. On this model, what Molfese picked up electrophysiologically was the result of brainstem-direct, "clerical" disposition of activation between the cerebral hemispheres, so that one side of the brain is more activated in a verbal context, the other in a musical context. That is why the left hemisphere usually achieves language dominance. It is unnecessary to suppose that it is better equipped in terms of its natural hookups. Rather, every time speech occurs or a verbal mental set is adopted, the left hemisphere is activated, whereas the right side, in the absence of activation, does not enrich its verbal repertoire (except at the relatively automatic level, for which little activation is required). If the left hemisphere is destroyed, then activation is diverted to the right hemisphere, and it shows a reasonable, if imperfect, language capability (Kinsbourne, 1971).

In summary, the lateral disposition of language skills is preprogrammed by means of a species-specific differential activation of the relevant part of the brain in verbal context. This is the brain basis for the process of adopting a verbal mental set. The activation pattern proper to verbal set is implemented before language skills are. Deviations from the customary anatomical pattern might be inherited or arise from anomalies early in embryogenesis. If the activation pattern is deviant, this in itself does not necessarily constitute a problem. Those people who have deviant patterns and also cognitive problems do not necessarily have cognitive problems because of the deviant patterns; rather, the antecedent cause of the deviant pattern also may be the antecedent of the cognitive problem.

REFERENCES

Bakan, P. (1971) Birth order and handedness. *Nature, 229,* 195.
Bakan, P. Dibb, G., & Reed, P. (1973) Handedness and birth stress. *Neuropsychologia, 11,* 363–366.
Bakwin, H. (1950) Psychiatric aspects of pediatrics: Lateral dominance right- and left-handedness. *Journal of Pediatrics, 36,* 385–391.
Basser, L.S. (1962) Hemiplegia of early onset and the faculty of speech with special reference to the effects of hemispherectomy. *Brain, 85,* 427–460.

Berlin, C.I., Hughes, L.F., Lowe-Bell, S.S., & Berlin, H.L. (1973) Dichotic right ear advantage in children 5 to 13. *Cortex, 9,* 394–402.

Bever, T.G. (1971) The nature of cerebral dominance in speech behavior of the child and adult. In R. Huxley & E. Ingram (Eds.), *Language acquisition: Models and methods.* London: Academic Press.

Bryden, M.P. (1970) Laterality effects in dichotic listening: Relations with handedness and reading ability in children. *Neuropsychologia, 8,* 443–450.

Bryden, M.P. (1972) Perceptual strategies, attention, and memory in dichotic listening. Research report #43, Univ. of Waterloo.

Bryden, M.P., & Allard, F. (1976) Dichotic listening and the development of linguistic processes. In M. Kinsbourne (Ed.), *Hemispheric asymmetries of function.* New York: Cambridge Univ. Press.

Buffery, A.W.H. (1971) Sex differences in the development of hemispheric asymmetry of function in the human brain. *Brain Research, 31,* 364–365.

Caplan, P.J., & Kinsbourne, M. (1976) Baby drops the rattle: Asymmetry of duration of grasp by infants. *Child Development, 47,* 532–534.

Doll, E.A. (1933) Psychological significance of cerebral birth lesions. *American Journal of Psychology, 45,* 444–452.

Ettlinger, G., Jackson, C.V., & Zangwill, O.L. (1956) Cerebral dominance in sinistrals. *Brain, 79,* 569–588.

Gardiner, M.F., & Walter, D.O. (1976) Evidence of hemispheric specialization from infant EEG. In S. Harnad, R.W. Doty, L. Goldstein, J. Jaynes, & G. Krauthmer (Eds.), *Lateralization in the Nervous System.* New York: Academic Press.

Gazzaniga, M.S. (1970) *The bisected brain.* New York: Appleton.

Geffner, D.S., & Hochberg, I. (1971) Ear laterality preference of children from low and middle socioeconomic levels on a verbal dichotic listening task. *Cortex, 7,* 193–203.

Gesell, A., & Ames, L.B. (1947) The development of handedness. *Journal of Genetic Psychology, 70,* 155–175.

Gilbert, J.H.V., & Climan, I. (1974) Dichotic studies in 2 and 3 year-olds: A preliminary report. *Speech Communication Seminar, Stockholm, Vol. 2.* Upsala: Almquist & Wiksell.

Goodglass, H., & Quadfasal, F.A. (1954) Language laterality in left-handed aphasics. *Brain, 77,* 521–548.

Gordon, H. (1920) Left-handedness and mirrorwriting especially among defective children, *Brain, 43,* 313–368.

Hécaen, H. (1976) Acquired asphasia in children and the ontogenesis of hemispherical functional specialization. *Brain and Language, 3,* 114–134.

Hécaen, H., & Piercy, M. (1956) Paroxysmal dysphasia and the problem of cerebral dominance. *Journal of Neurology, Neurosurgery and Psychiatry, 19,* 194–201.

Hécaen, H., & Sauget, J. (1971) Cerebral dominance in left-handed subjects. *Cortex, 7,* 19–48.

Hicks, R.E. (1975) Intrahemispheric response competition between vocal and unimanual performance in normal adult human males. *Journal of Comparative and Physiological Psychology, 89,* 50–60.

Hicks, R.E., & Kinsbourne, M. (1977) Human handedness. In M. Kinsbourne (Ed.), *The asymmetrical function of the brain.* New York: Cambridge Univ. Press.

Hiscock, M., & Kinsbourne, M. (1977a) Selective listening asymmetry in preschool children. *Developmental Psychology.*

Hiscock, M., & Kinsbourne, M. (1977b) Ontogeny of cerebral dominance: Evidence from time-sharing asymmetry in children.

Hubbard, G.I. (1971) Handedness not a function of birth order. *Nature, 232,* 276–277.

Humphrey, M.E., & Zangwill, O.L. (1952) Dysphasia in left-handed patients with unilateral brain lesions. *Journal of Neurology, Neurosurgery and Psychiatry, 15,* 184–193.

Ingram, D. (1975) Cerebral speech lateralization in young children. *Neuropsychologia, 13,* 103–105.

Isaacson, R. (Ed.) 1968. *The neuropsychology of development*. New York: Wiley.

Kimura, D. (1961) Cerebral dominance and the perception of verbal stimuli. *Canadian Journal of Psychology, 15*, 166–171.

Kimura, D. (1963) Speech lateralization in young children as determined by an auditory test. *Journal of Comparative and Physiological Psychology, 56*, 899–902.

Kimura, D. (1966) Dual functional asymmetry of the brain in visual perception. *Neuropsychologia, 4*, 275–285.

Kimura, D. (1967) Functional asymmetry of the brain in dichotic listening. *Cortex, 3*, 163–178.

Kinsbourne, M. (1971) The minor cerebral hemisphere as a source of aphasic speech. *Archives of Neurology, 25*, 302–306.

Kinsbourne, M. (1972) Eye and head turning indicates cerebral lateralization. *Science, 176*, 539–541.

Kinsbourne, M. (1974) Direction of gaze and distribution of cerebral thought processes. *Neuropsychologia, 12*, 279–281.

Kinsbourne, M. (1975) The ontogeny of cerebral dominance. *Annals of the New York Academy of Sciences, 263*, 244–250.

Kinsbourne, M., & Cook, J. (1971) Generalized and lateralized effect of concurrent verbalization on a unimanual skill. *Quarterly Journal of Experimental Psychology, 23*, 341–343.

Kinsbourne, M., Hotch, D., & Sessions, T. (1974) Auditory search through dichotic digits by preschool children.

Kinsbourne, M., & Jardno, E. (1974) Direction of lateral gaze and mental set in preschool children.

Kinsbourne, M., & McMurray, J. (1975) The effect of cerebral dominance on time sharing between speaking and tapping by preschool children. *Child Development, 46*, 240–242.

Knox, C., & Kimura, D. (1970) Cerebral processing of nonverbal sounds in boys and girls. *Neuropsychologia, 8*, 227–237.

Kohn, B., & Dennis, M. (1974) Patterns of hemispheric specialization after hemidecortication for infantile hemiplegia. In M. Kinsbourne & W.L. Smith (Eds.), *Hemispheric disconnection and cerebral function*. Springfield, Illinois: Thomas.

Krashen, S. (1972) Language and the left hemisphere. *Working Papers in Phonetics, 24*, University of California at Los Angeles.

Kuhn, G.M. (1973) The phi coefficient as an index of ear differences in dichotic listening. *Cortex, 9*, 450–456.

Lenneberg, E. (1967) *Biological foundations of language*. New York: Wiley.

Levy, J. (1969) Possible basis for the evolution of lateral specialization of the human brain. *Nature, 224*, 614–615.

Maccoby, E.E., & Jacklin, C.N. (1974) *The psychology of sex differences*. Stanford, California: Stanford Univ. Press.

Miller, E.A., Goldman, P.S., & Rosvold, H.E. (1973) Delayed recovery of function following orbital prefrontal lesion in infant monkeys. *Science, 182*, 304–306.

Milner, B., Branch, C., & Rasmussen, T. (1964) Observations on cerebral dominance. In A.V.S. de Rueck & M. O'Conner (Eds.), *Ciba Foundation Symposium on disorders of language*. London: Churchill.

Molfese, D.L. (1973) Central asymmetry in infants, children and adults: Auditory evoked responses to speech and music. *Journal of the Acoustical Society of America, 53*, 363–373.

Molfese, D.L., Freeman, R.B. Jr., & Palermo, D. (1975) The ontogeny of brain lateralization for speech and nonspeech stimuli. *Brain and Language, 2*, 356–368.

Nagafuchi, M. (1970) Development of dichotic and monaural hearing abilities in young children. *Acta Otolaryngologica, 69*, 409–414.

Oldfield, R.C. (1971) The assessment and analysis of handedness: The Edinburgh Inventory. *Neuropsychologia, 9*, 97–113.

Rasmussen, T., & Milner, B. (1976) Clinical and surgical studies of the cerebral speech areas in man. In K.J. Zülch, O Creutzfeldt & G. Galbraith (Eds.), *Otfrid Foerster Symposium on cerebral localization*. Heidelberg: Springer.

Richardson, J.T.E. (1976) How to measure laterality. *Neuropsychologia, 14*, 135–136.

Roberts, L. (1969) Aphasia, apraxia and agnosia in abnormal states of cerebral dominance. In P.J. Vinken & G.W. Bruyn (Eds.), *Handbook of clinical neurology*, Vol. 4. Amsterdam: North-Holland.

Sarnat, H., & Netsky, M.G. (1974) *Evolution of the nervous system*. New York: Oxford University Press.

Satz, P. (1972) Pathological left handedness: An explanatory model. *Cortex, 8*, 121–135.

Satz, P., Bakker, D.J., Teunissen, J. Goebel, R., & Van Der Vlugt, H. (1975) Developmental parameters of the ear asymmetry: A multivariate approach. *Brain and Language, 2*, 171–185.

Schwartz, M. (in press) Left-handedness and high-risk preganacy. *Neuropsychologia*.

Semmes, J. (1968) Hemispheric specialization: A possible clue to mechanism. *Neuropsychologia, 6*, 11–26.

Shankweiler, D., & Studdert-Kennedy, M. (1975) A continuum of lateralization for speech perception? *Brain and Language, 2*, 212–225.

Siqueland, E.R., & Lipsitt, L.P. (1966) Conditioned head turning in human newborns. *Journal of Experimental Child Psychology, 4*, 356–357.

Treisman, A., & Geffen, G. (1968) Selective attention and cerebral dominance in perceiving and responding to speech messages. *Quarterly Journal of Experimental Psychology, 20*, 139–150.

Turkewitz, G., Gordon, B.W., & Birch, M.G. (1968) Head turning in the human neonate: effect of prandial condition and lateral preference. *Journal of Comparative and Physiological Psychology, 59*, 189–192.

Wada, J., & Rasmussen, T. (1960) Intracarotid injection of sodium amytal for the lateralization of cerebral speech dominance. *Journal of Neurosurgery, 17*, 266–282.

Wechsler, D. (1944) *The measurement of adult intelligence*. Baltimore: Williams & Wilkins.

White, M.J. (1969) Laterality differences in perception: A review. *Psychological Bulletin, 72*, 387–405.

Zangwill, O.L. (1960) *Cerebral dominance and its relation to psychological function*. Edinburgh: Oliver & Boyd.

Zangwill, O.L. (1967) Speech and the minor hemisphere. *Acta Neurologica et Psychiatrica Belgica, 67*, 1013–1020.

15

The Development of Lateralization of Language Functions and Its Relation to Cognitive and Linguistic Development: A Review and Some Theoretical Speculations

MORRIS MOSCOVITCH

Research on the development of cerebral dominance for language has been concerned primarily with two questions: (1) How and when does this dominance develop? and (2) What is the relation between the process of language lateralization and the development of linguistic and nonlinguistic skills associated with the mature left and right hemisphere, respectively? Because the two questions are closely related, many investigators have simply assumed that if the time at which lateralization appears in normal children were known, then such knowledge would provide some information about the relation between the development of cerebral dominance and cognitive processes. Straightforward and simple as this strategy may sound, the results of the research it has generated have been complex and often contradictory. It is only recently that a number of lines of evidence have converged on a solution to the question of when does cerebral dominance for language develop. The first section of this chapter briefly reviews the literature concerned with this issue and summarizes what I believe to be the current consensus. The second section examines some unsolved problems related to the development of laterality and its relation to cognition, proposes a number of solutions to these problems, and discusses the implications of these solutions for future research.

A BRIEF HISTORY

Despite a good deal of historical evidence to the contrary (Chapter 8, this volume; Hécaen, 1976), recent theories regarding the development of hemispheric specialization for language have been strongly influenced by one major piece of evidence—the contrast between the effect of early and late cortical damage on language processes (Basser, 1962; Bever, 1971; Bryden, 1970; Bryden & Allard, 1975; Gazzanniga, 1975; Lenneberg, 1967; Krashen, 1973; Satz, Bakker, Teunissen, Goebel, & van der Vlugt, 1975; Selnes, 1974). As is well known, the likelihood that left-hemisphere damage in adulthood will lead to permanent language deficits is very high, particularly if the damage encroaches on the classical language areas. Lesions to the right hemisphere, however, rarely produce any language disorders except those related to general cognitive impairments (Eisenson, 1962; Goodglass & Quadfasel, 1954; Hebb, 1942; Luria, 1970; Zangwill, 1960; Weisenberg & McBride, 1935). It has been claimed that recovery of language after left-hemisphere damage in childhood is usually rapid and relatively complete, so that the child's ultimate linguistic performance is close to normal (Lenneberg, 1967; Milner, 1974). In addition, the occurrence of language disorders following right-hemisphere damage in childhood is quite common and recovery is particularly rapid (Hécaen, 1976; Lenneberg, 1967).

The gross differences between the effects of early and late brain damage were so striking that they formed the basis of the most popular theory regarding the development of hemispheric dominance. Lenneberg (1967), who best articulated that theory, claimed that at birth and during early childhood, the hemispheres are equipotential in their ability to mediate language. As the child grows, maturational and environmental factors—in particular, the child's exposure to language and his use of it—cause linguistic processes to become gradually lateralized to the left hemisphere. This process of lateralization, in turn, aids and nurtures linguistic growth. The period during which lateralization develops was viewed by Lenneberg as being a period of relative neural plasticity for structures subserving language, as indicated by the rapid and complete recovery of language functions following cortical damage. Consequently, he regarded this period of neural plasticity as critical or optimal for language growth. On the basis of his own and Basser's data on the ages at which there is substantial recovery of language following cortical damage, Lenneberg estimated that the process of lateralization is rapid between the ages of 2 or 3 to 5, and then proceeds more slowly until puberty, by which time it is complete. Thus, this period coincides reasonably well with the periods of rapid growth and consolidation of language in normal children.

Attractive as Lenneberg's theory might be, more recent research and a closer examination of the early lesion data indicate that the principle of early hemispheric equipotentiality on which this theory rests is probably overstated, if not false. In some sense, the attack on Lenneberg's theory began even before he published it. In 1963, Kimura reported that children as young as 4 years of age showed a REA in recalling dicotichally presented numbers, which indicated a left-hemisphere dominance for language. Moreover, neither she, nor a number of others since then were able to find a reliable increase in the REA with age (Geffner & Dorman, 1976; Hiscock & Kinsbourne, 1976; Ingram, 1975(b); Nagafuchi, 1970; see Porter and Berlin, 1975, for review). More recently, Entus (Chapter 6) adapted the dichotic listening techniques for use with infants 4 to 16 weeks old and found that they, too, showed a REA for speech and a LEA for music. Although it is too soon to know whether Entus's study can be replicated, the substantial number of studies showing a REA in young children suggests that the failure of some investigators to find this effect (Bryden & Allard, 1975; Satz et al., 1975) is due either to an artifact in their testing procedure (see Bryden & Allard, 1975, for review) or to the possibility that they were testing for lateralization of functions that were not yet fully developed (see Porter and Berlin, 1975).

In addition to dichotic listening, a number of other tasks that are correlated with left-hemisphere dominance for language have revealed evidence of lateralization in infants and young children. Ingram (1975a) found that children as young as 3 gesture more with the right than the left hand while speaking, a pattern of activity similar to that found in adults with left-hemisphere dominance (Kimura, 1973). Kinsbourne and McMurray (1975) and Hiscock and Kinsbourne (1976 and Chapter 14) showed that speaking interferes with simultaneous finger tapping of the right hand more than the left in children as young as 3. Finally, Molfese (Chapter 2; Molfese, Freeman, & Palermo, 1975) found that the pattern of evoked potentials to speech and nonspeech stimuli indicated that hemispheric differences in processing these stimuli were already present in infants. Molfese's and Entus' evidence for the existence of functional hemispheric asymmetries in infants receives some indirect support from a number of studies showing that, at birth, the region of the planum temporale, an area that encompasses the posterior speech zones, is larger in the left hemisphere than in the right (Teszner, Tzavaras, Grunes, & Hécaen, 1972; Wada, Clark, & Hamm, 1975; Witelson & Pallie, 1973). This corresponds to similar structural asymmetries found in adult brains (Geschwind & Levitsky, 1968).

The finding that both structural and functional asymmetries exist in early infancy seems to be inconsistent with the lesion data that purport to demonstrate that the two hemispheres are equipotential at least until middle childhood. This discrepancy, however, may be more apparent than real. Dennis and Whitaker (Chapter 8) and Hécaen (1976) have carefully reviewed the literature on the effects of early cortical damage on language development and have concluded that language deficits on linguistic tasks are more common and longer lasting following left- rather than right-hemisphere lesions. Since these reviews are quite thorough, I wish only to examine Basser's (1962) findings by way of illustration, since it is his study that has been most widely quoted as evidence for the equipotentiality hypothesis. Basser investigated over 100 cases of hemiplegia of early onset and claimed to have found no differences in IQ or language development between left and right hemiplegics. However, if we examine only those patients who incurred damage following the appearance of language, we find that of the 20 that showed speech arrest for 2 weeks or longer, 13 had left-hemisphere lesions, whereas of the 10 who showed no language loss after brain damage, only 2 had left-hemisphere lesions. Even Basser's study, then, suggests that the left hemisphere is likely to be dominant for language once speech production is evident. Failure to find similar relationships between the side of damage and language development in individuals who sustained damage prior to speech onset may have been due, in part, to the extreme severity of such damage in Basser's population. This impression is confirmed both by Basser's admission that the lesions incurred in infancy had such devastating effects that the IQ of the majority of such cases could not even be tested and, in those cases where it could be, it was extremely low. A more recent, better-controlled study by Annett (1973) found that even in patients with unilateral brain damage sustained prior to speech onset, the probability of occurrence of language deficits was 30% for individuals with left-hemisphere damage compared to 15% for those with right-hemisphere damage.

This brief review indicates that there is converging evidence from neurological, electrophysiological, behavioral, and anatomical studies for the existence of early functional and structural differences between the hemispheres. Although this evidence argues against the equipotentiality hypothesis, it should be remembered that it does not deny the possibility that some of the differences found in infancy may become more pronounced or that new differences may emerge as the child matures. In short, there may yet be a process of developing lateralization. The present evidence does not tell us very much about lateralization. Moreover, the present evidence does not tell us very much about the relation between lateralization of function and the development of linguistic and nonlinguistic skills. The remaining sections of this chapter will address these issues. Because the studies on them are scanty, often contradictory, and, therefore, inconclusive, I will make no serious attempt to synthesize the available material and offer a comprehensive theory. Rather, I will focus on a number of problems and outline some theoretical or research approaches that may serve as frameworks for further investigations.

THE RESTITUTION OF LANGUAGE IN THE RIGHT
HEMISPHERE FOLLOWING LEFT-HEMISPHERE DAMAGE

As indicated earlier, the extent of restitution of language functions following left-hemisphere damage at various ages has been used to determine the temporal course of lateralization of language functions. So long as no claims are made regarding the equipotentiality of the hemispheres, this evidence can still be used to argue in favour of a process of increasing lateralization in which an initial left-hemisphere superiority in infancy is magnified during the first 5 to 10 years of life. An alternative interpretation of these findings is that they provide an index of the relative plasticity of the language areas on the left as well as the right hemisphere at the time of damage. Milner (1974) and Hécaen (1976) have noted that in some cases of early damage to the left hemisphere, restitution of language functions is mediated by the undamaged tissue on the left. More often, however, if the primary language zones are damaged, it is the right hemisphere that assumes the dominant linguistic role. The right hemisphere's ability to do so may not be an indication that lateralization to the left has not occurred, but rather that the homologous areas on the right side are either relatively immature or uncommitted with regard to function (see Hécaen, 1976; Lansdell, 1969; Moscovitch, 1972, 1973; Goldman, 1974, regarding frontal functions in monkeys). That is, the homologous areas on the right hemisphere may lag in development, or they may not be as fully differentiated with regard to this function as the left; in either case, these areas on the right side may be freer to assume the role necessary for recovery of language functions. This assumption is supported by Waber's (1976) finding that the development of spatial skills presumed to be mediated by the right hemisphere occurs late in relation to the development of verbal skills and appears to be associated with hormonal changes that occur at puberty.

Two predictions follow from this account. The first is that since the areas on the right had not been designated, at birth, to play the leading linguistic role, they are unlikely to perform linguistic functions as competently as those on the left. Second, since the structures on the right might ordinarily serve primarily nonlinguistic functions, the transfer of language dominance to the right will probably be at the expense of these nonlinguistic functions. There is evidence to support both predictions. A number of investigators (Dennis & Kohn, 1975; Dennis & Whitaker, Chapter 8, this volume; Lansdell, 1969; Milner, 1974; Teuber, 1974) have found that, on the average, patients whose language is mediated by the right hemisphere as a result of early left-sided damage, will show small, but noticeable, verbal deficits in adulthood. Moreover, their performance of nonverbal tasks that are typically mediated by the right hemisphere may even be inferior to their verbal performance relative to normal controls, despite the fact that they have a healthy right hemisphere (Lansdell, 1969; Teuber, 1974). Although this latter evidence supports the notion that transfer of language dominance to the right is at the expense of nonverbal functions, there is some question about the universality of this finding (Kohn & Dennis, 1974).

The present interpretation, therefore, emphasizes that it is right hemisphere plasticity, rather than hemispheric equipotentiality, that accounts for the right hemisphere's capacity to mediate language recovery following early left-hemisphere damage. This is not to imply that under normal conditions the right hemisphere fails to develop any linguistic skill. On the contrary, there is much evidence from studies of split-brain and hemispherectomized people to suggest that even when the left hemisphere develops normally, the right hemisphere attains some limited linguistic skills. The "plasticity" interpretation suggests further that the right hemisphere's linguistic capacities will remain relatively impoverished unless early damage to the left hemisphere enables the right to develop and extend its linguistic skills.

In earlier papers (Moscovitch, 1971, 1973, 1976), I suggested that the impoverishment of right-hemisphere language was occasioned by the left hemisphere actively suppressing the linguistic performance of the right via interhemispheric pathways. In early childhood, this interhemispheric process may lead not only to the suppression of linguistic development in the right hemisphere, but also to the differentiation of structures on the right from those that are potentially linguistic in function to those that are primarily nonlinguistic. Damage to the language areas of the left hemisphere may reduce their ability to control the right hemisphere thereby allowing the right hemisphere to develop into the linguistically dominant one (see Milner, 1974; Sperry, 1974, and Teuber, 1974, for similar suggestions).

It follows from this account that the congenital absence of the interhemispheric pathways by which the left hemisphere exerts its control over the right, or early damage to them, should have similar effects on right-hemisphere development as would early damage to the left hemisphere (Moscovitch, 1971, 1973, 1976; Selnes, 1974). Suggestive evidence for this view is available from studies of hemispheric specialization in people with agenesis of the corpus callosum. Although the presence of a variety of other disturbances makes it difficult to interpret the results of these studies, many of the individuals, especially those whose neurological deficits are minimal (Bryden & Zurif, 1970; Netley, Chapter 11, this volume; Saul & Sperry, 1968; Sperry, 1974), show small perceptual asymmetries or no asymmetries for verbal material, suggesting bilateral representation of language. By selectively anesthetizing one hemisphere at a time with sodium amytal, Saul and Gott (1973) confirmed that speech was bilaterally represented in the agenesis patient studied by Saul and Sperry. Another indication that speech was bilaterally represented in that patient was that her performance on nonlanguage tests was quite poor and inferior to her verbal skills, a pattern similar to that found in many people in whom early left-sided damage caused a reorganization of language on the right (Sperry, 1970, 1974). Further investigation of other relatively intact patients with agenesis of the corpus callosum would be necessary to establish that the depression of this nonverbal performance is a common phenomenon. In addition, if the evidence regarding the inherent, potential verbal superiority of the left hemisphere is upheld, then it should be possible to show that even people with callosal agenesis exhibit hemispheric asymmetries with regard to language. Although their right hemisphere is free to develop linguistically, it should still not attain the level of proficiency reached by the left hemisphere. To demonstrate this, however, it may be necessary to use perceptual asymmetry tasks requiring a level of skill that tests the limits of right-hemisphere performance.

THE NATURE OF RIGHT-HEMISPHERE LANGUAGE

Another question related to the development of language by the right hemisphere concerns the nature of language processes on the right. Are the processes underlying language on the right similar, but inferior, to those on the left, or is the difference between them more fundamental? It has been proposed by a number of investigators that the general cognitive mode in which the right hemisphere operates is different from that of the left. The right hemisphere has been characterized as a holistic, parallel, Gestalt processor, whereas the left is considered to operate in an analytic, linear, and sequential mode (Bogen, 1969; Cohen, 1973; Levy, 1974; Ornstein, 1972). Thus, it has been shown that each hemisphere is likely to process the same information according to its unique mode of operation (Bever & Chiarello, 1974; Levy, 1974). This suggests that as a consequence of their different modes of operation, each hemisphere will adopt different strategies in acquiring language and that the language so acquired will be represented differently in each hemisphere. There is already some indication from Zaidel's (1973) work with split-brain and hemispherectomized people that right-hemisphere language is qualitatively different from the left. He suggested that the right hemisphere processes language in global, holistic ways and relies much more heavily than the left on contextual and semantic cues. Thus, the right hemisphere has difficulty interpreting utterances or concepts that must be analysed into their constituent components if they are to be understood properly. However, Zaidel only tested people whose right hemisphere had developed under the influence of a dominant left hemisphere. It is, therefore, still not known whether right-hemisphere language would display similar characteristics if it developed from an early age in relative freedom from a competing, language dominant left hemisphere (see Chapter 8 for more information on this issue).

The only indication in the literature that right-hemisphere language would be qualitatively different from the left even under those circumstances comes from studying Genie, a girl who had been raised in almost total isolation from about 20 months until she was almost 14-years old. According to Fromkin, Krashen, Curtiss and Rigter (1974), Genie had not yet acquired language when she emerged from isolation. Her subsequent linguistic development was similar to that of a normal child in many respects, but very different in others. One of the more striking differences noted by Fromkin *et al.* was that after a few months of exposure to the real world, her general cognitive skills far exceeded her verbal skills and, within the domain of verbal skills, her vocabulary was much larger than that of children whose syntactic development was comparable to hers. This pattern of development is reminiscent of observations of the split-brain right hemisphere and of Dennis and Whitaker's observation that a lag in syntactic development, but not single word utterances, is characteristic of children whose language functions have been transferred to the right. Consistent with the speculation of a right-hemisphere pattern of language acquisition, is Genie's performance on dichotic listening tasks. Despite being right-handed, Genie showed a strong LEA, suggesting right-hemisphere dominance for speech. In fact, she did not report any items from the right ear, a pattern typical of hemispherectomized or split-brain patients who extinguish on items ipsilateral to the reporting hemisphere and one that also suggests a left hemisphere whose language skills are severely impaired.

Although a single case, particularly one as extraordinary as Genie, cannot serve as the basis for generalizing about the course of development of right-hemisphere language, it does offer an example of the possibility of tracing the linguistic development of children with early left or right-sided damage from the time the damage occurred. Will the pattern of linguistic development differ in the two groups? What kind of differences, other than a lag in development, might one look for? It is difficult to predict the differences that might emerge. However, a research strategy that might be successful in attacking this problem is one that is currently being used by many psychologists to study early language development in normal children (see the relevant papers in Moore, 1973; Lenneberg & Lenneberg, 1975). An example of this kind of theoretical and empirical approach is found in the work of Katherine Nelson (1973, 1975). By collecting the earliest utterances of children and the context in which the utterances appeared, as well as by giving a series of cognitive tasks that revealed the nature of the child's semantic concepts, Nelson found that normal children could be differentiated on the basis of the strategies they adopted in acquiring language.[1] Although a detailed presentation of her findings is not possible, I have referred to her work merely to call attention to the kind of theoretical and empirical analysis that is capable of revealing differences between children with left- and right-sided damage in cognitive development and language acquisition strategies. Ultimately, such research may help to give us a better notion about the nature of linguistic and cognitive representation in the two hemispheres.

SOME SPECULATION ON THE CAUSES OF DYSPHASIA FOLLOWING EARLY RIGHT-SIDED DAMAGE

Why is dysphasia more common if damage to the right hemisphere occurs in childhood than if it occurs in adulthood? Prior to the age of 5, the incidence of right-hemisphere dysphasia is about 10% to 35%, whereas in adulthood it is less than 1%. The traditional answer to this question has been that at an early age both hemispheres contribute to linguistic performance, though probably not to an equal extent since even in childhood the incidence of dysphasia is higher following left-sided, than right-sided, lesions. Moreover, it has also typically been assumed that the right hemisphere's contribution to linguistic performance is similar, but perhaps inferior, to that of the left—that is, it mediates the phonetic, syntactic, and semantic processes necessary for the production and comprehension of speech. Although there is no evidence to refute this notion, there is also, to my knowledge, no strong evidence to support it. Consequently, I wish to offer two alternatives against which the traditional ideas may be tested.

---

[1] Briefly stated, Nelson found that children could be classified into one of two types, referential or expressive, depending on the nature of their early linguistic utterances and on the cognitive strategics they presumably adopted in learning to speak. The referential group learned principally nouns at the beginning and progressed clearly in stages from one-word to multiword utterances. On the other hand, the expressive group acquired other word classes more frequently (verbs, adjectives, function words, and expressive phrases), used a large number of phrases and sentences early in language acquisition, and did not seem to progress systematically from one- to two- to three-word utterances. This reference to Nelson's work is not meant to imply that categories such as those found by Nelson will distinguish children with damage to the left hemisphere from those with damage to the right, although such an outcome is possible.

The first alternative is that the data concerning the incidence of dysphasia following early right-sided damage may reveal as much about the general vulnerability of the maturing nervous system as about early involvement of the right hemisphere in language acquisition. The general trauma caused by right-sided damage may, in some circumstances, disturb some processes in the still fragile and developing left hemisphere, thus disrupting the linguistic skills that are still very rudimentary. Once these skills have been mastered, right-sided damage has little effect. Thus, according to this view, dysphasia does not result directly from damage to the right hemisphere, but indirectly through trauma to the left. If this is true, it follows that the converse should hold, that is, early left-sided damage, in addition to causing dysphasia, should also lead, in about 30% of the cases, to a loss of skills mediated by the right hemisphere. At present this prediction is difficult, if not impossible, to test. Loss of language, even in a 2-year-old, is an event that is so striking that it will rarely escape the parents' notice. However, it is not at all clear how anyone would determine which right-hemisphere functions are lost at that age since, to my knowledge, it is not known which functions, if any, are mediated primarily by the right-hemisphere in a 2-year-old. At present, our knowledge of right-hemisphere functions in very young children is very limited and in much the same state as was our knowledge of these functions in adults 25 years ago. As a starting point for deriving much-needed information about right-hemisphere function in children, one might test those with early left- or right-sided damage, shortly after the time of this damage, on a variety of spatial and visual tasks. Those tasks that would be affected primarily by right-sided damage could then serve as a reliable behavioral index of right-hemisphere function (see Milner, 1974, for a similar suggestion).

The second alternative is to view the occasional dysphasia that results from early right-hemisphere damage as arising from the disruption of general cognitive structures or schemes on the right, rather than being caused by the impairment of structures that are specifically linguistic. This view, although highly speculative, is consistent with current research on language development in normal children, which suggests that the child's first utterances derive from and reflect the cognitive structures—the system of concepts, relations, and operations—that he had acquired during the sensorimotor stages of development (Bloom, 1970; Bowerman, 1973; Brown, 1973; McNamara, 1972; Nelson, 1974; Piaget, 1952; Schlesinger, 1971; Sinclair, 1971; Slobin, 1973; see also relevant chapters in Moore, 1973; Lenneberg and Lenneberg, 1975). Being sensorimotor in nature, it is reasonable to assume that at least some of these structures may be represented bilaterally or in the right hemisphere, while others may be represented in the left, depending on the compatibility of the structures with the mode of operation of the hemispheres. In the early stages of language acquisition, the child's language, the organization of the sensorimotor conceptual system from which it stems, and the relation between them, seem labile and fragile as is indicated by the instability of the concepts expressed in language. The very lability of the organization of the conceptual system suggests that it is likely to be especially vulnerable to disruption, which, if it occurs, might lead to the loss or extreme modification of a variety of concepts and relations without which language cannot exist. Thus, even damage to the right hemisphere, whose contributions to language functions may be minimal later in development, may have sufficiently disruptive effects on the organization of the child's developing conceptual system to lead to dysphasia or even mutism. This explanation for the dysphasia that occasionally accompanies early right-hemisphere damage, like the alternative offered earlier, is difficult to test in the absence of adequate information about early right-hemisphere functions. Nonetheless, I have proposed this explanation in order to call attention to the possibility that the contribution of the right hemisphere in language development may be in a domain that is not, strictly speaking, linguistic, but is rather more broadly cognitive and conceptual. If this view has merit, it suggests that research on the development of lateralization of language must take account of the role played by nonlinguistic cognitive functions, as well as linguistic ones. This issue is dealt with more fully in the next section.

THE PROCESS OF LATERALIZATION OF LANGUAGE TO THE LEFT HEMISPHERE AND ITS RELATION TO NORMAL COGNITIVE DEVELOPMENT

The Phonetic–Phonological System

Until very recently, many people investigating the development of cerebral dominance in normal people focused on very simple linguistic tasks—such as the detection of stop consonants, or numbers, or single words—since it was only these tasks that were amenable to testing in a dichotic situation. Not surprisingly, so long as memory factors were kept to a minimum (see Porter & Berlin, 1975; Hiscock & Kinsbourne, 1976), performance on these tasks revealed a REA even at 2 months of age (see Chapter 6), suggesting early left-hemisphere specialization for language. The reason it is not surprising to obtain evidence of early left-hemisphere specialization is that these tests usually tap the very lowest level of processing that could still be called "linguistic," namely, the phonetic level. The experiments of Eimas and his colleagues (Eimas, Siqueland, Jusczyk, & Vigorito, 1971; Eimas, 1974) suggest that even infants are sensitive to phonetic distinctions in speech stimuli, in much the same way that adults are. It is likely, therefore, that they would also have the specialized analyzers or mechanisms necessary for speech perception and that these mechanisms would reside primarily in the left hemisphere. One can take this point further. If the environmental conditions are such that the development of the phonetic system can be sustained, then lateralization of at least that system will be present early in most individuals, regardless of whatever other language deficits they may have, so long as there is no evidence of focal cortical damage or collosal agenesis. Thus, it has been shown that lateralization of language, as measured by dichotic listening tests that primarily tap phonetic functions, is present in dyslexics (Witelson, 1975; McKeever & Van Deventer, 1975), in stutterers (Dorman & Porter, 1975), in children from underprivileged backgrounds (Geffner & Dorman, 1976), and even in mongoloids (Reinhart, 1976).[2] However, if the phonetic system does not develop normally, as is the case for the congenitally deaf, lateralization of function must presumably await the development of another symbol system that can sustain language. Partial support for this view comes from Neville's finding (Chapter 10) that only those deaf children who have acquired a sign-language system show marginal hemispheric asymmetries as measured by electroencephelography, whereas even such marginal differences are absent in deaf children who are not "signers." This evidence is consistent with the observation that sign-language "dysphasia" in deaf people, though seemingly not as severe as comparable dysphasias in speaking people, have always resulted from a left-sided lesion in the handful of cases reported in the literature (Critchley, 1938; Douglas & Richardson, 1959; Sarno, Swisher, & Sarno, 1969, and references therein; Tureen, Smolik, & Tritt, 1951).

Contrary to this evidence, McKeever, Hoemann, Florian, and Van Deventer (1976) have found that college-educated, congenitally deaf adults show minimal

[2] Whether other language functions are similarly lateralized in these individuals is a matter of controversy. There are indications that when tests of perceptual asymmetry include a mnemonic, syntactic, or graphemic component, then "normal" children show greater left-hemisphere lateralization than do poor readers or children from a low socioeconomic background (Bryden, 1970; Kimura, 1967; Marcel & Rajan, 1975; Satz, Rurdin, & Ross, 1971). Using these higher-level tests, some investigators find an increase in laterality with age in normal individuals (Bever, 1971; Bryden, 1970; Satz et al., 1975). Even in this regard, the evidence is not conclusive, since other investigators, using similar tasks, failed to replicate their results whether with normal children (Kimura, 1963), children from low socioeconomic backgrounds (Geffner & Hochberg, 1971), or poor readers (McKeever & Van Deventer, 1975; Witelson, 1975; Yeni-Komshian, Isenberg, & Goldberg, 1975).

Witelson (1975) has suggested that at least with regard to dyslexia it may be that right, and not left, hemisphere functions are poorly lateralized. Intriguing as her idea might be, it is not universally supported. The only other published study that bears directly on this point has shown that poor readers display a normal right-hemisphere dominance for face recognition (Marcel & Rajan, 1975). Moreover, by Witelson's own account, normal females without reading disorders are as poorly lateralized in this regard as dyslexic boys.

The premise underlying many studies on lateralization in people with some kinds of developmental language disorders seems to be that the normal pattern of hemispheric dominance is the ideal condition for good linguistic performance. Any deviation from the ideal, therefore, is likely to lead to language problems or, conversely, deficits in language are likely to be indicative of poor lateralization. To my knowledge, there is no solid evidence that lateralization of function is predictive of superior or normal performance with regard to the function that is lateralized. Indeed, there is some evidence that individuals with bilateral representation of language, such as left-handers (Levy, 1974) or females (McGlone & Davidson, 1973) may have better than average verbal abilities.

Rather than take the view that developmental language disorders are associated with poorly lateralized functions, an alternative hypothesis should be considered, namely, that children with poor performance on some language tasks show normal lateralization of function but that those lateralized functions are impaired. Thus, developmental dyslexics often show a normal pattern of left-hemisphere lateralization for language as determined by tests of perceptual asymmetry, but a worse than average overall performance on those tests (McKeever & Van Deventer, 1975; Witelson, 1975; Yeni-Komshian et al., 1975; Zurif & Carson, 1970). The same case could, of course, be made for mongoloids and children from impoverished linguistic backgrounds. Whether this pattern holds for children with other linguistic or nonlinguistic disorders remains to be seen.

perceptual asymmetries on a variety of tachistoscopic tasks, suggesting that the absence of a normally developed phonetic system may permanently affect the process of lateralization for other functions as well. The hypothesis that lateralization of phonetic processes is a prerequisite for normal lateralization of other functions seems to receive little support from the lesion literature or from Neville's work. As McKeever *et al.* note, however, the dearth of reports of deaf people with dysphasia due to brain damage (and, one might add, the marginal asymmetries reported by Neville) suggest that if language is lateralized to the left in deaf people, the extent of lateralization is much weaker than in hearing people. Further research will hopefully clarify the issues regarding the role of hearing on the development of lateralization of function.

Although the experiments cited in this section are valuable in that they tell us that some language functions—namely, those related to phonetic perception—are functionally lateralized at an early age, their focus is too narrow in that they tell us very little about the lateralization of such higher-level linguistic processes as syntax and semantics. A similar argument may be made against studies on early brain damage. If damage to the left hemisphere impairs the phonetic and phonological processing mechanisms on that side, then speech will not be sustained, regardless of whatever other processes relevant to language might reside on the right. As Porter and Berlin (1975) rightly observe, different linguistic processes may become lateralized at different ages. But so long as the majority of current tests tap only the lowest level of linguistic processing, we are not likely to observe these changes. Whether higher order linguistic processes do indeed become progressively more lateralized with age is open to debate. The remainder of the chapter addresses this issue.

The Syntactic and Semantic Systems

Before the child emits his first meaningful linguistic utterances, both his phonological and cognitive capacities must have developed sufficiently to sustain speech and language. By virtue of its association with the speech—perception system, the phonological system is assumed to be lateralized in the left hemisphere (see Studdert-Kennedy, 1975, for an interesting discussion on this point). It is not known, however, which hemisphere embodies the sensorimotor cognitive structures that are believed to mediate the syntactic and semantic content of the child's first utterances. Nor, to my knowledge, is it known whether a child who is acquiring language possesses syntactic and semantic systems that are separate from, but dependent on, these general cognitive structures. Given this state of ignorance, any thoughts about the developing lateralization of these higher-order linguistic systems or structures must necessarily be highly speculative. Nonetheless, I will outline two views of the process of lateralization.

In an earlier section I suggested that at least some of the cognitive structures which are presumed to underlie the child's first utterances are represented in the right hemisphere. The majority of such structures, however, will be assumed to reside in the left hemisphere. In some instances, the participation of these right-hemisphere structures in the child's early linguistic output is quite critical, since their loss following right hemisphere damage might occasionally lead to dysphasia or mutism. Later in development, right-hemisphere cognitive representations seem either to play only a peripheral role in maintaining language or, they may have migrated to the left; that is, some of the originally right-hemisphere cognitive representations may have been transformed and integrated into the representational system of the left hemisphere. The result, in either case, is that the incidence of dysphasia is very low following right-hemisphere damage in adulthood. According to this view, there is a gradual process of lateralization in which the cognitive system underlying language gradually becomes lateralized to the left.

The other possibility is that all language functions, once they develop sufficiently to be observed, are lateralized to the left. That is, not only the phonetic and phonological systems but also the sensorimotor representations on which the syntactic and semantic systems depend are already lateralized to the left hemisphere before language is observed. This may occur because the left hemisphere mediates those aspects of sensorimotor development that serve as the immediate precursors of language; or it may occur as a result of a process by which the left hemisphere transforms sensorimotor representations into a cognitive mode that is compatible with speech (Levy, 1974). In either event, according to this second view, syntactic and semantic processes in language would be mediated by the left hemisphere from the very beginning.

There is very little evidence to help in deciding between the two alternatives. Bever (1971), on the basis of rather weak evidence, cautiously suggests that the lateralization of perceptual strategies in sentence comprehension, which involves syntactic and semantic processes, develops with age in response to external experience. Thus, according to Bever, the left hemisphere will become the locus of these strategies earlier in middle-class children than in children raised in a more impoverished linguistic environment. A study reported by Bishop (1967), however, indicates that the lateralization of semantic and syntactic systems is already apparent, if not complete, between the second and third years. Bishop studied language acquisition in infantile hemiplegics with left- or right-hemisphere damage and found that that those with left-hemisphere damage were delayed in acquiring word combinations but not single words. This finding suggests that the cognitive or semantic systems mediating single-word utterances may be bilaterally represented, but that these systems are already lateralized to the left once two-word utterances are acquired.

Clearly, more information is needed to decide which of the two alterantives, if either, provides even a reasonable account of the lateralization of higher order language functions. One possible approach that might yield more information is .c study the development of language and cognition in children with early left- or right-hemisphere damage with the method currently being used so successfully by developmental psycholinguists (see p. 200). Another approach might be to try to determine whether there are developmental changes in hemispheric asymmetries of different components of the evoked potential to meaningful language stimuli

(Chapters 2 and 10) and whether these changes correspond to comparable changes in psychological processes. Thus, it would be necessary to know with which psychological processes the components of the evoked potential are correlated before one can make meaningful psychological sense of the results. A third might look for perceptual asymmetries in tasks in which the response is contingent on a syntactic or semantic decision.

The suggestions for future research as well as the two views of the process of lateralization of languages that I have proposed are not meant to be comprehensive. A number of important issues have not been considered in either: the development and lateralization of structures mediating short-term verbal memory that are critical for supporting normal linguistic performance (Milner, 1974; Tallal, 1975; Warrington & Shallice, 1969; Zaidel, 1973), sex differences in lateralization of function (Lake & Bryden, 1976; McGlone & Davidson, 1973; Witelson, 1976); and the influence of the developing left hemisphere on right-hemisphere language functions (Moscovitch, 1973, 1976). Nonetheless, I have offered these sketchy and speculative views to try to shift the focus of inquiry on language lateralization away from an overly strong and long concern with the phonetic and the phonological system and toward a consideration of cognitive, syntactic, and semantic systems. In both alternatives that I have outlined, the phonological system is assumed to be lateralized very early in normal people, certainly before speech begins; the only question that remains is whether other functions critical to language develop initially on the left or whether they are first bilaterally represented. Even if it should turn out that the phonological system takes longer to lateralize than I have assumed, it would still be useful to gain information about the lateralization of other linguistic processes.

SUMMARY

The question "Does lateralization of language develop?" is too broad for a simple answer. In this chapter I have tried to call attention to the fact that the development of lateralization of language is a process that involves a variety of functions each of which may develop at different rates and may become lateralized in different ways and at different times (see also Lenneberg, 1967; Lenneberg & Lenneberg, 1975; Milner, 1974). Thus, although the evidence presented in this chapter favors the notion that hemispheric differences in structure and function are apparent very early in development, it does not follow that the process of lateralization is complete at this early stage. I have argued that lateralization of certain low-level linguistic functions, such as phonetic and phonological ones, is probably complete by the first year of life so long as the structures mediating those functions receive sufficient stimulation from the environment. Because the majority of studies on the development of laterality have used tests that are directed primarily at the phonetic and phonological level, one can only guess about the process of lateralization for other linguistic functions, such as those related to syntax, semantics, and verbal memory. I have suggested that the sensorimotor cognitive structures that presumably underlie the child's early use of syntax and semantics are represented in both hemispheres and, consequently, at this early stage, his meaningful linguistic utterances will be mediated by both hemispheres, although perhaps not to the same degree. This may account for the occasional dysphasias following early right-hemisphere damage. As his linguistic and cognitive skills develop, language becomes more strongly lateralized to the left hemisphere. The alternative to this view of a process of gradual lateralization is that syntactic and semantic functions, or their sensorimotor precursors, are already completely lateralized by the time the child utters his first words. According to the second alternative, experience and maturation affect only the development of language in the left hemisphere, but not the process of lateralization. Hopefully, a broader view of language and lateralization will lead to the development of new techniques and research strategies that will allow us to decide which of these two alternatives—or some other one not yet proposed—provides the best account of the process of lateralization.

ACKNOWLEDGMENTS

I wish to thank Sandra Trehub and Jill Moscovitch for their incisive comments on earlier versions of this chapter. Some valuable conversations with Walter Hindemith helped me greatly in organizing my views on the problems discussed in this chapter.

REFERENCES

Annett, M. (1973) Laterality of childhood hemiplegia and the growth of speech and intelligence. *Cortex, 9,* 4–33.

Basser, L.S. (1962) Hemiplegia of early onset and the faculty of speech with special reference to the effects of hemispherectomy. *Brain, 85,* 427–460.

Bever, T.G. (1971) The nature of cerebral dominance in speech behaviour of the child and adult. In R. Huxley & E. Ingram (Eds.), *Language acquisition: Models and methods.* New York: Academic.

Bever, T.G., & Chiarello, R. (1974) Cerebral dominance in musicians and nonmusicians. *Science, 185,* 537–539.

Bloom, L.M. (1970 *Language development: Form and function in emerging grammars.* Cambridge, Massachusetts: M.I.T. Press.

Bogen, J.E. (1969) The other side of the brain I: Dysgraphia and dyscopia following cerebral commissurotomy. *Bulletin of the Los Angeles Neurological Societies, 34,* 73–105.

Bowerman, M. (1973) Structural relationships in children's utterances: Syntactic or semantic? In T.E. Moore (Ed.), *Cognitive development and the acquisition of language.* New York: Academic.

Brown, R.W. (1973) *A first language: The early stages.* Cambridge, Massachusetts: Harvard Univ. Press.

Bryden, M.P. (1970) Laterality effects in dichotic listening: Relations with handedness and reading ability in children. *Neuropsychologia, 8,* 443–450.

Bryden, M.P., & Allard, F. (1975) Dichotic listening and the development of linguistic processes. In M. Kinsbourne (Ed.), *Hemispheric asymmetries of function.* New York: Cambridge Univ. Press.

Bryden, M.P., & Zurif, E.B. (1970) Dichotic listening performance in a case of agenesis of the corpus callosum. *Neuropsychologia, 8,* 371–377.

Cohen, G. (1973) Hemispheric differences in serial versus parallel processing. *Journal of Experimental Psychology, 97,* 349–356.

Critchley, M. (1938) Aphasia in a partial deaf-mute. *Brain, 61,* 163–169.

Dennis, M., & Kohn, B. (1975) Comprehension of syntax in infantile hemiplegics after cerebral hemidecortication: Left hemisphere superiority. *Brain and Language, 2,* 475–486.

Dorman, M.F., & Porter, R.J. (1975) Hemispheric lateralization for speech perception in stutterers. *Cortex, 11,* 181–185.

Douglass, E., & Richardson, J.C. (1959) Aphasia in a congenital deaf-mute. *Brain, 82,* 68–80.

Eimas, P.D. (1974) Auditory and linguistic processing of cues for place of articulation by infants. *Perception and psychophysics, 16,* 513–521.

Eimas, P.D., Siqueland, E.R., Jusczyk, P., & Vigorito, J. (1971) Speech perception in infants. *Science, 171,* 303–306.

Eisenson, J. (1962) Language and intellectual modifications associated with right cerebral damage. *Language and speech, 5,* 49–53.

Fromkin, V.A., Krashen, S., Curtiss, D.R., & Rigter, M. (1974) The development of language in Genie: A case of language acquisition beyond the critical period. *Brain and Language, 1,* 81–108.

Gazzaniga, M.S. (1970) *The bisected brain.* New York: Appleton.

Geffner, D.S., & Dorman, M.F. (1976) Hemispheric specialization for speech perception in four-year-old children from low and middle socio-economic classes. *Cortex, 12,* 71–73.

Geffner, D.S., & Hochberg, I. (1971) Ear laterality performance of children from low and middle socio-economic levels on a verbal dichotic listening task. *Cortex, 7,* 193–203.

Geschwind, N. and Levitsky, W. (1968) Human brain; left-right asymmetries in temporal speech region. *Science, 161,* 186–187.

Goldman, P. (1974) An alternative to developmental plasticity: Heterology of CNS structures in infants and adults. In D.G. Stein, J.J. Rosen, & N. Butters (Eds.), *Plasticity and recovery of function in the central nervous system.* New York: Academic.

Goodglass, H., & Quadfasel, F. (1954) Language laterality in left-handed aphasics. *Brain, 77,* 521–48.

Hebb, D.O. (1942) The effects of early and late brain injury upon test scores and the nature of normal adult intelligence. *Proceedings of the American Philosophical Society, 85,* 275–292.

Hécaen, H. (1976) Acquired aphasia in children and the ontogenesis of hemispheric functional specialization. *Brain and Language, 3,* 114–134.

Hiscock, M., & Kinsbourne, M. (1976) Perceptual and motor measures of cerebral lateralization in children. Paper presented at the Canadian Psychological Association. Toronto.

Ingram, D. (1975a) Motor asymmetries in young children. *Neuropsychologia, 13,* 95–102.

Ingram, D. (1975b) Cerebral speech lateralization in young children. *Neuropsychologia, 13,* 103–106.

Kimura, D. (1963) Speech lateralization in young children as determined by an auditory test. *Journal of Comparative and Physiological Psychology, 56,* 899–902.

Kimura, D. (1967) Functional asymmetry of the brain in dichotic listening. *Cortex, 3,* 163–178.

Kimura, D. (1973) Manual activity during speaking–I. Right-handers. *Neuropsychologia, 11,* 45–50.

Kinsbourne, M., & McMurray, J. (1975) The effect of cerebral dominance on time sharing between speaking and tapping by preschool children. *Child Development, 46,* 240–242.

Kohn, B., & Dennis, M. (1974) Selective impairments of visuo-spatial abilities in infantile hemiplegics after right hemidecortication. *Neuropsychologia, 12,* 505–512.

Krashen, S. (1973) Lateralization, language learning, and the critical period: Some new evidence. *Language Learning, 23,* 63–74.

Lake, D.H., & Bryden, M.P. (1976) Handedness and sex differences in hemispheric asymmetry. *Brain and Language, 3,* 266–282.

Lansdell, H. (1969) Verbal and nonverbal factors in right-hemisphere speech: relations to early neurological history. *Journal of Comparative and Physiological Psychology, 69,* 734–738.

Lenneberg, E.H. (1967) *Biological foundations of language.* New York: Wiley.

Lenneberg, E.H., & Lenneberg, E. (Eds.) (1975) *Foundations of language development.* New York: Academic.

Levy, J. (1974) Psychobiological implications of bilateral asymmetry. In S.J. Dimond & G. Beaumont (Eds.), *Hemisphere function in the human brain.* London: Elek Scientific Books.

Luria, A.R. (1970) *Traumatic aphasia.* The Hague: Mouton.

Marcel, T., & Rajan, P. (1975) Lateral specialization for recognition of words and faces in good and poor readers. *Neuropsychologia, 13,* 489–497.

McGlone, J., & Davidson, W. (1973) The relation between cerebral speech laterality and spatial ability with special reference to sex and hand preference. *Neuropsychologia, 11,* 105–113.

McKeever, W.F., Hoemann, H.W., Florian, V., & Van Deventer, A.D. (1976) Evidence of minimal cerebral asymmetries for the processing of English words and American sign language in the congenitally deaf. *Neuropsychologia, 14,* 413–424.

McKeever, W.F., & Van Deventer, A.D. (1975) Dyslexic adolescents: Evidence of impaired visual and auditory language processing associated with normal lateralization and visual responsivity. *Cortex, 11,* 361–378.

McNamara, J. (1972) Cognitive basis of language learning in infants. *Psychological Review, 79,* 1–13.

Milner, B. (1974) Hemispheric specialization: Scope and limits. In F.O. Schmitt & F.G. Worden (Eds.), *The neurosciences: Third study program.* Cambridge, Massachusetts: M.I.T. Press.

Molfese, D., Freeman, R.B. Jr., & Palermo, D.S. (1975) The ontogeny of brain lateralization for speech and nonspeech stimuli. *Brain and Language, 3,* 356–368.

Moore, T.E. (Ed.) (1973) *Cognitive development and the acquisition of language.* New York: Academic.

Moscovitch, M. (1972) Reaction-time studies assessing the verbal behaviour of the minor hemisphere in normal right-handed, adult humans *or* What does someone in his right mind know? Unpublished doctoral dissertation, Univ. of Pennsylvania.

Moscovitch, M. (1973) Language and the cerebral hemispheres: Reaction-time studies and their implications for models of cerebral dominance. In P. Pliner, T. Alloway, & L. Krames (Eds.), *Communication and affect: Language and thought.* New York: Academic. Pp. 89–126.

Moscovitch, M. (1976) On the representation of language in the right hemisphere of right-handed people. *Brain and Language, 3,* 47–71.

Nagafuchi, M. (1970) Development of dichotic and monaural hearing abilities in young children. *Acta Oto-Laryngology, 69,* 409–414.

Nelson, K. (1973) Structure and strategy in learning to talk. *Monograph of the Society for Research in Child Development, 38,* (1–2, Serial No. 149).

Nelson, K. (1974) Concept, word, and sentence: Interrelations in acquisition and development. *Psychological Review, 81,* 267–285.

Nelson, K. (1975) The nominal shift in semantic-syntactic development. *Cognitive Psychology, 7,* 461–479.

Ornstein, R.E. (1972) *The psychology of consciousness.* San Francisco: Freeman.

Piaget, J. (1952) *The origins of intelligence in children.* New York: International Universities Press.

Porter, R.J., & Berlin, C.I. (1975) On interpreting developmental changes in the dichotic right-ear advantage. *Brain and Language, 2,* 186–200.

Reinhart, C. (1976) The cerebral laterlization of speech processes in Down's Syndrome and normal individuals. Paper presented at the Canadian Psychological Association Meeting, Toronto, June.

Sarno, J.E., Swisher, L.P., & Sarno, M.T. (1969) Aphasia in a congenitally deaf man. *Cortex, 5,* 398–414.

Satz, P., Bakker, D.J., Teunissen, J., Goebel, R., & van der Vlugt, H. (1975) Developmental parameters of ear asymmetry: A multivariate approach. *Brain and Language, 2,* 171–185.

Satz, P., Rurdin, D., & Ross, J. (1971) An evaluation of a theory of specific developmental dyslexia. *Child Development, 42,* 2009–2021.

Saul, R.E., & Gott, P.S. (1973) Compensatory mechanisms in agenesis of the corpus callosum. *Neurology, 23* (4), Abstract 13T 68.

Saul, R., & Sperry, R.W. (1968) Absence of commissurotomy symptoms with agenesis of the corpus callosum. *Neurology, 18,* 307.

Schlesinger, I.M. (1971) Production of utterances and language acquisition. In D.I. Slobin (Ed.), *The ontogenesis of grammar.* New York: Academic.

Selnes, O.A. (1974) The corpus callosum: Some anatomical and functional considerations with special reference to language. *Brain and Language, 1,* 111–139.

Sinclair, H. (1971) Sensorimotor action patterns as a condition for the acquisition of syntax. In R. Huxley & E. Ingram (Eds.), *Language acquisition: Models and methods.* New York: Academic.

Slobin, D.I. (1966) Comments on "developmental psycholinguistics". In F. Smith & G.A. Miller (Eds.), *The genesis of language.* Cambridge, Massachusetts: M.I.T. Press.

Slobin, D.I. (1973) Cognitive prerequisites for the development of grammar. In C.A. Ferguson & D.I. Slobin (Eds.), *Studies in child language development.* New York: Holt.

Slorach, N., & Noehr, B. (1973) Dichotic listening in stuttering and dyslalic children. *Cortex, 9,* 295–300.

Sperry, R.W. (1970) Cerebral dominance in perception. In F.A. Young & D.B. Lindsley (Eds.), *Early experience in visual information processing in perceptual and reading disorders.* Washington, D.C.: National Academy of Sciences.

Sperry, R.W. (1974) Lateral specialization in the surgically separated hemispheres. In F.O. Schmitt & F.G. Worden (Eds.), *The neurosciences: Third study program.* Cambridge, Massachusetts: M.I.T. Press.

Studdert-Kennedy, M. (1975) The nature and function of phonetic categories. In R.M. Shiffrin, N.J. Castellan, H. Lindan, D. Pisoni, and F. Restle (Eds.) *Cognitive Theory,* Vol. 1, Potomac, Md.: Erlbaum Assoc.

Tallal, P. (1975) Perceptual and linguistic factors in the language impairment of developmental dysphasics: An experimental investigation with the Token Test. *Cortex, 11,* 196–205.

Teszner, D., Tzavaras, A., Grunere, J., and Hécaen, H. (1972) L'asymetrie droite-gauche due planum temporale. Apropos de l'etude anatomique de 100 cerveaux *Revue neurologique, 126,* 444–449.

Teuber, H-L. (1974) Why two brains? In F.O. Schmitt & F.G. Worden (Eds.), *The neurosciences: third study program.* Cambridge, Massachusetts: M.I.T. Press.

Tureen, L.L., Smolik, E.A., & Tritt, J.H. (1951) Aphasia in a deaf-mute. *Neurology, 1,* 237–249.

Vygotsky, L.S. (1962) *Thought and language.* Cambridge, Massachusetts: M.I.T. Press.

Wada, J., Clark, R., & Hamm, A. 1975. Cerebral hemispheric asymmetry in humans. *Archives of Neurology, 32,* 239–246.

Warrington, E.K., & Shallice, T. (1969) The selective impairment of auditory verbal short-term memory. *Brain, 92,* 885–96.

Weisenberg, T., & McBride, K.E. (1935) *Aphasia: A clinical and psychological study.* New York: Commonwealth Fund.

Witelson, S.F. (1975) Abnormal right hemisphere specialization in developmental dyslexia.

Paper presented at N.A.T.D. Conference on The Neuropsychology of Learning Disorders, Korsor, Denmark.

Witelson, S.F., & Pallie, W. (1973) Left hemisphere specialization for language in the newborn: Neuroanatomical evidence of asymmetry. *Brain, 96,* 641–646.

Yeni-Komshian, G.G., Isenberg, D., & Goldberg, H. (1975) Cerebral dominance and reading disability: Left visual field deficit in poor readers. *Neuropsychologia, 13,* 83–94.

Zaidel, E. (1973) Linguistic competence and related functions in the right cerebral hemisphere of man following commissurotomy and hemispherectomy. Unpublished doctoral dissertation, California Institute of Technology, Pasadena, California.

Zangwill, O.L. (1960) *Cerebral dominance and its relations to psychological function.* Edinburgh: Oliver and Boyd.

Zurif, E.B. & Carson, G. (1970) Dyslexia in relation to cerebral dominance and temporal analysis. *Neuropsychologia, 8,* 351–361.

Waber, D.P. (1976) Sex differences in cognition: A function of maturation rate? *Science, 192,* 572–574.

16

Early Hemisphere Specialization and Interhemisphere Plasticity: An Empirical and Theoretical Review

SANDRA F. WITELSON

OUTLINE OF CHAPTER

The possible existence of hemisphere specialization during childhood and the phenomena of early hemisphere equipotentiality and interhemisphere transfer of speech and language functions are issues that have received long-standing consideration in terms of their implications both for theories of brain—behavior relationships during development and for clinical issues. There have been numerous comprehensive summaries of data and theoretical statements concerning hemisphere specialization in adults (e.g., Dimond & Beaumont, 1974; Kinsbourne & W. Smith, 1974; Mountcastle, 1962; M. White, 1969). To summarize briefly the situation in adults, each hemisphere appears dominant or specialized for specific cognitive functions. The distinctiveness of the hemispheres lies not so much in what functions each hemisphere mediates, that is, what stimuli or tasks each processes, as in how the information is processed, that is, what cognitive mode each hemisphere uses. For most individuals, the left hemisphere may be described as processing in a sequential, analytic, linguistic mode, and the right in a parallel, holistic, spatial, nonlinguistic mode.

Whether the dichotomy between the hemispheres is complete or whether each hemisphere is able to process information to some degree in the alternate mode is still to be determined. Although traditionally cerebral dominance has been considered an all-or-nothing phenomenon, the alternative that each hemisphere has a mechanism for each cognitive mode, although to markedly different degrees, would appear to be of adaptive value since the two hemispheres must communicate with each other and some common "language" or processing mode would be useful. Accordingly, any particular behavioral or cognitive function may be mediated predominantly by one hemisphere but possibly also minimally by the other. It also appears that some cognitive tasks may be processed, at least to some extent, in different modes and in this respect may also be mediated by either hemisphere, masking the manifestation of hemisphere specialization to some degree.

There are fewer summaries and theoretical reports concerning hemisphere specialization during development. The earliest reviews are based on reports of language deficits in brain-damaged children (e.g., Basser, 1962; Freud, 1968; McFie, 1961a; Zangwill, 1964; and more recently, Hécaen, 1976) and, in general, conclude that there is bilateral representation of language in the early years of life. The first comprehensive theoretical statement is probably that of Lenneberg (1967), who theorized that during the first two years of life there is bilateral representation of language, that left-hemisphere specialization for language develops during childhood, and that it is not complete until puberty, at which time plasticity is lost and primary language learning is no longer possible. There have been a few more recent reviews, but these generally have restricted themselves to more specific topics. Krashen (1972, 1975) suggested that development of left-hemisphere specialization is complete by about 5 years of age, which he suggests is the end of the critical period for first language acquisition and related cognitive development and of hemisphere equipotentiality for speech and language functions. Several other reports have reviewed the evidence for left-hemisphere specialization in early childhood based on the performance of normal children on verbal dichotic stimulation tests and have argued either for an increase in left-hemisphere specialization with age (Bryden & Allard, 1976b; Satz, Bakker, Teunissen, Goebel, & Van der Vlugt, 1975) or for no change in degree of specialization in at least some linguistic functions (Porter & C. Berlin, 1975). Kinsbourne (1975) has hypothesized that left-hemisphere specialization exists at birth and does not undergo any subsequent change. It is interesting to note that although the existence of hemisphere specialization in children is still being investigated, Orton hypothesized, as early as 1928, that the neural substrate of various developmental language disorders may be an absence of aspects of cerebral dominance, the implicit assumption being that lateralization of function is present in normal children.

A more general review of hemisphere specialization in childhood and related issues seems warranted, particularly at this time. Within the last few years, several new strategies and procedures to study early hemisphere specialization have been developed. They have generated considerable data which have increased our information particularly for the early years and for right-hemisphere specialization. Some of these results challenge and also may help clarify some of the existing conceptualizations in the field.

Several major issues emerge for consideration. It is probably misleading to talk of the development or ontogeny of hemisphere specialization, as is frequently done, since such labels carry the implicit assumption that hemisphere specialization develops; in other words, that there is a change from some nonexistent or less marked condition of specialization to one of greater specialization such as that which exists at maturity. That such a change occurs is not known. In fact, questions as to whether left-hemisphere specialization is indeed present at the time of birth and whether it increases during development are currently major issues.

The possible existence of left-hemisphere specialization at birth is inextricably linked with two other issues. First, if left-hemisphere specialization exists at birth, how is this compatible with the data that indicate a greater role of the right (non-language-dominant) hemisphere for speech functions in early life than at maturity? Second, if left-hemisphere specialization exists at birth, how can this be reconciled with the evidence indicative of hemisphere equipotentiality in subserving speech and language functions, and the documented ability of these functions to transfer to the right hemisphere after damage to crucial areas in the left hemisphere, at least in early life? Another issue involves the nature of left-hemisphere specialization during development. Is it similar to that of adults in that it represents a predominance of the left hemisphere for sequential, analytic, linguistic processing?

Finally, what is the situation in the other half of the brain? Is there right-hemisphere specialization for spatial, holistic, nonlinguistic processing during development? In addition, what interdependence, if any, exists between the hemispheres in their roles as different types of processors? And what relationship may specialization of the right hemisphere for its own functions have to early right-hemisphere participation in language, and to the time-limited transferability of speech from the left to the right hemisphere?

Within the context of these issues, the purpose of this paper is (1) to review the methods presently available for the study of hemisphere specialization in children, and to indicate their associated methodological and conceptual difficulties; (2) to summarize, and to indicate and possibly to reconcile some of the inconsistent results of, the three subsets of data relevant to left-hemisphere specialization in childhood: first, the evidence for very early left-hemisphere specialization for language functions; second, the data concerning the role of the right hemisphere in language functions in childhood; and third, the evidence for early hemisphere equipotentiality for and transferability of speech and language functions; (3) to summarize the data concerning specialization of the right hemisphere during childhood, an issue which has received relatively little attention; and (4) to present a possible theoretical framework of early cerebral organization that proposes functioning—not only potential—specialization of the left and right hemispheres for their respective cognitive functions at the time of birth; and that allows for such specialization to be coexistent with early participation of the right hemisphere in speech and language functions and with interhemisphere plasticity for speech and language functions, and to be subject to environmental factors and individual differences.

METHODS OF STUDYING HEMISPHERE SPECIALIZATION IN CHILDREN

Study of Children with Brain Damage

As in the study of all aspects of hemisphere specialization—whether of the left or right hemisphere and whether in adults or in children—the initial information has come from studying the behavioral and cognitive deficits in brain-damaged individuals. With children, as with adults, there have been phenomenological or naturalistic observations of behavior (e.g., Basser, 1962) as well as more objective experimental studies following unilateral brain trauma (e.g., Annett, 1973; Goodglass, 1967; Rudel, Teuber, & Twitchell, 1974).

Such studies of brain-damaged children, however, are often associated with one of two possible logical errors in interpretation of the results. In such studies, in order to obtain data relevant to the existence of hemisphere specialization at the time of the early lesion, it is imperative for behavior to be assessed as soon as possible after the trauma. If the behavioral or cognitive measures are not obtained until months or years later, recovery of function may have occurred and will therefore obscure any immediate loss of function. In many studies behavior had to be assessed years later because the subjects were obtained retrospectively (e.g., Annett, 1973; Rudel, Teuber, & Twitchell, 1974) or could only be tested years after the original lesion (e.g., Dennis & Kohn, 1975). The observation in such situations of no loss of function may lead to incorrect conclusions concerning hemisphere specialization. What such data may reflect is the plasticity of the immature brain, rather than a lack of hemisphere specialization.

More frequently, the results of such studies indicate an association between verbal and spatial deficits at the time of testing and the lateralization of the early lesion. Such results are indicative of hemisphere specialization. However, even though the lesion may have been sustained in infancy, the data indicate only that the hemispheres are functioning differentially at the time of testing and, furthermore, that there was the potential for such hemisphere specialization as early as the time of the original lesion. Such data do not provide evidence that there was actual differential processing by the hemispheres, that is, hemisphere specialization, in the years prior to testing. This, however, is how many such studies have been interpreted in various reports. In view of these considerations, in order for the study of brain-damaged children to provide data relevant to early hemisphere specialization, the behavior and cognition of the children must be tested immediately following brain damage. This has rarely been done and presents a more difficult situation than in adults, since the behavioral repertoire of young children is relatively limited and thus presents a challenge to devise tests to assess possible deficits.

The study of brain-damaged children is limited in still another way. In adults there exist cases with well-defined unilateral neurosurgical ablations associated with such clinical conditions as epilepsy, tumors, aneurysms and abscesses. And there exist associated presurgical tests, such as direct cortical electrical stimulation (Penfield & Roberts, 1959) and the possible associated clinical testing (e.g., Fedio & Van Buren, 1974); intracarotid sodium amytal injections for speech lateralization (Wada & Rasmussen, 1960) and its possible associated cognitive testing (e.g., Fedio & Weinberg, 1971); and, more recently, computerized study of regional blood flow changes associated with various mental activities (Risberg, Halsey, Wills, & Wilson, 1975). However, such surgery and the associated presurgical tests are much less frequent in children. In addition, the very powerful strategy of studying commissurotomized individuals—individuals in whom the interhemisphere commissures are sectioned for the treatment of epilepsy (Sperry, Gazzaniga, & Bogen, 1969)—is limited with children due to the lack of such cases. As a result, there are relatively few cases involving children which provide data based on precisely defined cortical ablations and the associated direct neurological measures. Consequently, the available data for children are limited in both quantity and quality.

Noninvasive Techniques with Neurologically Intact Children

Inference of neural localization of functions which is based on the association of cognitive deficits with known cortical lesions has some logical limitations. This is so in the case of adults; it is of even more concern with children, as the maximal extent of their lesions, usually of a nonsurgical nature, is less certain. On the basis of the study of brain-damaged individuals, all that one strictly may conclude is that the remaining intact neural structures, in the presence or absence of the dysfunctioning tissue, is insufficient to mediate effectively that function which is impaired. More direct support for the conclusion that the dysfunctioning tissue is necessary for a particular function, and for the exclusion of general intellectual, attentional, or motivational factors as the source of the poor performance, comes from results indicating a double dissociation effect. This refers to the situation where Lesion A is found to be associated with impairment in Function X but not in Function Y, whereas Lesion B is associated with impairment in Function Y but not in Function X. Such situations are difficult to obtain without the kinds of experimental studies that are possible with nonhuman species (see P. Milner, 1970) and in the absence of studies of groups of cases with known ablations in various cortical areas, such as are available for adult neurological patients (e.g., B. Milner, 1962). For this reason, the study of brain—behavior relationships in normal children is particularly important, to obtain data that complement those from the study of brain-damaged children. However, the interpretations that follow from the techniques available for normal individuals are necessarily inferential and have imperfect validity (see Satz, 1976). Therefore the importance of the availability of different techniques to assess the same hypothetical neural patterns and possibly to obtain converging results cannot be overestimated.

Tests of Perceptual Asymmetry

Several test paradigms which involve no medical intervention have been developed for use with normal adults, and many of these have been or can be adapted for use with normal children. The procedure common to the various tests is the comparison of the perception of stimuli presented in the left and right sensory fields. The basic rationale of these tests is based upon the fact that stimulation may be lateralized so that it is initially transmitted predominantly (as in the auditory and somesthetic modalities) or solely (as in the visual modality) to the contralateral hemisphere (see Figure 1). Consequently, any asymmetry in accuracy or reaction time in the perception of left versus right field stimuli may reflect the superiority of the contralateral hemisphere for the processing of that information.

In the auditory and tactual modalities, because there is some ipsilateral as well as contralateral transmission of information, techniques that involve simultaneous but different inputs to both sensory fields and that may elicit some competition in the neural system seem to be most effective in yielding perceptual asymmetries. In the auditory modality the dichotic stimulation procedure (Kimura, 1961a) is well known, and since its inception has been used frequently with children. The stimuli may vary from simple nonsense syllables to meaningful words to musical chords and may require linguistic, sequential, or holistic, parallel processing. Accordingly, the test may be used to reflect either left- or right-hemisphere superiority (e.g., C. Berlin & McNeil, 1976; H. Gordon, 1974a; Kimura, 1967; Studdert-Kennedy &

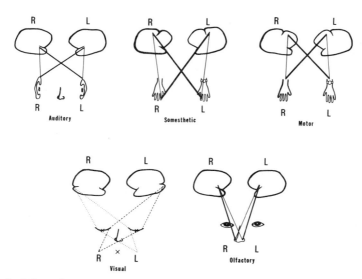

Figure 1. Schematic representation comparing the anatomical pathways in the various sensory and motor systems.

Shankweiler, 1970). Similarly, in the haptic modality (that is, active touch which involves tactile and proprioceptive stimulation), a technique of dichhaptic stimulation has been devised, in this case originally designed for use with children (Witelson, 1974, 1976a). In this tactile test the stimuli may also vary, reflecting either right-hemisphere specialization or in some cases a balance between left- and right-hemisphere processing (Witelson, 1974). The latter situation may occur, rather than left-hemisphere predominance, because haptic perception, even for tasks involving linguistic processing, may depend sufficiently on spatial processing by the right hemisphere that greater left-hemisphere participation is not observed (Witelson, 1974, 1976b). A somewhat similar technique involving competing stimuli in the tactual modality, so far used only with adults, involves bimanual tactile stimulation to the immobile hands. Stimulation may vary to require sequential or more spatial perception (Nachshon & Carmon, 1975).

In both the auditory and tactual modalities, however, it appears that if the task is made sufficiently difficult, some perceptual asymmetry may be observed even with monaural stimulation (e.g., Bakker, 1969; versus Jarvella, Herman, & Pisoni, 1970) or with unimanual stimulation (Benton, Levin, & Varney, 1973; Lechelt & Tanne, 1976).

At a lower level of processing, sensory thresholds for light touch have been reported to be lower for left than right fingers and hands, both in adults (e.g., Weinstein, 1968) and in children (Ghent, 1961). However, more recent studies, particularly one using a more precise method to assess pressure thresholds than is possible with the von Frey hair method of the previous studies, has failed to find any hand asymmetry (Carmon, Bilstrom, & Benton, 1969).

In the visual modality, because of the complete contralateral transmission from visual field to occipital cortex [except possibly for central vision involving part of the macular regions of the retinae (Pearlman, 1975)], unilateral rapid presentation of stimuli readily yields perceptual asymmetries. Some test paradigms have used different stimulation simultaneously to the two fields, referred to as dichoptic stimulation (e.g., Carmon, Kleiner, & Nachshon, 1975; McKeever & Huling, 1971). Simultaneous different inputs to the two lateral half-fields appears less crucial in eliciting hemisphere asymmetry in the visual system than in other sensory systems. Rapid or tachistoscopic stimulation (binocular or monocular) in the hemifields may involve various stimuli which again may reflect either left- or right-hemisphere superiority (e.g., Kimura & Durnford, 1974; M. White, 1969). Relatively little work has used tachistoscopic tasks with children, possibly because of the difficulty in obtaining central fixation in children which is crucial for these methods. Moreover, children vary greatly in the duration of the stimulus exposure that yields optimal accuracy to reflect hemisphere asymmetry, and thus they require the additional procedure of individual determination of exposure time (e.g., Witelson, 1975, 1976c). Other visual tasks which involve lateral apparent movement (Jasper, 1932; Spreen, C. Miller, & Benton, 1966) and fragmentation of lateralized stimuli (McKinney, 1967) have also been described and may have potential use in the study of hemisphere specialization in children.

Even the olfactory system has been used, although only with adult commissurotomized individuals to date (H. Gordon, 1974b). This technique may have potential for use with normal individuals and, more importantly, with children, since the association of oral labels to various odors may be a simple enough task for even the very young. Given the anatomy of the olfactory system, in which transmission from the receptors of each nasal cavity is predominantly to the ipsilateral hemisphere, but in which there is also a smaller decussating pathway (see Figure 1), it may be that stimulation to one nostril alone in normal individuals may not lead to perceptual asymmetry. Although there have been no such studies, perhaps tasks involving the perception of "dichnosmic" stimulation (that is, simultaneous but different stimulation to each nostril) and naming of the odors may reflect hemisphere specialization and thereby provide a means to study left hemisphere superiority for speech production in very young children, which has not yet been available to study by other means.

Tests of Motoric Asymmetry

A few motor tasks have been used with adults and, again, either have been or can be adapted for use with children. The direction of lateral eye gaze has been suggested to be an index of which hemisphere is more active during a particular cognitive task and may thus be used as an index of hemisphere specialization (e.g., Kinsbourne, 1972). To date there are no reports with young children, but conceivably this technique may prove useful, particularly for the study of right-hemisphere specialization for spatial processing in very young children.

Various motor tasks, such as rapid finger movements (e.g., Denckla, 1973; D. Ingram, 1975a) and hand predominance in the production of gestures associated with the act of speaking (D. Ingram, 1975a; Kimura, 1973) have been observed to yield right-hand superiority in adults and children and, by inference, suggest specialization of the left hemisphere for the execution of sequential patterns of movement. The anatomical substrate which allows for such motor asymmetries is the predominantly contralateral control of each hand (see Figure 1) and possibly only contralateral control of finger movement (Brinkman & Kuypers, 1972). Of course, related to this group of measures is hand preference for writing and for other unimanual tasks, probably the first behavioral measure suggested as an index of hemisphere asymmetry. However, hand preference has been shown to be only grossly correlated with speech lateralization (e.g., Branch, B. Milner, & Rasmussen, 1964; Hécaen & Sauguet, 1971). Almost all right-handed individuals and the majority of left-handed individuals have left-hemisphere representation of speech. Yet there is some correlation since more left- than right-handed individuals have reversed language lateralization, that is, right-hemisphere language. The variable of hand posture in writing, as recently described by Levy and Reid (1976a), may prove to be important in differentiating left handers according to cerebral organization.

Foot preference has also been suggested as an index of speech lateralization (e.g., A. Harris, 1958) but has yet to receive any validation. Eye preference as well has been implicated as an index of hemisphere specialization. However, as Walls (1951) has clearly indicated, eye dominance is not a simple phenomenon. He describes 25 different possible operational definitions of eye preference. Moreover, given that both eyes have bilateral motor and sensory innervation, it is not obvious how any aspect of dominance for one eye could be a result of asymmetrical hemisphere processing. In this context, the concept that "mixed" eye—hand dominance indicates atypical hemisphere lateralization of function is highly questionable. Furthermore, mixed eye—hand dominance was observed to be the rule rather than the exception (Belmont & Birch, 1963). A sensory asymmetry in vision may exist however—not between eyes but between hemiretinae—based on differential sensitivity of nasal and temporal hemiretinae, or on differential efficiency of the crossed and uncrossed optic pathways, respectively (e.g., McKinney, 1967; Polyak, 1957). Such possible asymmetry is an added "lateral asymmetry" variable in the visual system; it may serve to confound perceptual asymmetry in binocular viewing conditions which are typically used but may help to explain the observed eye differences in perceptual asymmetry with monocular viewing (e.g., Hayashi & Bryden, 1967).

Various tests of finger movement have been studied with concurrent independent activity such as speaking. This results in greater decrement of right- than left-hand performance in adults and in children (e.g., Hicks, Provenzano, & Rybstein, 1975; Kinsbourne & Cook, 1971; Kinsbourne & McMurray, 1975; Lomas & Kimura, 1976). The rationale is that right-hand performance suffers greater interference because it is mediated by the left hemisphere, the same hemisphere that mediates the concurrent independent activity of speech production.

Some aspects of hand performance, such as individual finger flexion in adults (Kimura & Vanderwolf, 1970) and copying hand positions in children (D. Ingram, 1975a), have been observed to yield left-hand superiority and, by inference, right-hemisphere specialization. One may conceptualize such tasks as involving spatial rather than sequential components.

The use of a right-left competing situation has also been adapted for motor tasks. Buffery and Gray (1972) reported left-hand superiority in the simultaneous drawing of different shapes by each hand in children, and Caplan and Kinsbourne (1976) reported right-hand superiority in a bimanual grasping task in infants. However, the behavioral and cognitive processes required in these tasks are not explicit and, in general, when this is so—as in the case of Braille reading, which is discussed in detail in a later section—inference as to hemisphere specialization is more equivocal.

Other early behavioral measures that may prove to be correlates of hemisphere specialization are asymmetry in direction of the tonic neck reflex in neonates, for which a preponderance of right-sided turns has been consistently observed (e.g., Turkewitz, E. Gordon, & Birch, 1965a), and directional orientation of the longitudinal (sagittal fissure) axis of the head of the fetus as it emerges from the birth canal (Churchill, Inga, & Senf, 1962).

It is only a matter of time and of experimenter ingenuity until further tasks are devised that combine the principles of the many test paradigms described here and the behavioral capabilities of the young child or infant. Such an example is described in a study by Entus (this volume, Chapter 6) that combines dichotic stimulation with the non-nutritive-sucking response in neonates to study hemisphere specialization.

Electrophysiological Measures

Various measures of electrophysiological activity of the cortex via scalp electrodes have yielded hemisphere differences for various stimuli and cognitive tasks. Some measures involve various analyses of ongoing electroencephalographic recordings, others involve time-locked cortical evoked potentials (for review, see Donchin, Kutas, & G. McCarthy, 1976). Both methods obviously have particularly important application for the study of infants and young children and have been used to date in several instances.

Neuroanatomical Study

An era of study of asymmetry in the gross morphology of the brain in postmortem specimens was initiated by the report of Geschwind and Levitsky (1968), which documented that the planum temporale, the superior surface of the temporal lobe posterior to Heschl's transverse gyrus and fissure, is markedly larger in the left than in the right hemisphere in most adults. This area is the superior surface of the core of the classical area of Wernicke, whose role in language comprehension is well documented. The facts (1) that consistent asymmetry is observed in precisely an area known to mediate language functions and (2) that the larger planum is observed to be in the left hemisphere (and there is precedence in neural organization for more intricately developed functions to be represented by larger areas, for example, sensory and motor cortical representations of the hand are markedly larger than those of the truck) provide evidence for a correlation between the temporal-lobe anatomical asymmetry and functional asymmetry. Stronger support for a correlation between anatomy and function such as might satisfy even the skeptics—those who are strongly influenced by the fact of functional equipotentiality of the hemispheres and who are more impressed with the infinite patterns of human cortical fissurization than with the possibility of one consistent asymmetry—would be the documentation of a correlation of different patterns of anatomical asymmetry with lateralization of speech or with patterns of cognitive abilities. It also remains to be determined whether there are histological or electronmicroscopic differences between the hemispheres in the temporal lobe speech areas.

It has been possible to extend the study of gross morphology in the temporal lobes to infants (e.g., Witelson & Pallie, 1973). It is important to note, however, that the existence of anatomical asymmetry in neonates suggests strictly only a preprogrammed bias in structure which may underlie subsequent functional asymmetry and a potential for eventual left-hemisphere specialization for language. The presence of anatomical asymmetry at birth does not necessarily indicate that asymmetrical neural functioning is operative at birth.

Other neural areas may also be found to have functionally relevant asymmetry (e.g., LeMay, 1976; Wada, 1976). In addition to direct morphological study, pneumoencephalograms (Dalby, 1975; McRae, Branch, & B. Milner, 1968), arteriograms (Hochberg & LeMay, 1975), and, more recently, computerized X-rays (LeMay, 1976) provide other means to study anatomical asymmetry, in these cases in the live individual. However, the relationship between any anatomical asymmetry and functional asymmetry is inferential and requires corroborating evidence as already noted.

The following four main sections present a review of data pertaining to early left-hemisphere specialization for language, early speech lateralization and the right hemisphere's role in language, early speech lateralization and interhemisphere transfer of speech, and early right-hemisphere specialization for spatial-holistic processing.

EARLY SPECIALIZATION OF THE LEFT HEMISPHERE FOR SPEECH AND LANGUAGE

Noninvasive Methods with Normal Children

Although the first relevant data for early left-hemisphere specialization came from studies of brain-damaged children, the most unequivocal evidence comes from the study of young normal children. Most of the work has used the dichotic stimulation test paradigm with various linguistic stimuli.

Dichotic Stimulation

A summary of the main results of all the studies of which I am aware that report data on left—right ear asymmetry for groups including at least 10 normal children who are designated as right handed and who are 7 years of age or younger (an arbitrary age selected on the basis of the distribution pattern of chronological age in the many studies), regardless of positive or negative results, is presented in Table 1. Numerous other studies have reported data only for children older than 7 years of age, usually not in direct study of normal children but as control groups for various clinical samples (Leong, 1976; Ling, 1971; Satz, Rardin, & Ross, 1971; Slorach & Noehr, 1973; Sobotka, 1974; Sparrow & Satz, 1970; L. Taylor, 1962; Witelson, 1962; Witelson & Rabinovitch, 1972; Yeni-Komshian, Isenberg, & Goldberg, 1975; Zurif & Carson, 1970). The large majority of studies in this latter group show significant right-ear superiority, the others show nearly significant differences and, by inference, left hemisphere specialization for language functions in school-age children. These results are not presented in detail here as they are less relevant to the issue of early lateralization.

TABLE 1 Summary of Results of Studies on Verbal Dichotic Stimulation Tests in Young Normal Children

Study	Subjects	Stimuli	Response	Score	Results
Kimura, 1963	4–9 years old $N = 145$ Girls (G) and Boys (B)	1, 2, and 3 pairs of digits	Free recall	Number correct per ear	All age–sex groups showed a significant REA, except 7- and 9-year-old girls.
Kimura, 1967	5–8 years old $N = 140$ Low to middle socioeconomic level (SE) G & B	1, 2, and 3 pairs of digits	Free recall	Number correct per ear	All age–sex groups showed REA, except 5-year-old boys.
Inglis & Sykes, 1967	5–10 years old $N = 120$ G & B	Sets of 1, 2, and 3 pairs of digits	Free recall	Number correct per ear	Only 6- and 9-year-old groups on 3-pair trials showed REA. When order of ear report considered, right-ear scores tended to be higher. No sex analysis.
Bryden, 1970	7, 9, 11 years old $N = 152$ G & B	2 and 3 pairs of digits	Free recall	Side of greater accuracy	Only about 58% of the 7-year-old group showed greater right- than left-ear scores and this proportion increased with age. No sex difference.
Knox & Kimura, 1970	5–8 years old $N = 80$ Low SE G & B	Experiment 1: 1, 2 and 3 pairs of digits	Free recall	Number correct per ear	All age–sex groups showed (probably significant) REA.

(continued)

TABLE 1 *(Continued)*

Study	Subjects	Stimuli	Response	Score	Results
	5–8 years old N = 120 Low SE G & B	Experiment 2: 1, 2, and 3 pairs of digits	Free recall	Number correct per ear	All age–sex groups showed (probably significant) REA.
	5–8 years old N = 120 Low SE G & B	Experiment 3: 1 pair of similar-sounding words	Point to one picture (of the word)	Number correct per ear	All age–sex groups showed (probably significant) REA.
	5–8 years old N = 120 Low SE G & B	Experiment 4: 2 pairs of words within a sentence	Place one object on one picture	Number correct per ear	All age–sex groups showed (probably significant) REA.
Nagafuchi, 1970	3–6 years old N = 80 G & B	Sets of 1 pair of 2- and 3-syllable words	Free recall	Number correct per ear	All age–sex groups showed REA in at least one condition, except 4- and 6-year-old girls.
Bever, 1971	2½–5 years old N = 195	2 pairs of animal names	Point to the animals	Proportion of right-ear responses	About 65% chose more right-than left-ear stimuli.
Geffner & Hochberg, 1971	4–7 years old N = 208 Low & middle SE G & B	2 pairs of digits	Free recall	Number correct per ear	All subgroups showed REA except the 4-, 5- and 6-year-old low SE groups. No sex difference.
Pizzamiglio & Cecchini, 1971	5–10 years old N = 192 Low & upper SE G & B	2 pairs of words and 3 pairs of digits	Free recall	Number correct per ear	All subgroups showed REA, except 5- and 6-year-old low SE groups.
Satz, Rardin, & Ross, 1971	7–8, 11–12 years old N = 20 B	3 pairs of digits	Free recall	Percentage correct per ear	Both age groups showed REA.

Sommers & Taylor, 1972	5–6 years old N = 10	1 pair of phonetically similar words, and 2 and 3 pairs of digits	Free recall	Number correct per ear	Each subject showed greater right-ear scores on both tests.
Berlin, Hughes, Lowe-Bell, & Berlin, 1973	5–13 years old N = 150 G & B	1 pair CV syllables	Recognize 2 written items (5-yr group, oral report)	Number of single-correct trials per ear	All age groups showed (probably significant) REA. No difference in size of REA with age. No sex difference.
Goodglass, 1973	6–12 years old N = 109 G & B	1 pair CVC words	Free recall	Number of competing consonants & vowels correct per ear	All age subgroups showed REA for both types of phonemes. No evidence for developmental progression. No sex analysis.
Yeni-Komshian, 1973	3–5 years old N = 42 G & B	1 pair 1-syllable boys' names	Free recall	$\dfrac{R-L}{R+L} \times 100$	Most age–sex subgroups showed REA, but not 4-year-old girls.
Dorman & Geffner, 1974	6 years old N = 52 Low & middle SE Caucasian & Negro groups	1 pair CV syllables	Report the one syllable heard	$\dfrac{R-L}{R+L} \times 100$	All SE–race subgroups showed REA.
Ingram, 1975b	3–5 years old N = 84 G & B	Experiment 1: 1 pair of similar-sounding words	Point to one picture	Number correct per ear	All age–sex groups showed REA, except 4-year-old girls.
		Experiment 2: 2 pairs of words within a sentence	Place one object on one picture	Number correct per ear	

(continued)

TABLE 1 *(Continued)*

Study	Subjects	Stimuli	Response	Score	Results
Satz, Bakker, Teunissen, Goebel, & Van der Vlugt, 1975	6–11 years old N = 198 G & B	4 pairs of digits	Free recall	Number correct per ear	REA found only in children 9 years old and older. No sex difference.
Borowy & Satz, 1973	5–11 years old N = 120	3 pairs of digits	Free recall	Number correct per ear	REA at all age levels.
Darby & Satz, 1973	5, 7, 12 years old N = 55	3 pairs of digits	Free recall	Number correct per ear	REA only at age 12.
Anderson & Barry, 1976	4, 5, 8, 11 years old N = 40 G & B	1, 2, and 3 pairs of digits Rate: 1 pr/sec	Free recall	Number correct per ear	All age groups showed REA except 4-year-olds. No sex analysis.
Bryden & Allard, 1976b	7–12 years old N = 72 G & B	2 and 3 pairs of digits	Free recall	Number correct per ear	REA at all age levels. No age or sex differences.
				Side of greater accuracy	Only oldest group had significantly more children with greater right- than left-ear scores.
Bryden, Allard, & Scarpino, 1973	6–14 years old N = 120 G & B	1 pair of CV syllables	Free recall	R–L (only first response scored)	Girls showed REA by age 9; boys only at a later age.
Hiscock & Kinsbourne, 1976	3–5 years old N = 42 G & B	3 pairs of digits	Precueing or postcueing of which ear to give attention to	Number correct per cued ear & N correct per ear regardless of instructions	REA in all age subgroups for both pre- and postcueing, and on both measures. No sex difference.
Kinsbourne & Hiscock, this volume, Chapter 14	3–12 years old N = 150 G & B	3 pairs of digits	Free recall	Number correct per ear.	All age groups showed REA, except 3- and 4-year-old groups. No sex difference.

Study	Subjects	Stimulus	Task	Measure	Result
Kinsbourne, Hotch, & Sessions, 1976	3–5 years old N = 20			Kuhn's phi coefficient.	With phi scores, no change in magnitude of REA with age observed.
		Experiment 1: 1 pair of digits	Indicate if "target" given	Number of errors per ear	REA observed.
	3 years old N = 16	Experiment 2: 1 pair of digits	Precueing of which ear to report	Number correct per ear	REA observed.
Geffner & Dorman, 1976	4 years old N = 44 Low & middle SE G & B	1 pair CV syllables	Report the one syllable heard	$\frac{R-L}{R+L} \times 100$	Both male SE groups showed REA. Neither female SE group showed REA.
Gilbert, 1976	$2\frac{1}{2}$–3 years old N = 12	1 pair CVC words	Free recall	Percentage correct per ear	REA observed.
Schulman-Galambos, 1976	6–10 years old N = 156 upper SE G & B	3 pairs of 1-syllable words	Free recall	Percentage correct per ear	All age subgroups showed REA. No change in magnitude of REA with age. No sex difference.
Witelson, 1976a, 1976c	6–14 years old N = 245 Middle SE G & B	2 and 3 pairs of digits	Free recall	Number correct per ear	REA observed for each age–sex subgroup.
Witelson, 1976d	3–5 years old N = 120 G & B	2 and 3 pairs of digits	Free recall	Number correct per ear	REA observed for each age–sex subgroup
Entus, this volume, Chapter 6	$1\frac{1}{2}$–3 months N = 48 G & B	1 pair of CV syllables	Nonnutritive sucking	Percentage change in number of sucks with stimulus change, per ear	REA observed. No sex difference.

[a]REA (right-ear advantage) refers only to a significant difference between ears.

Inspection of Table 1 reveals a marked consistency for greater right- than left-ear scores on verbal dichotic listening tests for children as young as 2 to 3 years of age. Of 36 experiments, 30, or about 83%, reported right-ear superiority for their youngest subgroups, and all found right-ear superiority in at least their older subgroups. Of all the perceptual tests used as indices of hemisphere specialization, the dichotic stimulation test has the most demonstrated construct validity based on external criteria. (1) Right-ear superiority is obtained only with stimuli that require linguistic or sequential processing, such as consonant—vowel syllables (e.g., Studdert-Kennedy & Shankweiler, 1970), simple words (e.g., Kimura, 1961a), and Morse code symbols (Papcun, Krashen, Terbeek, Remington, & Harshman, 1974), but not with nonlinguistic stimuli processed in a holistic, parallel mode, such as environmental sounds (e.g., Curry, 1967), chords (H. Gordon, 1970), and melodies (Bever & Chiarello, 1974). (2) Individuals known to have speech functions represented in the right hemisphere, on the basis of intracarotid sodium amytal testing, showed greater left- than right-ear scores on a verbal dichotic listening task (Kimura, 1961b). (3) Greater right-ear superiority is not due to the use of a verbal response, as a recognition response also yields greater right-ear scores (Broadbent & Gregory, 1964).

Within this background, the data in Table 1, which indicate consistent right-ear superiority and never left-ear superiority in numerous groups of children, provide strong support for greater participation of the left than the right hemisphere in various aspects of linguistic processing as early as 3 years of age, the youngest age repeatedly tested, and possibly as early as infancy.

It is difficult to compare specific aspects of the results of the different studies, since they differ on many dimensions that are possibly relevant to ear asymmetry: for example, various acoustic parameters of the dichotic stimuli, such as intensity level, signal-to-noise ratio, channel balance, rate of presentation of pairs of stimuli (see C. Berlin and Cullen, this volume, Chapter 7); and the type of stimuli and level of required linguistic processing, such as lower level processing for phonemic discrimination versus higher levels involving memory and semantic processing. These factors may affect the difficulty level of the different tests. Moreover, even the same test varies in difficulty level at different ages. This situation may lead to ceiling and floor effects in overall performance and thus obscure right—left differences. Some studies possibly involve an added attentional factor (e.g., Bryden, Allard, & Scarpino, 1973; Hiscock & Kinsbourne, 1976), which has been shown to be a relevant variable in studies of selective attention in dichotic listening with children (Clifton & Bogartz, 1968; Maccoby & Konrad, 1966). Finally, the groups differ in characteristics that may affect overall performance and indirectly right—left asymmetry, such as intelligence, social class, and demonstrated normal and equal hearing acuity in both ears.

The failure of the few studies to find significant right-ear superiority in their youngest subgroups (e.g., Anderson & Barry, 1976; Bryden, 1970; Bryden et al., 1973; Darby & Satz, 1973; Inglis & Sykes, 1967; Satz et al., 1975) may be due to the operation of some of the above factors: for example, a ceiling effect due to too easy a task (Inglis & Sykes, 1967); a floor effect possibly related to acoustic factors, resulting in low overall performance by the young subjects in the Bryden *et al.* (1973) study; and a floor effect due to too difficult a task associated with too large a memory component (e.g., Anderson & Barry, 1976; Satz *et al.*, 1975). However, in almost similar studies in the same laboratory (Borowy & Satz, 1973; Satz *et al.*, 1971) right-ear superiority was observed for young children. Perhaps the formal statistical model used in the 1975 Satz et al. study also contributed to the lack of significant right-ear superiority in the younger groups.

The few studies that found a lack of significant right-ear superiority in various age subgroups at apparently random ages (e.g., Nagafuchi, 1970) may be merely due to sampling error. The few reports indicating less ear asymmetry in low socioeconomic groups may have had lower overall accuracy (floor effect) operating as a confounding factor.

One current issue is not only whether left-hemisphere specialization exists in early life but whether left-hemisphere specialization increases in degree during development. This is difficult to assess on the basis of the available data. First, there is no reason to assume a priori that any dichotic test is sufficiently sensitive that the magnitude of ear difference is an index of the degree of hemisphere lateralization of function. The one investigation pertinent to this question (Shankweiler & Studdert-Kennedy, 1975) provides evidence of a moderate correlation between the magnitude of ear asymmetry and the degree of hand preference, and therefore, by inference, possibly of degree of hemisphere specialization. Second, as indicated above, the fact that the size of ear asymmetry may be related to overall accuracy—a factor that increases with age—confounds interpretation of the magnitude of left—right asymmetry at different ages as an index of change in hemisphere specialization. Krashen (1972) reanalyzed some of the earlier studies of dichotic listening in children using percentage of correct and percentage of error scores to partial out the effects of increasing and decreasing overall performance with age. On the basis of this analysis he found no evidence of a change in the size of ear asymmetry with age. Of the 36 studies reviewed here, only four suggest an increase in size of ear asymmetry with age (Bryden, 1970; Bryden *et al.*, 1973; Darby & Satz, 1973; Satz *et al.*, 1975). All used somewhat unusual response scores. The few studies which used scores of ear asymmetry that take into account overall accuracy (e.g., Kinsbourne & Hiscock, this volume, Chapter 14; Schulman-Galambos, 1976) provide no evidence of any change in magnitude of ear asymmetry. The study by C. Berlin, Hughes, Lowe-Bell, and H. Berlin (1973) was specifically designed to study possible developmental changes in magnitude of ear asymmetry, at least for simple levels of linguistic processing. They used an analysis of left-versus right-ear accuracy based on those trials in which only a single-correct response was given thereby disentangling the size of ear asymmetry from the increase in overall accuracy that occurs with age, which in their analysis is represented by the increasing number of trials with double-correct responses. They found no change in ear asymmetry for single-correct reports from 5 to 13 years of age, the entire age range studied. It is noted, however, that there are many aspects of language and cognition considered to be specific functions of the left hemisphere, but which have not or cannot be studied for lateralization via dichotic listening.

A comment on sex differences is warranted here. The data provide no evidence of greater left-hemisphere specialization for linguistic functions in girls than in boys, although this interpretation is prevalent in the general literature. In fact, of the few studies that did find sex differences, more found a lack of ear asymmetry in girls (five studies and most implicated age 4) than in boys (two studies). This inconsistency for right-ear superiority may again be a reflection of varying levels of overall performance in different studies. Speculation of greater laterality in girls is usually based on Kimura's studies. However, in her first study Kimura (1963) concludes, on the basis of clear data, that ear asymmetry occurred as early in boys as in girls. Identical results are reported in the several studies reported by Knox and Kimura (1970). Only in Kimura's (1967) study did the 5-year-old group of boys of low socioeconomic level show no right-ear superiority. But how much weight should be given to one such finding? Several studies found that some age subgroups, in the middle of the age range studied, did not show right-ear superiority (e.g., Nagafuchi, 1970). Such results were considered to reflect sampling error rather than specific meaning. Moreover, more studies observed a lack of asymmetry in girls (e.g., Geffner & Dorman, 1976; D. Ingram, 1975b; Nagafuchi, 1970). What Kimura (1963) did indicate as a sex difference was overall accuracy, which she suggested may reflect the earlier development of language skills in females. But this does not necessarily mean greater lateralization, as many subsequent authors have interpreted her report.

Lateral Tachistoscopic Stimulation

A few studies with children have attempted to investigate the issue of left-hemisphere specialization for language functions via lateral tachistoscopic presentation of linguistic stimuli. These reports, again for right-handed children, are summarized in Table 2. The results of these studies, in general, provide limited information for the issue of early left-hemisphere specialization. First, most of the reports used normal children only as control groups for the study of poor readers, and accordingly involved older (school-age) children. Second, and of greater consequence, is the necessarily equivocal nature of the interpretation of the observed right-field superiority in most of these studies. There is considerable evidence that normally written words, that is, words written in horizontal fashion, elicit post-exposure attentional scanning processes, resulting from the experience of left to right scanning in reading (Heron, 1957). In English, with unilateral presentation, this scanning factor leads to right-field superiority, as does left-hemisphere specialization for language. Because of this situation, subsequent studies with adults used single letters, vertically arranged words, mirror-image words, or Hebrew words with native Hebrew (right to left) readers (for review, see M. White, 1969, 1973), in an attempt to disentangle the effects of directional scanning and left-hemisphere specialization.

However, almost all of the studies with children used unilateral presentation of horizontally arranged words. This was the exact procedure used in the original study with children by Forgays in 1953, which was done almost a decade before unilateral tachistoscopic stimulation was adapted as an index of hemisphere specialization. The aim of the study was to determine whether right visual field superiority increased with age and, by inference, whether equipotentiality in the visual system decreased due to increased experience in reading. The expected results were obtained and were interpreted as supporting the hypothesis of decreasing equipotentiality. Only later was the role of cerebral dominance on such tasks noted. The more recent reports, however, although aimed at studying hemisphere specialization, used procedures similar to Forgays' which makes it difficult to interpret whether the observed right-field superiority is a result of directional scanning or of hemisphere specialization (Marcel, Katz, & M. Smith, 1974; Marcel & Rajan, 1975; McKeever & Huling, 1970; Olson, 1973; Reitsma, 1975). The likelihood of scanning factors being operative is supported by the fact that in most studies, except those of Marcel and colleagues, right-field superiority was observed only after Grade 2 and increased with age, possibly reflecting increased reading experience. The confounding of factors is highlighted by the studies of L. Miller and Turner (1973) and Reitsma (1975), which used almost identical procedures and obtained almost identical results. However, the purpose and conclusion of each study differed: the former concluded that internalized scanning of written language increases with age, and the latter concluded that left-hemisphere specialization for language was observed only in the older groups because only they used linguistic rather than spatial processing of words.

The study by Yeni-Komshian et al. (1975) used single digits as well as vertically arranged words, both of which should rule out the effects of scanning. However, greater accuracy for stimuli presented in the right visual field was not obtained for either material used in this study. Reitsma (1975) also used digits and did not find right-field superiority except for his youngest group, aged 7 years—an age not studied in the Yeni-Komshian et al. study. It is possible that the naming of Arabic digits requires only low-level linguistic processing for older school-age children and for this reason no right-field superiority was obtained with older children in either study. It is more difficult to explain the lack of a right-field superiority for the vertically presented words in the Yeni-Komshian et al. study. No ceiling or floor effect was evident. One post hoc explanation may be that the words used were names of digits, which are very familiar and finite in number, and that the perceptual strategy used may have involved considerable visual-holistic processing in these older (10–13 years) school-age children. It is also possible that the exposure duration used (189 msec) for both tasks was sufficiently large to allow eye movements to bring the stimuli into central vision.

In a study in my laboratory, unilateral presentation of pairs of same or different, vertically arranged, uppercase letters was used, and the response required was "same" or "different." These stimuli were so designed as to help rule out possible scanning

TABLE 2 Summary of Results of Studies on Lateral Tachistoscopic Stimulation with Linguistic Stimuli in Normal Children

Study	Subjects	Stimuli	Response and score	Results
Forgays, 1953	7–16 years old N = 108 Girls (G) & Boys (B)	3- or 4-letter words, horizontally arranged (H), unilateral presentation (U)	Verbal recall. Number of words correct per field	Significantly greater accuracy for stimuli presented in the right visual field (RVF) only from about age 12 and older. No sex difference.
McKeever & Huling, 1970	13 years old N = 10	4-letter familiar nouns, H, U	Verbal recall. Number of words correct per field	RVF obtained. 8/10 subjects showed greater right-field accuracy.
Miller & Turner, 1973	8, 10, 12 years old N = 45 G & B	4- and 5-letter familiar words, H, U	Verbal recall. Number of words correct per field	RVF observed in only 10- and 12-year-old age groups. No sex analysis.
Olson, 1973	7–11 years old N = 50 G & B	3- and 4-letter familiar nouns, H, unilateral & bilateral (dichoptic) presentation	Verbal recall. Number of words correct per field	Total group showed RVF for both conditions. No sex difference.
Marcel, Katz, & Smith, 1974	7–8 years old N = 20 G & B	5-letter familiar words, H, U	Verbal recall. Number of words and number of letters correct per field	RVF obtained for both scores. Boys showed greater RVF.

Study	Age / N / Group	Stimuli	Measure	Results
Marcel & Rajan, 1975	7–9 years old, N = 20, G & B	5-letter familiar words, H, U	Verbal recall. Number of words and number of letters correct per field	RVF obtained for both scores. No sex difference.
Reitsma, 1975	8, 10, 12 years old, N = 60, G & B	Experiment 1: 3-letter words, H, U	Verbal recall. Number of words correct per field	RVF obtained only in 10- and 12-year old subgroups. No sex analysis.
	6, 7, 8 years old, N = 60	Experiment 2: Arabic digits, U	Verbal recall. Number of digits correct per field	RVF obtained only for 6-year subgroup.
Yeni-Komshian, Isenberg, & Goldberg, 1975	10–13 years old, N = 19, G & B	Experiment 1: Arabic digits, U	Verbal recall. Percentage correct	No RVF obtained.
		Experiment 2: words (numbers), vertically arranged, U		No RVF obtained. No sex difference in either experiment.
Witelson, 1977	6–14 years old, N = 86, B	Pairs of same or different, uppercase, vertically arranged letters, U	Distinguish same or different. Number of pairs correct per field	RVF obtained only in 6–7-year-old subgroup.

[a]RVF (right visual field) refers only to a significant superiority for right-visual-field stimuli.

influences. An additional objective was to have a task that did not involve naming of letters, so that the task could be applicable to dyslexic children, who are often not able to read simple words or even name letters. A significant right visual field superiority in normal children was observed; but only for the youngest (6 to 7 year) subgroup. Thereafter, until age 14, there was no visual field difference (Witelson, 1977). Unfortunately, this study was started when I was not aware of the work (Cohen, 1972; Geffen, Bradshaw, & Nettleton, 1972; Posner & Mitchell, 1967) indicating the possibility of making a "physical match" of "linguistic stimuli" without the use of linguistic processing, even though the experimenter may consider the stimuli as linguistic. One possible but post hoc interpretation of these data is that at early ages, when the alphabet has just been learned, children tend to associate the visual letters with their phonetic names, and therefore considerable linguistic processing may be involved, resulting in right-field superiority. With age, the cognitive process may change and come to depend more on a lower-level process of physical matching, resulting in no difference in accuracy between visual fields. This speculation is somewhat supported by the finding that, on the same task, young dyslexics did not show right-field superiority but did show a trend toward greater right-field accuracy with increasing age, presumably as they learn the alphabet and its phonetic code. In contrast, they do show right-ear superiority on a dichotic digit stimulation task at all ages (Witelson, 1976c, 1977). The importance of defining the cognitive processing required in tasks used to assess hemisphere specialization is again underlined in a study with school-age children by Neville (1975) in which a comparable difficulty appears to be operating. Line drawings of objects were unilaterally presented in the left or right visual fields with the expectation that greater accuracy would be observed for left-field stimuli. However, the response necessitated not a physical match but a conceptual match to a different picture depicting the same object as the stimulus. No field differences were observed.

In summary, it is reasonable to conclude that not one tachistoscopic study of left-hemisphere specialization in children is free of methodological difficulty or provides unequivocal results.

Lateral Motoric Tasks

Numerous studies have used a variety of motoric tasks as indices of aspects of hemisphere specialization. Table 3 presents a summary of such studies involving normal right-handed children of 7 years of age or younger. The number of different motor tasks used is almost as great as the number of studies. For most tasks the dimension of motor performance that may be relevant to left-hemisphere specialization was not explicitly stated in the description of the task nor even in the post hoc interpretations of the results. The results are quite consistent, however, in that right-hand or right-side superiority was observed in the large majority of the 34 studies.

The following post hoc conceptual scheme is offered for those aspects of motor performance as observed in these reports that may be related to left-hemisphere

TABLE 3 Summary of Results of Studies on Various Lateral Motoric Tests with Normal Children

Study	Subjects	Task	Response & score	Results
Gesell & Ames, 1947	2 months–10 years old N = 12–45 at each age level	Observation of hand behavior to objects presented in midline	Prehension and manipulation of objects by each hand	At 4–5 months, left-hand preference observed, followed by periods of bilateral and of right or left unilateral preference until 8 years old, when majority of individuals show right-hand preference.
Belmont & Birch, 1963	5–12 years old N = 148 Girls (G) & Boys (B)	Experiment 1: Hand preference on 4 tasks	Hand preference defined as 100% preference for one hand	Consistent right-hand preference for about 80% of children observed by age 9. No sex difference.
		Experiment 2: Foot preference on 2 tasks	Foot preference defined as preference for same side on both tasks	Consistent right-foot preference for about 80% of children observed by age 5. No sex analysis.
Cohen, 1966	8 months N = 100 G & B	Reaching for presented objects	Hand preference defined as at least 9/12 reaches with one hand	Greater frequency for right-hand preference. No sex analysis.
Knights & Moule, 1967	5–14 years old N = 169 G & B	Unilateral hand and unilateral foot tapping	Speed of tapping in 10-sec period	Dominant hand tapped faster than nondominant hand. Dominant foot tapped faster than nondominant foot. No sex difference.
Turkewitz, Gordon, & Birch, 1965b	3 days postnatal N = 75	Head turning in spontaneous and in tactile perioral stimulation conditions	Number of turns to each side	Significantly more head turns to the right, with and without stimulation.
Annett, 1970	3½–15 years old N = 152	Experiment 1: Hand preference on 5–7 unimanual skills	Right-hand preference defined as 100% preference	Approximately 70% of children showed consistent right-hand preference.
		Experiment 2: Speed of fine movements on a pegboard	Mean time for task per hand	Right hand exhibited faster performance at all age levels. Females showed greater right-hand superiority on both tasks.

(continued)

TABLE 3 *(Continued)*

Study	Subjects	Task	Response & score	Results
Reitan, 1971	5–8 years old $N = 26$	Name writing	Speed of name writing per hand	Faster speed with right hand.
Buffery, 1970	3–11 years old $N = 80$ G & B	Bimanual simultaneous drawing of square and circle (Conflict Drawing Test)	Number of subjects better drawn right- or left-hand squares	22/40 boys and 28/40 girls drew better squares with their left hand. There was a nonsignificant tendency for left-hand superiority and for earlier occurrence in girls.
Buffery, 1971; Buffery & Gray, 1972	3–11 years old $N = 160$ G & B	Bimanual simultaneous drawing of square and circle (Conflict Drawing Test)	Number of subjects better drawn right- or left-hand squares	Hand asymmetry observed for girls. Significant majority of girls showed left-hand superiority by at least age 5. No significant hand asymmetry observed for boys. Although significantly more boys showed right-hand superiority in the 3–5-year-old subgroup, thereafter only a tendency for more frequent right-hand preference, and subsequently no hand difference. These results constitute a sex difference.
Kinsbourne, 1972	5–6 years old $N = 108$	Unimanual "stick-dropping" test: 3 sticks between 4 fingers	Drop designated stick	No hand difference.
Denkla, 1973	5–7 years old $N = 237$ G & B	Unimanual repetitive and unilateral successive finger movements	Time for 20 movements	Significantly faster right-hand performance on repetitive task only. No sex difference in laterality on this task.
Seth, 1973	5–12 months $N = 19$ G & B	Monthly observations of infants' behavior in response to presentation of an object	Frequency of hand use under guidance by the eye, of use as the master hand, and of success with each hand	Left-hand preference exhibited at 5 months on all measures and gives way to right-hand preference by approx. 6–9 months.

Condon & Sander, 1974	median = 2 days N = 16	Observation of spontaneous movements associated with speech of caretaker	Analysis of segments of movements	Synchrony of organized correspondence between neonatal body movement and articulatory segments of adult speech
Denkla, 1974	5–10 years old N = 168 G & B	Experiment 1. Repetitive finger movements	Rate of movements	Faster right-side performance on all tasks except successive finger movements. Magnitude of asymmetry decreases with age. Girls show greater asymmetry, but only for toe tapping and hand pronation–supination at ages 5 and 6.
		Experiment 2. Successive finger movements		
		Experiment 3. Repetitive hand patting		
		Experiment 4. Alternating hand pronation–supination		
		Experiment 5. Alternating hand flexion–extension		
		Experiment 6. Repetitive foot tapping		
		Experiment 7. Alternating heel–toe tapping		
Trevarthen, 1974a,b	Birth to 6 months N = 5	Observation of spontaneous behavior with toy or with mother	Analysis of rudimentary forms of higher cognitive behavior	Spontaneous gesture-like activity and "prespeech" movements of lips and tongue present by 2 months.
Turkewitz & Creighton, 1974	0–72 hours postnatal N = 70	Observation of head turns from midline position	Number of spontaneous head turns to each side	Infants older than 12 hours made more right than left turns.
Ingram, 1975a	3, 4, 5 years old N = 84 G & B	Experiment 1. Hand strength	Pound force per hand	Right hand stronger for total group. Girls showed greater asymmetry.
		Experiment 2. Unimanual finger tapping	Number of taps per 10 sec	Significantly faster right-hand performance for total group. No sex difference in laterality.

(continued)

TABLE 3 *(Continued)*

Study	Subjects	Task	Response & score	Results
		Experiment 3. Copy hand postures of deaf alphabet	Scored for accuracy of posture	Significantly better left-hand performance for total group. No sex difference in laterality.
		Experiment 4. Copy finger spacing of a hand position	Scored for accuracy of posture	Significantly better left-hand performance for total group. No sex difference in laterality.
		Experiment 5. Lift individual fingers (from Rey test)	Number correct per hand	No hand difference.
		Experiment 6. Manual activity associated with speaking	Number of gesture and grooming movements per hand	More gesture-like movements made with right hand. No hand difference for grooming-type movements. No sex difference in laterality.
Kinsbourne & McMurray, 1975	5 years old $N = 48$ G & B	Unimanual finger tapping with and without concurrent verbal activity	Rate of tapping. Amount of decrement per hand while speaking	Significantly faster right-hand performance. Significantly greater interference with right-hand performance. No sex difference.
Caplan & Kinsbourne, 1976	1–4 months $\bar{X} = 2.7$ months $N = 21$ G & B	Unimanual grasp. Bimanual grasp of rattles, one in each hand	Frequency of longer grasps per hand. Duration of grasp per hand	Right-hand superiority on both measures for unimanual condition, and on frequency of longer grasps in bimanual condition. No sex difference.
Hiscock & Kinsbourne, 1976	3–11 years old $N = 151$	Unimanual finger tapping with and without concurrent verbal activity	Rate of tapping. Ratio of decrease to base rate	Significantly faster right-hand performance at all age levels. Significantly greater interference with right-hand performance at all age levels.
Wolff & Hurwitz, 1976	5–16 years old $N = 468$ G & B	Alternate tapping of left and right index fingers to rhythms	Deviation of tapping from model, per hand	More accurate right-hand performance until age 12. No sex difference in laterality.

specialization. Sequential processing of information in general (e.g., Carmon, 1975) and, in particular, the execution of sequences of motor behavior (Liepmann, 1908; Kimura, 1976) have been related to left-hemisphere specialization in adults. The lateralization of speech and language functions to the left hemisphere may be associated with a sequential dimension in terms of the production of sequences of articulatory sounds in oral speech, and the processing of sequential information of syntactic structures in language comprehension. Many of the motor tasks that yielded right-hand superiority in children and, by inference, indicated left-hemisphere specialization, involve aspects of sequential movements: finger tapping, alternating finger or arm movements, foot tapping (e.g., Annett, 1970; Denkla, 1973, 1974; D. Ingram, 1975a; Knights & Moule, 1967; Wolff & Hurwitz, 1976). This conceptualization is corroborated by the finding that impairment in copying movement sequences with either hand is associated in adults with left-hemisphere lesions, but not with right-hemisphere lesions (Kimura, 1976). Furthermore, left-hemisphere predominance in mediating such behavior is supported by the observation of greater interference in right- than in left-hand performance with concurrent speech production (Hiscock & Kinsbourne, 1976; Kinsbourne & McMurray, 1975), suggesting that the neural structures involved in mediating speech and such motor behavior of the right hand are closely related, either functionally or anatomically or both. The rationale is that concurrent execution of independent activities which are dependent on related neural structures results in interference in one of the behaviors.

Gesture-like movements, particularly with the right hand, have been observed to increase in frequency in association with speech production in adults (Kimura, 1973) and now this finding has been demonstrated for children as well (D. Ingram, 1975a). In this case the two behaviors, speech and hand gestures, are considered to be not independent but related—both manifestations of the same neural functioning. Therefore, the occurrence of one behavior may increase the frequency of the other.

The observations (1) of right-hand superiority in various sequential motor tasks, (2) of greater decrement of right-hand performance on some tasks while speaking, and (3) of right-hand predominance in the production of gesture-like movements while speaking, in each case as early as 3 years of age, suggest that the production of motor sequences and speech-related movements may be lateralized to the left hemisphere as early as age 3.

The studies of Condon and Sander (1974) and Trevarthen (1974a, b) may be of relevance here. Although they are not studies of lateral asymmetry, they both indicate the existence of very early and possibly innately preprogrammed complex motor sequences, in each case associated in some fashion with speech. It remains to be determined whether these behaviors are mediated mainly by the left hemisphere in infancy. If this were the case, it would provide evidence for actual asymmetrical functioning of the two hemispheres for aspects of motor sequencing associated with speech in infancy, which would be consistent with the finding of left-hemisphere lateralization of phonemic discrimination suggested by Entus (this volume, Chapter 6).

It is more difficult to define what some of the other motor behaviors reflect. Predominance of head turning to the right has been consistently reported for neonates (Turkewitz & Creighton, 1974; Turkewitz, Gordon, & Birch, 1965b). More frequent reaching by the right hand has been reported for children as young as 8 months (A. Cohen, 1966; Seth, 1973). Perhaps these behaviors are also examples of motor sequences. Possibly they are early correlates or manifestations of subsequent right-hand preference. But how then can one incorporate the results of the several studies that have reported more frequent reaching with the left hand at about 4 to 5 months of age (Gesell & Ames, 1947; Seth, 1973), which then disappears? Moreover, consistent right-hand preference in the majority of children is not observed until much later, by about 8 to 9 years of age (Belmont & Birch, 1963; Gesell & Ames, 1947). At this point there are insufficient data to make selection possible among the various alternatives.

Caplan and Kinsbourne (1976) noted a longer duration for grasping objects by the right hand in infants who ranged in age from 1 to 4 months, just below the age for which more frequent left-hand reaching has been observed. If both duration of grasp and frequency of reaching are manifestations of the same central lateral phenomenon, then perhaps longer grasping would be observed for the left hand in children older than 4 months. Or perhaps reaching and grasp maintaining reflect different behaviors and have different neural substrates. Then, the longer grasp by the right hand may indirectly reflect the infant's tendency to use the left hand more frequently for reaching at that stage of development, which may be why "the left hand drops the rattle first." Perhaps all these early measures (head turning, reaching, grasp maintaining) reflect an attentional bias to the contralateral field, similar to that described by Kinsbourne (1973), which, in infants, may vary in the early stages of development.

The few lateral motoric tests that did not show right-hand superiority but yielded either left-hand superiority or no asymmetry may have relevance to right-hemisphere specialization, which will be further discussed in general in a later section. These particular tests may be conceptualized as involving spatial perception and individual discrete finger movements, both of which have been related to right-hemisphere specialization in adults (e.g., Kimura & Durnford, 1974; Kimura & Vanderwolf, 1970). The relevant tasks in children are the individual stick-dropping (Kinsbourne, 1972) and individual finger lifting tasks (D. Ingram, 1975a), which appear to involve individual finger movements comparable to the task in the Kimura and Vanderwolf (1970) study. The left-hand superiority on the two tasks of copying hand postures (D. Ingram, 1975a) may involve spatial components similar to those underlying right-hand dyscopia (Bogen, 1969) and constructional apraxia (Warrington, 1969) associated with right-hemisphere lesions. It is notable that there are no reports that demonstrate hand asymmetry either in executing motor sequences or in copying postures in normal adults, but such asymmetry has been observed in normal children (e.g., D. Ingram, 1975a). This raises the question of whether aspects of hemisphere specialization manifested in the motor system may be greater in children than in adults. There is some evidence to support such a decrease in asymmetry with age (Denckla, 1974; Wolff & Hurwitz, 1976). This group of reports indicating left-hand superiority suggests that some aspects of right-hemisphere specialization may be functionally present in children again as young as 3 years of age.

Finally there are the results showing left-hand superiority in a bimanual drawing task (Conflict Drawing Test), at least for girls in one of the two studies reported by Buffery (1970, 1971). These results are very difficult to interpret. Buffery suggests that the results indicate right-hemisphere specialization for this task and earlier such specialization in girls than in boys. Although the girls did show more frequent left-hand superiority on this task, the boys never did show significantly more frequent better left- than right-hand drawings, either as a total group or at any age subgroup. In contrast, a recent study using this task with adults (unspecified as to sex) reports a strong tendency for better drawing of squares by the right hand (Clyma & Clarke, 1973). Even in the eventuality of clear left behavioral superiority, what does the task measure and what is it that is more lateralized to the right hemisphere? This is a particularly clear example of a difficulty in research in brain—behavior relationships and the inevitable circularity that may occur in brain—behavior theorizing: The processes of the task are not specified, behavioral asymmetry is observed, asymmetrical hemisphere functioning is postulated, the task is then described in terms of functions known to be lateralized to that hemisphere, and then the hemisphere is said to be specialized for that function. At best, hemisphere lateralization is inferential, so at the least there must be a clear independent variable to serve as the anchor point. Then, the availability of several such converging sets of data, all indicative of the same hypothesis, increases the validity of any inference.

Buffery reports that, following the theorizing of Lukianowicz who devised the task, hemisphere asymmetry is reflected on this task because "proprioceptive feedback from each hand is processed initially by the contralateral hemisphere." Does this mean that the aspect of the task that is lateralized is somesthetic perception? If so, then why is there superiority in the left-hand right-hemisphere system? All the motor tasks discussed involve proprioception and yet many yielded right-hand superiority. Another possible interpretation is that the task involves sequential motor performance in the drawing of a geometrical shape. But, if so, why not right-hand superiority, as in the other reports indicated above? The 3 to 5 year subgroup of boys did show significantly more frequent right-hand superiority, but this was not stressed in the report. In this connection, it may be relevant to note Bogen's (1969) report, which suggests that shapes such as squares may be drawn using either of two cognitive strategies, an analytic one mediated by the right-hand left-hemisphere system, and a holistic one mediated by the left-hand right-hemisphere system, as is clearly observable in commissurotomized individuals.

Could different strategies have been used with different hands in the Conflict Drawing Test? Analytic processing may be more likely with a square, because of its reference points, than with a circle (e.g., Kimura, 1969). The question arises whether any hand difference exists on this task for drawing circles. These results are not given. Finally, the task may reflect spatial processing, and perhaps this is why left-hand superiority was observed at least for girls. But why in girls and not in boys? The direction of this sex difference is inconsistent with the literature. In those reports in which significant sex differences were observed, it has usually been the males who show greater hemisphere specialization: for right-hemisphere functions such as tactile—spatial processing in children (Witelson, 1976a), visuo—spatial processing (Kimura, 1969; Lansdell, 1962; Levy & Reid, 1976a; McGlone & Davidson, 1973) and the perception of musical chords (H. Gordon, 1976) in adults; and for left-hemisphere functions such as linguistic processing (Lake & Bryden, 1976). In conclusion, the purpose of this detailed analysis is to indicate the difficulty in interpreting results of studies which have no "givens" or independent variables.

The motor system may provide a fruitful means for the study of very early lateralization. Lateral eye gaze in infants has not yet been used as an index of hemisphere specialization. It is difficult to measure perception, memory, and, of course, speech and language in the infant, but motor behavior is predominant in their repertoire. It is for this reason that motor skills are a major component of infant intelligence tests (e.g., Bayley, 1969; Cattell, 1950; Gesell & Amatruda, 1940).

Electrophysiological Measures

Several studies have used electrophysiological measures to study hemisphere specialization in young children. Molfese, Freeman, and Palermo (1975) observed larger amplitudes in evoked potentials to phonemic stimuli over the left than right temporal lobe regions in infants. In further studies with neonates (Molfese, 1976; Molfese, Nunez, Seibert, & Ramanaiah, 1976), the acoustic parameters of the linguistic stimuli that elicit differential hemisphere activity and the associated components of the auditory evoked potential (AEP) were investigated. Bandwidth and number of formants, rather than transitional elements, appear to be critical acoustic factors. Another laboratory has also reported greater amplitude of AEPs in the left hemisphere for speech stimuli in infants (Barnet, Vicentini, & Campos, 1974). M. Gardiner, Schulman, and Walter (1974) and M. Gardiner and Walter (1976) reported hemisphere difference in EEG power distributions to continuous speech versus nonspeech stimulation in infants. Černáček and Podivinský (1971) observed that in those infants and young children who demonstrated right-hand preference, the amplitude of the cortical somatosensory evoked potential (SEP) was higher in the hemisphere (left) contralateral to the preferred hand than in the ipsilateral hemisphere; and the ipsilateral SEPs were larger for the "dominant" hand than for the nonpreferred hand. These results further support the existence of left-hemisphere specialization for aspects of hand dominance and possibly for speech within the first year of life.

Neuroanatomical Studies

Following Geschwind and Levitsky's (1968) lead that there is anatomical asymmetry in language-mediating areas in the temporal lobes in adults, several studies have been done with neonates and infants. The results are summarized in Table 4. The cortical area in question is the posterior part of the superior surface of the temporal lobe. Fortunately for researchers, the planum temporale is one of the few cortical areas that has clearly defined anatomical boundaries as well as well-documented asymmetrically represented cognitive functions. The results of these studies provide strong evidence for the existence of a reliably larger left than right planum in neonates. Note (in Table 4) the marked similarity in relative size of right to left planum in the Witelson and Pallie (1973) and Wada, Clarke, and Hamm (1975) studies, even though they were done independently and vary greatly in sample size. However, the percentage of neonates (56%) with a larger left planum is relatively low in the Wada et al. study compared to all other studies—both of infants and of adults.

The data indicate a preprogrammed morphological asymmetry and a correlation between anatomical and functional asymmetry of the hemispheres. However, that there is a meaningful or causal relationship between the two asymmetries remains to be demonstrated. Even if the anatomical and functional asymmetries are related, anatomical asymmetry in neonates can indicate at most a biologically pre-programmed potential for language to become lateralized to the left hemisphere. The hypothesis of an innate potential for the left hemisphere to mediate language implies that random learning or the effects of hand preference (as suggested by Gazzaniga, 1970) are at most only secondary factors in determining the pattern of hemisphere specialization. The fact that almost all right-handed and the majority of left-handed individuals have speech represented in the left hemisphere also suggests that the greater use of one hand is unlikely to be a critical factor in the determination of speech lateralization.

The anatomical results may suggest a potential for functional asymmetry but they do not necessarily indicate that there is actual functioning asymmetry at birth. However, recent cognitive studies have demonstrated that neonates are capable of phonemic discrimination (e.g., Eimas, Siqueland, Jusczyk, & Vigorito, 1971); behavioral and electrophysiological asymmetries have been observed in neonates on tasks involving such phonemic discrimination (e.g., Entus, this volume, Chapter 6; Molfese et al., 1975); and the cortical area likely involved in mediating these linguistic discriminations, namely Wernicke's area, has been consistently observed to have left-sided anatomical bias in neonates as in adults. These findings suggest that the neuroanatomical asymmetry is likely correlated with functional asymmetry, and that it may be a morphological substrate of the functional asymmetry of the hemispheres.

TABLE: 4 Summary of Results of Studies of Anatomical Asymmetry in the Planum Temporale in Infants

Study	Sample size	Age	Measure	Mean Size			Number of cases[a]		
				Left	Right	R/L ratio	L > R	Same	R > L
Teszner, Tzavaras, Gruner, & Hécaen, 1972	1 specimen and 7 iconographs	7–9 months gestational	Length	–	–		6 (75)	1 (12.5)	1 (12.5)
Witelson & Pallie, 1973	14 specimens	1 day–3 months postnatal, (median = 12 days)	Length (cm)	1.9	.9	.57	12 (86)	0	2 (14)
			Area (cm²)	1.9	1.1	.61	11 (79)	3 (21)	0
Wada, Clarke, & Hamm, 1975	100 specimens	Approx. 7 months gestational to 18 months postnatal, ($\bar{X} \doteq 3$ months postnatal)	Area (planimetric units)	20.7	11.7	.67	56 (56) (0 ± 5 units)	32 (32)	12 (12)

[a]Figures in parentheses are percentage of cases.

Studies with Brain-Damaged Children

The first evidence to suggest that speech and language functions are more dependent on left- than right-hemisphere functioning comes from the observation of speech and language functions after apparent unilateral brain damage in childhood. There have been numerous individual reports and summaries of such cases. In general, the study of these children has been of a phenomenological nature, so that details of severity, duration, and type of the aphasic symptoms are usually not documented. However, the reports do consistently indicate a greater frequency of speech loss associated with left- than with right-hemisphere lesions in childhood (e.g., Alajouanine & Lhermitte, 1965; Annett, 1973; Basser, 1962; Byers & McLean, 1962; Dunsdon, 1952; Guttman, 1942; Hécaen, 1976; T. Ingram, 1964; J. McCarthy, 1963). Some of these reports have been reviewed elsewhere (e.g., Hécaen, 1976; Krashen, 1972; and most recently by Dennis & Whitaker, this volume, Chapter 8) this latter chapter also presenting a review of similar but less-known nineteenth-century reports; for further references see NIH Bibliography: Childhood Aphasia, 1973). The studies vary greatly in many respects such as characteristics of the subjects, age at which the lesion was sustained, and the nature and timing of the language assessment. However, a rough estimate of the combined results is that speech loss in childhood is associated more than twice as frequently with left than with right lesions (about 75% versus 30%). These results suggest a greater role of the left hemisphere in mediating speech and language, at least as early as the chronological age at which the earliest language assessments were done, which is approximately 2 years. It is on the basis of such data that Lenneberg (1967, pp. 151, 153) concluded that there must be some left-hemisphere specialization for language by age 2, a speculation that has been frequently overlooked by recent theorists. Lenneberg's other postulate, that left-hemisphere specialization for language is fully developed or firmly established only by puberty, has been given more attention and interpreted by some authors to mean that Lenneberg ruled out the existence of early left-hemisphere specialization, which he did not. These result of greater participation of the left than right hemisphere in speech functions by about 2 years of age, based on the study of brain-damaged children, are consistent with the more recent data based on the newer strategies of studying hemisphere specialization in normal children, as reviewed earlier.

But what of the situation before age 2? In regard to this issue the method of observing speech functions in brain-damaged children is limited and, perhaps because of this, has led to misinterpretation. If there is little or no speech to be interfered with as is usually the case with children before the age of 2, and if objective testing of language comprehension in pre-2-year olds who have sustained brain damage is not done, as is the case in these observational studies, then it is impossible on the basis of such study to determine whether one hemisphere is more involved than the other in language functions at that early stage of development. Given this situation, the most precise conclusion is that there are no data available to indicate whether there is or is not functioning left-hemisphere specialization for language functions prior to age 2. This situation was confounded by the availability of data concerning the status at maturity of speech and language functions of individuals who sustained unilateral lesions before the onset of speech. On the basis of gross observations of adult language in such cases, the results indicated that it made no difference which hemisphere originally sustained the early lesion (e.g., Basser, 1962; Carlson, Netley, Hendrick, & Prichard, 1968; K. Fitzhugh, L. Fitzhugh, & Reitan, 1962; McFie, 1961a). These studies were interpreted as indicating equipotentiality of the two hemispheres for subserving speech, which is logically correct. However, factually it does turn out to be only partially correct, as this equipotentiality appears to have limitations when more precise language analyses are done, as will be discussed in a later section. But these findings were also interpreted to indicate that the left hemisphere was not predominant in mediating language in the first 2 years of life and that there must then be bilateral representation. It is this conclusion that does not necessarily follow. If comparable levels of speech functions are observed later in life, regardless of the side of the early lesion, this finding has relevance for the plasticity of the brain but not for what the functioning neural organization was at the time of the injury. These two situations likely led to the unwarranted hypothesis by Lenneberg (1967, p. 151) and others that left-hemisphere specialization is not present, that is, not operative, in the first years of life. However, the recent studies reported with normal children are providing a beginning for the lacking data for the period from birth to 2 years of age. And so far most of this evidence indicates functioning hemisphere asymmetry from the time of neonatal life.

So, what have been the data that supported the popular notion of no left-hemisphere predominance for speech and language functions in at least the early years of childhood? There are three main sets of data: (1) evidence of a greater role of the right hemisphere in mediating language in early life than at maturity, (2) the apparent equipotentiality of the two hemispheres to eventually subserve speech and language functions following early brain damage, and (3) the ability of speech and language functions to transfer to the right hemisphere following damage to the left hemisphere within some period of childhood but not at maturity. These three hypotheses have been interpreted by many individuals as indicating that functioning left-hemisphere specialization for speech and language functions early in life is impossible. Some have even gone further, saying that the recently observed neonatal anatomical asymmetry in the temporal lobes cannot underlie even potential functional asymmetry in view of the documented hemisphere equipotentiality for and transferability of speech and language functions.

Summary

The data from the various types of studies, involving auditory perception, visual perception, motor performance, and electrophysiological measures, consistently indicate a greater role of the left hemisphere for speech and language functions and for aspects of motor performance in children as young as 3 years of age and possibly even in infancy. In particular, the results from the dichotic and the motor tasks, in terms of both consistency and quantity, provide strong evidence for functioning left-hemisphere specialization at least by age 3, the earliest age repeatedly tested. Further study of children younger than age 3 is clearly needed.

The results from the study of brain-damaged children also suggest that by about 2 years the left hemisphere plays a greater role than the right in speech and language functions. The neuroanatomical data cannot provide information about actual functioning dominance, but they are consistent with the suggestion of very early left hemisphere specialization and do suggest that the potential for left lateralization of language is present at the time of birth.

Considerable attention is currently being given to the issue of what basic cognitive processes constitute the functional specialization of the left hemisphere, for example, linguistic processing (Studdert-Kennedy & Shankweiler, 1970), motor sequencing (Kimura, 1976), analytic processing (Bever, 1975), and sequential processing (Carmon, 1975). What is the nature of left-hemisphere specialization in children? To date the design of most studies with children has been to demonstrate the existence of lateralization, rather than to discern what cognitive process it is that is lateralized. On the basis of the available data it appears that the mediation of phonemic discrimination, speech production, and language functions in general, and the production of motor sequences constitute, at least in part, left-hemisphere specialization in childhood. Further exploration of lateralization of sequential processing in nonmotor tasks and of analytic processing remains to be done.

Greater left- than right-hemisphere functioning for linguistic processing and motor sequencing is certainly present in early childhood and may be present at birth. The question still remains whether this left-hemisphere specialization increases with age, as indicated by Lenneberg (1967) and subsequent theorists. Neonates have been shown to be capable of phonemic discriminations (e.g., Eimas et al., 1971; Trehub & Rabinovitch, 1972) and of speech-associated sequential movements (Condon & Sander, 1974). Once such behavioral and cognitive functions are manifest, they may be asymmetrically processed by the left hemisphere even in neonatal life. It is meaningless, however, to consider lateralization of a function which is not yet in the behavioral and cognitive repertoire of a child as, for example, speech production within the first months of life. Speech develops usually around 1 year, and may then be shown to be mediated predominantly by the left hemisphere. To conclude from this that left-hemisphere specialization was not present during the first year of life is a distortion. What has developed is a cognitive skill and the possibility for its neural lateralization. Obviously what does increase during childhood is the repertoire of cognitive skills acquired by the child. As a cognitive function becomes part of the child's repertoire, if it is mainly dependent on linguistic and sequential processing—considered to be specific functions of the left hemisphere—then that cognitive function may be mediated, at least predominantly, by the left hemisphere. Thus, what develops primarily is cognition, and as more cognitive functions are available to be lateralized to the left hemisphere, they are. In this analysis, then, left-hemisphere specialization does increase in some fashion, but only as a secondary manifestation of cognitive development.

ROLE OF THE RIGHT HEMISPHERE IN THE EARLY
MEDIATION OF SPEECH AND LANGUAGE

As indicated above there are numerous studies reporting more frequent speech loss with left- than with right-sided lesions in children, as is the case with adults. However, the studies also indicate that the child and adult situations are different. Language deficits associated with right-sided damage occur more frequently in children than in adults, approximately 30% in children versus 5 to 10% in adults [calculated from data presented by Zangwill (1967)]. This observed incidence in adults is quite similar to that inferred on the basis of the pattern of speech lateralization in right- and left-handed adults determined by intracarotid sodium amytal testing (B. Milner, 1974; B. Milner, Branch, & Rasmussen, 1964). The difference between children and adults led to the inference that the right hemisphere plays a greater role in language functions in children than in adults. This, in turn, led to the further hypothesis that there is bilateral representation of language in children, at least during some early period of development.

These data derive from the study of clinical cases which by their nature necessarily usually involve imprecise localization of lesions and nonrigorous cognitive testing. The results are of theoretical importance, however, and accordingly deserve critical evaluation. In order to yield unequivocal results concerning early lateralization of speech and language, such data must meet several criteria, some of which have been noted previously by Kinsbourne (1975).

Considerations in the Study of Clinical Cases

Avoiding Bias in the Selection of Cases

There must be an unbiased selection of the cases studied. Summaries of individual case reports found in the literature may be biased, since it is the unusual rather than the expected case which more often is reported. This being so, any estimate of the incidence of children who suffer aphasic symptoms following right-hemisphere damage that is based on such data would be quite invalid. However, the crucial comparison for the present discussion is the relative frequency of such cases in children and in adults. If there is a bias toward reporting unusual cases, there is no reason why this should not also be the case with adults. One might, in fact, expect a greater bias in the case of adults. There are more cases of brain damage in adults than in children that are available for study. Moreover, language loss associated with right-sided lesions at maturity is more unexpected than such loss during childhood. In this connection, note the attention given the report of a right-handed adult who developed some speech (possibly not even propositional speech) subsequent to left hemispherectomy done at maturity due to a late-occurring lesion (A. Smith & Burkland, 1966). There is no reason to assume that any bias in reporting the unexpected is greater for children than for adults. In this context, the data may be used to suggest a greater role of the right hemisphere for language in children than adults.

One approach to circumvent directly any such bias is to study consecutive cases from medical files or unselected cases as they present at a clinic. The few reports that selected their samples in unbiased fashion still report more frequent speech loss associated with right-sided lesions in children than is reported for adults (e.g., Annett, 1973; Byers & McLean, 1962; Hécaen, 1976).

Classifying Side of Lesion

The true extent of the lesion in brain-damaged children is often difficult to define precisely, as it usually is a result of trauma, rather than neurosurgical ablation, and may involve diffuse damage and undiagnosed contracoup. One might suggest that the cases considered to have right-hemisphere lesions also involve left-hemisphere damage and it is the latter factor that is responsible for speech loss. However, the same uncertainty must rest with lesions labeled "left-hemisphere" as "right-hemisphere." The case could just as logically be made that right-sided damage exists in all cases and that right-hemisphere damage is the crucial factor. There is no reason to assume a bias in misclassification of side of lesion, and one remains, therefore, with data, imperfect as they may be, that indicate a greater incidence of speech loss associated with right hemisphere lesions in children than in adults.

Immediacy of Cognitive Assessment

Only the assessment of speech and language functions made immediately following the brain insult can indicate whether the damaged area was involved in mediating speech at the time of the injury and whether hemisphere specialization existed at the age at which the lesion occurred. Many of the reports of speech loss in children do involve immediate assessment (e.g., Alajouanine & Lhermitte, 1965; Basser, 1962; Hécaen, 1976) and thus provide unequivocal evidence that the right hemisphere was, in fact, involved in language functions at the time of the injury. If assessment is made years or even months subsequent to the injury, one possible result is that no deficits will be observed. Such results, however, may reflect the rapid and excellent recovery and the neural plasticity that are possible in children (e.g., McFie, 1961a; Riese & Collison, 1964). They do not provide unequivocal information concerning early neural lateralization of function. This issue is highlighted in the latter study, in which the authors state, and I think incorrectly, that transient language disorders in children cannot be used to indicate cerebral localization of language because recovery is "natural" and "it is the lasting or residual defects which alone indicate cerebral localization [p. 294]." I suggest that it is only

252 Sandra F. Witelson

the transient deficits which may provide evidence of early lateralization of language, and that the lasting deficits indicate cerebral lateralization but, more importantly, the limits of plasticity.

The other possibile result is that, years after the original lesion, an asymmetrical pattern of deficits associated with different lesions may be observed. Such results only indicate that there is functioning asymmetry of the brain at the time of the testing, whether it is during childhood or at maturity, and that there was potential specialization or potential difference between the hemispheres at the time of the original lesion. They do not indicate whether there was functioning hemisphere specialization at the time of the original lesion. Furthermore, if the observed asymmetry is less than that observed in individuals with lesions sustained at maturity, it does not necessarily follow that there is less hemisphere asymmetry in childhood. Rather, the results may reflect the greater plasticity of the younger brain. Studies of this type are exemplified by those of Annett (1973), Kohn and Dennis (1974a), McFie (1961b), and Rudel, Teuber, & Twitchell (1974). However, many authors have incorrectly interpreted these studies as indicating functioning lateralization of cognitive functions as early as the age of the original lesion, which does not necessarily follow.

The Problem of Undeveloped Hand Preference

Handedness has been demonstrated to be correlated at least to some degree with speech lateralization. The patterns of bilateral and right-hemisphere speech representation are more frequent among non-right-handed than among right-handed individuals (e.g., Hécaen & Sauguet, 1971; B. Milner, Branch, & Rasmussen, 1964, 1966). When young children are involved, it is likely too early to discern their hand preference, as indicated in the studies of hand preference reviewed in the previous section. Therefore, there is more chance of including non-right-handed cases in groups of children than in adults. However, the incidence of speech loss associated with right-hemisphere damage in young children is considerably higher than the incidence of right-hemisphere speech in adults. Therefore, it is unlikely that most of the children showing speech loss with right-hemisphere damage are cases of potential right-hemisphere speech representation at maturity.

The Inferences to Be Drawn From Expressive versus Receptive Language Loss

The strongest case for a greater role of the right hemisphere in language in children than in adults may be made by focusing on an analysis of loss of speech production, regardless of any other aphasic impairments that may or may not be present. This is so because in adults, speech production appears to be that aspect of language which is most completely lateralized to the left hemisphere (Gazzaniga & Sperry, 1967; Levy, Nebes, & Sperry, 1971). If one considers the clinical data in this framework, one finds clear evidence of speech loss in many cases of children with right-sided lesions, but, in contrast, speech loss is rarely observed following right-hemisphere damage in right-handed adults. It is usually receptive language loss. Moreover, adults with left-hemisphere damage may show profound and persistent inability to speak even though their right hemisphere is intact (Luria, 1970); and in commissurotomized individuals, the right hemisphere cannot produce any oral speech.

There may be more right-hemisphere participation for receptive language also in children compared to adults. Classically it was thought that receptive language is lateralized to the left hemisphere as completely as is speech production. It has become a challenge to demonstrate any language deficits in right-handed adults that are associated with right-hemisphere lesions sustained at maturity and are not attributable to a general intellectual impairment. However, some evidence is accumulating that even in right-handed adults, the right hemisphere may have some role, albeit limited, in mediating receptive language, not only when it is disconnected from the left hemisphere (Gazzaniga & Hillyard, 1971; Zaidel, 1976a, b), but also in neurologically impaired, but noncommissurotomized individuals (e.g., Brown & Wilson, 1973; Kinsbourne, 1971; Ulatowska & Baker, 1974). And, if the right hemisphere is involved to some degree in receptive language in adults, then why not in children?

It may be, however, that in normal adults only the potential for some language comprehension is present, and that it is not expressed unless an inhibitory effect of the left hemisphere via the corpus collosum is removed (Moscovitch, 1976). Even so, giving the right hemisphere of adults some role or potential role in receptive language the fact remains that, immediately following early damage to the left hemisphere, the child usually has a level of linguistic competence that is higher than that observed for right-handed adults with left-hemisphere damage but with an intact right hemisphere (e.g., Luria, 1970; Penfield & Roberts, 1959) or for adults with a disconnected and intact right hemisphere (Zaidel, 1976a, b).

Summary

There is cause for concern about the possible equivocal nature of the clinical data that indicate greater participation of the right hemisphere in language functions in children than in adults. Nevertheless, in spite of the imperfections of the data, I suggest that there is sufficient evidence to support the position that the right hemisphere has a greater role in processing speech and language functions in children than it has in adults. But its role is less than that of the left hemisphere even in childhood. One remains, therefore, with the position that the left hemisphere is predominant in mediating language functions in the early years, although it is a case of only relative dominance, rather than one of complete dominance. However, hemisphere specialization, in general, may only be a matter of relative predominance of one hemisphere over the other. Remember that in adults for whom left-hemisphere specialization for language is well documented, there also is the possibility that the right hemisphere has some role, albeit limited, in the mediation of some language functions. These data, for both children and adults, support the hypothesis that hemisphere specialization is compatible with bilateral, although unequal, participation of the two hemispheres in processing specific cognitive functions.

The Possibility of Developmental Changes in
Cerebral Organization

If the role of the right hemisphere in mediating language is greater in children than in adults, then this suggests the hypothesis that the functioning neural substrate of language may change with age, specifically, may decrease and become more focused in one hemisphere or, as Kinsbourne and Hiscock (this volume, Chapter 14) have termed such a situation, "shrinkage." Kinsbourne suggests that such a neural event is highly improbable. However, that the neural substrate of a function may change with age, perhaps even decrease with age, is not without precedence. A clear example comes from experimental work with rhesus monkeys. Bilateral lesions made at maturity in the orbital pre-frontal cortex lead to impaired performance on several discrimination—learning tasks. When the same lesions are made in infancy, and in this case specifically in female monkeys, no test deficits are observed in infancy, which suggests that at least at this stage of development, the ablated areas are not necessary for normal performance on this task. However, when these early-lesioned animals reach adolescence (18 months), without any further intervention, they begin to show deficits on these tasks and the deficits persist to maturity (Goldman, Crawford, Stokes, Galkin, & Rosvold, 1974). In similar studies, monkeys of both sexes who sustained bilateral dorsolateral pre-frontal lesions made in infancy do not exhibit such learning deficits until they reach about 2 years of age (Miller, Goldman, & Rosvold, 1973). The results from both of these studies suggest that the early ablated cortex is only necessary for normal performance on these tasks at maturity, and that whatever neural structures mediated the tasks in infancy are no longer sufficient. The neural substrate has changed and possibly decreased. And that is what Lenneberg (1967) suggested for the neural substrate of language between early childhood and adolescence.

EARLY HEMISPHERE EQUIPOTENTIALITY AND
INTERHEMISPHERE TRANSFER OF
SPEECH AND LANGUAGE

Two other sets of data have been interpreted as counterindicative of early left-hemisphere specialization. One is the apparent lack of association between the laterality of early cerebral lesions and language ability at maturity, particularly for those cases in which the lesion occurs before the onset of speech (e.g., Basser, 1962; Carlson et al., 1968; K. Fitzhugh et al., 1962; McFie, 1961a). These results suggest that, at least within the first year of life, there is neural equipotentiality for speech and language functions. Whether it is intrahemisphere or interhemisphere equipo-tentiality is not possible to determine except in those cases in which there is subsequent hemispherectomy. Such plasticity, however, is only one instance of the greater neural plasticity of the immature than mature brain observable in all species (e.g., Kling & Tucker, 1968; Sperry, 1971). However, as previously indicated, the inference that either hemisphere may be able to subserve speech and language functions adequately after early cerebral lesions does not rule out the possibility that there is left-hemisphere lateralization of linguistic functions, albeit very elementary functions, at the time of the injury.

It is noteworthy that, although there is generally considered to be greater plasticity in the immature than mature brain, this is likely so only for certain, probably specific, functions. In some instances, earlier lesions may lead to greater deficits than do later lesions as, for example, for general intelligence or learning ability (Hebb, 1942; Teuber & Rudel, 1962; Witelson, 1966).

The other set of data concerns the phenomenon of the ability of speech and language functions to transfer to the right hemisphere. Most of the evidence comes from cases of children who sustained early brain damage which was followed by therapeutic hemispherectomy usually performed in adolescence. The remarkable phenomenon is that, regardless of whether it is the left or the right hemisphere which is excised, speech and language functions are usually not interfered with at all. Moreover, speech and language functions are often within the normal range. These results provide unequivocal evidence of transfer of speech and language functions to the right hemisphere in individuals who likely would have had left-hemisphere dominance for language had the trauma not occurred (Basser, 1962; Dennis & Kohn, 1975; McFie, 1961a; H. White, 1961). Other relevant data are presented by Rasmussen (1964) based on intracarotid sodium amytal testing in a series of children who suffered speech loss following unilateral left-hemisphere lesions sustained from 2 to 8 years of age. The speech loss provides clearcut proof of at least some left-hemisphere mediation of language at the time of the injury. Years later, after speech functions were regained, the Wada test was done and speech functions were found to be mediated by the right hemisphere in at least some cases, thus providing direct evidence of a shift of language functions to the right hemisphere in these cases.

Some of these reports have been summarized by Krashen (1972). Transfer of speech functions to the right hemisphere definitely may occur. The remaining question is until what age such transfer is possible. Krashen indicates that there is evidence for complete transfer at least until 5 years of age, but that the upper age limit for the occurrence of any transfer is still undetermined. The definitive answer to this question resides in the study of cases that are still too few in number to provide sufficient information. Such cases would entail the following criteria: (1) that the individual be right-handed and have only right-handed family members; (2) that the original lesion occur in the left hemisphere after age 5 but before puberty, the age indicated as critical by Lenneberg (1967); (3) that speech loss follow the lesion, ensuring that the left hemisphere was involved in mediating speech; (4) that speech be regained; and (5) that left hemispherectomy be subsequently carried out. The crucial result would be whether language functions are disrupted or not by the hemispherectomy. The few cases available, which unfortunately do not fulfill all of the above criteria, are discussed by Krashen (e.g., W. Gardiner, Karnosh, McClure, & A. Gardiner, 1955; Hillier, 1954; Obrador, 1964; H. White, 1961). These cases tend to show either no or only some loss of speech following hemispherectomy, but never complete aphasia, suggesting that transfer of at least some speech functions to the right hemisphere is possible after age 5. A more recent report (Van der Vlugt, 1975) indicates that in a case of severe aphasia following left-sided damage in a 14-year-old right-handed boy, excellent recovery occurred over the subsequent year with eventually only a slight receptive disturbance remaining. No peripheral hearing impairment was observed. Coupled with this recovery was a gradual increase in left-ear scores and no change in the relatively lower right-ear scores on verbal dichotic stimulation tasks, suggesting the possibility of right-hemisphere takeover of language functions well after age 5.

Given, however, that transfer of speech is indisputable until at least age 5, how has this been interpreted as evidence incompatible with early left-hemisphere specialization? There may appear to be some face validity to the idea that, if such interhemisphere equipotentiality is not present in adults when specialization is known to exist, then perhaps when such plasticity is operative there is no functioning hemisphere specialization. It is likely that such speculation was considered to receive support from the data indicative of some right-hemisphere representation of language functions in the early years as reviewed earlier. However, a functional relationship, or even a correlation, between hemisphere specialization and interhemisphere equipotentiality is not a conceptual necessity. Yet it has been considered to be such. For example, Krashen states that "very little can be concluded about the ability of the minor hemisphere to assume the language function . . . and thus little about the development of lateralization [1972, p. 25]."

When one considers all the data, such a relationship is not only conceptually unnecessary, but likely also incorrect. Interhemisphere transfer of language functions is clearly possible at least until age 5, yet left-hemisphere specialization, that is, greater participation of the left hemisphere in mediating language and the performance of motor sequences, is clearly and consistently indicated for children as young as 3 years of age and possibly for infants as well. In fact, in the first study of hemisphere specialization in normal young children, Kimura (1963) suggested that the finding of left-hemisphere predominance for speech functions in such young children is not necessarily incompatible with the phenomenon of transferability of speech. There can be functioning specialization as well as plasticity. Even neural systems that are fully developed and well organized by birth, such as the cortical systems for sensory and motor functions, have some plasticity in early life. Recovery of function is greater following early than late lesions in these cortical areas in nonhuman species (e.g., Kennard, 1942) and in humans, as evidenced in the motor deficits associated with cerebral palsy (Towbin, 1960) versus the profound deficits resulting from later brain trauma, and in the paucity of sensory deficits associated with early lesions (Rudel, Teuber, & Twitchell, 1974). However, such recovery may be due to either intrahemisphere plasticity or interhemisphere plasticity associated with greater use of ipsilateral pathways.

The phenomena of transferability of speech and associated interhemisphere plasticity provide crucial sets of data which lie at the bases of the theoretical statements of Lenneberg (1967) and Krashen (1972) concerning the age by which left hemisphere specialization is developed, that is, by puberty or by age 5 years, respectively. Their speculations may well be consistent with more recent data if what was really meant by their terms "lateralization" or "developed lateralization" was, more precisely, firmly established lateralization of speech and language functions to the left hemisphere. Lenneberg (1967, p. 178) did in fact sometimes use the term "firmly established." This term implies a lack of interhemisphere plasticity, which does appear to be the case at some point in development; it does not necessarily imply a lack of prior hemisphere specialization of function, which is not the case.

Transferability of speech may also appear incompatible with the findings of neonatal anatomical asymmetry that indicate more frequent and larger cortical areas in potential language-mediating areas in the left hemisphere (e.g., Witelson & Pallie, 1973). Such anatomical asymmetry indicates, at the least, the possibility of biological preprogramming of and potential for left-hemisphere specialization for language or some cognitive skills; or, at the most, greater participation of the left hemisphere very early in life. In either case, the anatomical asymmetry is not necessarily incompatible with transferability of speech. However, such anatomical asymmetry raises the possibility that interhemisphere equipotentiality for speech and language functions may not be without limits (see Witelson & Pallie, 1973). Zangwill (1964) also suggested this on the basis of clinical behavioral data. Specifically, the prediction is that when the right hemisphere assumes the functions of speech and language subsequent to left-hemisphere damage, the level of its processing may be limited. In contrast, it is generally accepted that language skills are normal in such cases. The conclusion of normal language in such individuals is based on the observations that their speech and language functions appear normal in casual observation and that their verbal IQ scores are often within the normal range—or at least commensurate with their overall intellectual ability. Such verbal assessments are obviously at a gross level, and finer analyses may reveal difficulties. Given what we know about the specific functions of the left hemisphere, one might expect difficulties not so much in size of vocabulary or general verbal comprehension as in the comprehension of syntactic structures that depend largely on sequential analysis.

The position that further language assessment in such cases is not fruitful has typically been based on the fact that it is impossible to determine what the individual's level of language skills would have been without brain damage, therefore ruling out the possibility of any baseline level against which to evaluate any possible deficits. In one approach to this general problem, the performance of each brain-damaged patient was compared to that of his own sibling nearest in age (Woods & Teuber, 1973). Another strategy that allows for investigation of this issue is the study of speech and language functions in comparable groups of individuals with right or left hemispherectomy. In a series of studies, such hemispherectomy patients were carefully assessed for many linguistic skills, including the ability to process the syntactic aspects of language (Dennis & Kohn, 1975; Dennis & Whitaker, 1976, this volume, Chap. 8). Although both groups obtained grossly normal and comparable verbal IQ scores, the individuals who had only a right hemisphere showed more difficulty in the aquisition of word relationships and in syntax than did individuals who had only a left hemisphere. These results suggest that the right hemisphere cannot mediate some aspects of language as well as the left hemisphere, even subsequent to very early transfer of language functions. Therefore, interhemisphere plasticity or equipotentiality for language processing may have some limits, and perhaps one of the limiting factors is different innate biological preprogramming of the language areas, as is evidenced in the gross morphological asymmetry in the temporal lobes.

If transferability of speech does coexist with early left hemisphere specialization, what other factors, if any, may be related to the early existence and the eventual decrease of interhemisphere plasticity? One possible factor may be the role the right hemisphere plays in processing language early in life, which subsequently decreases with age. Another factor may be the specialization of the right hemisphere for its unique cognitive functions, that is, the processing of information in a parallel, holistic, spatial mode. Little attention has been given to early right-hemisphere specialization and even less to the possible interdependence of the two hemispheres in respect to their functional specialization. The decrease of the right hemisphere's role in processing language in early life may be related to a change in the role of the right hemisphere's mediation of its specific type of cognitive processing. Right-hemisphere specialization also likely becomes firmly established by some age, and perhaps then it is no longer able to assume the different and perhaps incompatible cognitive mode for processing language functions. The same neural area may not be able to process information in different modes, that is, have two different types of mechanisms (Lashley, 1937; Levy, 1969). In fact it may be that "cerebral localization is determined by the separation of such incompatible mechanisms [Lashley, 1937, p. 384]."

EARLY SPECIALIZATION OF THE RIGHT HEMISPHERE FOR SPATIAL–HOLISTIC PROCESSING

Specialization of the right hemisphere has been investigated later and given less attention than has specialization of the left hemisphere both in the study of adults and particularly in the study of children.

Studies with Brain-Damaged Children

Deficits in form and space perception are much less obvious than is, for example, speech loss in the daily repertoire of hospital behavior in children after brain damage. Accordingly, phenomenological studies have yielded limited information concerning lateralization of spatial, holistic processing. A few experimental studies have used objective testing to assess spatial deficits in brain-damaged children. However, in all of these studies testing was done many years after the injury, usually in late childhood or adolescence, and therefore the results can only indicate whether right hemisphere specialization for spatial processing was present at the time of testing.

Rudel, Teuber, and Twitchell (1974) observed that a group of 34 children presumed to have early right-hemisphere lesions was more impaired on a spatial task of visual route finding than a comparable group of 11 children with left-sided lesions, all of whom were tested between 7 to 18 years of age. That the spatial deficits were not merely due to a difference in overall intelligence was indicated by a reversed difference between groups on verbal tasks. These results suggest that there is functioning right-hemisphere specialization for aspects of spatial processing at least by the age of testing—but not necessarily within the first year of life as the authors suggest. In another study (Woods & Teuber, 1973), a similar pattern of imparied performance on visual–spatial tasks and better performance on verbal tasks was observed for a group of 17 individuals with known right-hemisphere lesions compared to a group of 19 with known left-hemisphere lesions. The range of age of injury was prenatal to 15 years, and testing was done in each case at least 5 years subsequent to the injury. Therefore, once again the results provide evidence for functioning right-hemisphere specialization by school age at the earliest, but only a potential for such specialization earlier in life.

Kohn and Dennis (1974b) studied a different type of clinic population, individuals who suffered infantile hemiplegia and who subsequently had the diseased hemisphere removed. Testing was usually done at adolescence. They found that those individuals who remained with only a left hemisphere were able to do some spatial tasks but were impaired on later-developing spatial tasks (those that usually develop after age 10) compared to individuals who had only a right hemisphere; similarly, when only the right hemisphere remained, it was some linguistic skills that were deficient (e.g., Dennis & Kohn, 1975). These results clearly indicate the very early potential specialization of the right hemisphere for spatial processing. The issue of functioning right-hemisphere specialization in infancy cannot be answered by the Kohn and Dennis (1974b) study either. But this report is one of the few which demonstrates that interhemisphere plasticity also exists from right to left, that is, that the left hemisphere may assume right hemisphere functions to some degree. However, the results clearly indicate that, again, there are limits to hemisphere equipotentiality: for the left, limits on spatial functions; for the right, limits on language functions, as previously discussed.

Noninvasive Methods with Normal Children

Most of the information concerning specialization of the right hemisphere in children, and the only information concerning the early years of life, comes from recent studies with various tests of lateral perception and electrophysiological

TABLE 5   Summary of Results of Perceptual and Electrophysiological Studies of Right Hemisphere Specialization in Normal Children

Study	Subjects	Stimuli	Response	Score	Results[a]
Nonlinguistic auditory perception					
A. Dichotic stimulation					
Knox & Kimura, 1970	5–8 years old $N = 80$ Girls (G) & Boys (B)	Experiment 1: 1 pair of familiar environmental sounds of 4 sec duration	Free recall. Verbal identification	Number correct per ear	Significant LEA for total group. For individual age–sex subgroups, LEA obtained only for 6- and 7-year-old girls and 7- and 8-year-old boys. No sex difference in laterality.
	5–8 years old $N = 120$ G & B	Experiment 2: 1 pair of familiar environmental sounds of 4 sec duration	Free recall. Verbal identification	Number correct per ear	LEA for total group. Each age–sex subgroup showed greater (but not indicated if significant) left-ear scores except 5-year-old girls. No sex difference in laterality.
		Experiment 3: 1 pair of familiar animal sounds of 4 sec duration	Free recall. Verbal identification	Number correct per ear	Nonsignificant tendency for greater left-ear scores for total group and for all age–sex subgroups except 7-year-old girls and 8-year-old boys. No sex difference in laterality.
Anderson & Barry, 1976	4, 5, 8, and 11 years old $N = 40$ G & B	1 pair of familiar environmental sounds. Length of stimulus not given	Verbal identification of 2 sounds	Number correct per ear. No. of subjects with greater left- or right-ear scores	No ear difference at any age on either measure. No sex analysis.
MacFarlane & Witelson, 1976	9–11 years old $\bar{X} = 10.4$ $N = 28$ G & B	2 pairs of familiar environmental sounds of 200 msec duration; rate = 2 pr/1.2 sec	Point to the pictures of the sounds	Number correct per ear	LEA obtained for the total group. LEA obtained for boys. No ear difference for girls.

Entus, this volume, Chapter 6	$1\frac{1}{2}$–3 months $N = 48$ G & B	1 pair of tones (440 Hz) on piano, viola, bassoon, or cello, of 500 msec duration	Nonnutritive sucking	LEA observed. No sex difference.

B. Monaural stimulation

Bakker, 1967	6–12 years old $N = 120$ G & B	Morse-like sound patterns of 3 to 5 elements	Reproduction of pattern with a buzzer	Significantly more children showed greater left-ear scores. No sex difference in laterality. LEA disappeared by age 10.

C. Electrophysiological measures

Barnet, Vicentini, & Campos, 1974	5–12 months $\overline{X} = 8$ months $N = 16$	Clicks	Amplitude of auditory evoked potentials AEPs recorded from C_3 and C_4 positions	Greater right AEPs observed.
Molfese, Freeman, & Palermo, 1975	Infants $\overline{X} = 5.8$ months $N = 10$ G & B	C-major piano chord, a burst of noise (250–4000 Hz); each 500 msec in duration	Amplitude shift from N_1 to P_2 of AEP from T_3 and T_4	Each of the 10 infants showed a larger right AEP to both stimuli.
	4–11 years old $N = 11$ G & B			Each of the 11 children showed a larger right AEP to the chord, and 9/11 to the noise stimulus.
Gardiner & Walter, 1976	6 months $N = 4$	Continuous segments of music	Power spectral analysis of EEGs from P_3, P_4 and W_1, W_2.	Power spectrum decreased between 3 and 5 Hz for the right hemisphere during music condition.

(continued)

TABLE 5 *(Continued)*

Study	Subjects	Stimuli	Response	Score	Results[a]
Molfese, Nunez, Seibert, & Ramanaiah, 1976	$\overline{X}$ = 48 hours N = 14 G & B	2 speech syllables; 3 nonspeech stimuli including a 500-Hz tone	AEPs from T_3 and T_4 over a 900-msec period		In general, greater AEPs in right hemisphere for nonspeech stimuli and greater AEPs in left hemisphere for speech stimuli.

Form and space perception

A. Haptic modality

Study	Subjects	Stimuli	Response	Score	Results[a]
Witelson, 1974	6–14 years old $\overline{X}$ = 10.7 N = 26 B	1 dichhaptic pair of meaningless shapes	Visual recognition of the 2 shapes	Number correct per hand	Significantly greater accuracy for left-hand objects, (left-hand advantage, LHA) was obtained for total group, but only when subjects not tested previously with a "linguistic" dichhaptic test.
Witelson, 1976a	6–13 years old $\overline{X}$ = 10.5 N = 200 G & B	1 dichhaptic pair of meaningless shapes	Visual recognition of the 2 shapes	Number correct per hand	LHA observed for total group of boys, and for all age subgroups, including the youngest (6–7), except the 8–9 subgroup. LHA not observed for girls of any age subgroup.
Levy & Reid, 1976b	5–8 years old G & B	1 dichhaptic pair of meaningless shapes, as in Witelson, 1974; 1976a	Visual recognition of the 2 shapes	Number correct per hand	LHA observed for boys as early as age 5. LHA not observed for girls until age 8 when a greater left-hand score (significant?) was observed.
Witelson & Gibson, 1976	4–5 years old N = 18 14 B	Unilateral guided stimulation of a circle enclosing a	Match haptic perception to a visual choice	Number correct per hand	No hand difference. No suggestion of any sex difference.

B. Visual modality

Marcel & Rajan, 1975	7–9 years old $N = 20$ G & B	Faces at different exposure durations below 150 msec. Unilateral presentation (U)	Recognition of stimulus from 2 choices	Lowest exposure duration for 3 successive correct responses per field	Significantly briefer exposures obtained for left visual field. Possible sex difference in laterality.
Reitsma, 1975	6, 7, 8 years old $N = 60$	Slanted lines, U	Visual recognition of the correct line	Number correct per field	No field difference.
Witelson, 1976a	6–13 years old $N = 85$ B	Pair of same or different vertically arranged $6mm^2$ pictures of human figures, U	Distinguish same or different	Number pairs correct per field	Significantly greater accuracy for stimuli in left-field obtained for the total group.
Witelson, 1976e	6–14 years old $N = 84$ B	Groups of 3 to 6 dots, U	Oral response. Dot enumeration	Number correct per field	Tendency for greater accuracy for left-field stimuli ($.10 > p > .05$).

C. Electrophysiological Measures

Crowell, Jones, Kapuniai, & Nakagawa, 1973	Newborns $N = 97$ G & B	Binocular stimulation with repetitive light flashes (3/sec)	EEGs from O_1 and O_2 positions	Spectral analysis for photic driving at 3 Hz	Only 36 infants showed photic driving; 18 bilateral, and 18 unilateral, but more (16 versus 2) showed a right-hemisphere response. No sex difference.

[a]LEA (left-ear advantage) and LHA (left-hand advantage) refer only to a significant difference.

measures. Studies with adults have indicated that the special functions of the right hemisphere are manifest in two types of tasks—those requiring the perception of nonlinguistic, holistic, auditory stimuli and those involving spatial, holistic process-ing in the visual and somesthetic modalities. The studies with children, relevant to the right hemisphere, vary greatly in method; they are summarized in Table 5.

Nonlinguistic Auditory Perception

The few studies of dichotic "nonlinguistic" auditory perception in school-age children vary greatly in the stimuli and responses used. The one consistent finding is that right-ear superiority is never observed. In one study (Knox & Kimura, 1970) left-ear superiority was observed, even with stimuli of such long duration that unilateral attention to each channel is quite possible and with the use of a response that required verbal identification. In another apparently similar study (Anderson & Barry, 1976), no ear difference was observed. A third study differed considerably in that the stimuli used were of very short duration (comparable to that of consonant-vowel (CV) syllables) and, therefore, bilateral attention was more likely and a nonverbal response was used. In this case, greater accuracy for left-ear stimuli was again observed, but only for boys (MacFarlane & Witelson, 1976). Left-ear superiority may have been attenuated to some degree in this study, however, due to the time parameters of the presentation of the stimuli. When pairs of stimuli are presented at a rate such that the time between the offset and onset of successive pairs is less than that of the stimulus itself (as is the case in the typical rate of presentation of sets of dichotic digits: two pairs per second with a digit being of about 400 msec duration), the typical response is an ear order of report—that is, first one ear is reported, then the other—maximizing possible ear asymmetry. This has been demonstrated for adults (Bryden, 1962) and for children (Witelson & Rabinovitch, 1971). In the MacFarlane and Witelson (1976) study, the time between pairs (325 msec) was longer than the stimulus duration (200 msec), and, as a result, temporal orders of response—that is, pair by pair—tended to be given, thereby possibly reducing ear asymmetry.

The only other study with school-age children was again very different and used monaural presentation of Morse-like patterns of sounds (Bakker, 1967). A signifi-cant left-ear superiority was observed, but only in the younger boys. Left-ear superiority may be surprising for any subgroup if one considers Morse-code patterns as involving sequential processing and that adults who are naive in the use of Morse code showed right-ear superiority for patterns up to 7 elements in length (Papçun *et al.,* 1974). When longer patterns were used, however, these adults showed a left-ear superiority, suggesting right-hemisphere predominance and holistic processing of the task. Similarly it is possible that the stimuli used in the children's study (3 to 5 elements) were difficult, particularly for the younger boys, and, accordingly, they used a right-hemisphere holistic approach to the task, which was reflected in a left-ear superiority. With age, however, the task may become less difficult and the children may possibly use an analytic approach, as did the adults with simpler stimuli in the Papçun et al. study; then, the left-ear superiority is attenuated. The possible interpretation offered here is of course post hoc, but it once again underlines the difficulty involved when cognitive tasks relevant to left- and right-hemisphere processing are used to assess hemisphere specialization but are not defined a priori as to the cognitive processes involved.

The five studies with infants (one perceptual, four electrophysiological) all report evidence of right-hemisphere specialization for nonlinguistic auditory processing.

Form and Space Perception

The studies of form and space perception in the visual and haptic modalities generally indicate right-hemisphere specialization in children at least as young as 6 years of age, and possibly even in newborns (Crowell, Jones, Kapuniai, & Nakagawa, 1973). Of the nine studies, six reported left-field superiority. Three studies did not find left-field superiority, and in two cases this may have been due to a floor effect. The Witelson and Gibson (1976) study was the last in a series of many pilot studies that attempted to devise a task patterned after dichhaptic stimulation (Witelson, 1974, 1976a) that was simple enough for 3- to 5-year-olds. The final task used, however, was still too difficult, as several children unexpectedly performed at chance level. And in order to make the task sufficiently simple, we resorted to unimanual stimulation, which may be less sensitive than dichhaptic stimulation in reflecting hemisphere differences for those children who did perform above chance level. The task in Reitsma's (1975) study was also very difficult, and performance was just above chance level. In the third study (Witelson, 1976e) a dot enumeration task was used patterned after Kimura's (1966) task with adults, and a left-field superiority was observed which fell just short of the .05 level of significance. However, this task may not be a sufficiently sensitive measure of right-hemisphere specialization, as results with adults have been inconsistent (e.g., Kimura, 1966; McGlone & Davidson, 1973; versus Bryden, 1976).

Sex Differences in Lateralization

Whether a sex difference in laterality for nonlinguistic auditory processing exists is not clear. Knox and Kimura (1970) did not observe any sex differences in laterality although they did find that overall performance was superior for boys than for girls. As in the similar but reversed situation with their verbal dichotic tasks, these findings have been erroneously interpreted as greater right-hemisphere specialization in boys. However, a marked sex difference in laterality was observed in the MacFarlane and Witelson (1976) study, suggesting right-hemisphere specialization for boys but not for girls, comparable to the results of several studies of right-hemisphere specialization for spatial-holistic processing in the visual and tactual modalities.

A sex difference indicating right-hemisphere specialization only in boys, or to a greater extent in boys than in girls, was found in several studies of form perception

(Levy & Reid, 1976b; Witelson, 1976a, and likely in Marcel & Rajan, 1975), although not in the several other studies which looked at the sexes separately. In contrast to the situation for left-hemisphere specialization for language functions, there may be marked sex differences, at least during development, in the neural representation of nonlinguistic, spatial, holistic processing. This situation is somewhat similar to that of adults, in which there is evidence to suggest a lack of right-hemisphere specialization in women for several cognitive tasks (H. Gordon, 1976; Kimura, 1969; Lansdell, 1962; McGlone & Davidson, 1973). A sex difference in left-hemisphere specialization has been observed for adults, but it has been of less magnitude and more a matter of degree (Lake & Bryden, 1976).

Summary

To summarize the situation of right hemisphere specialization during childhood, the evidence strongly indicates greater participation of the right hemisphere in both nonlinguistic auditory perception and visual and haptic spatial perception by at least age 6, and possibly in infancy. Remember also the few studies of motoric asymmetry (see Table 3) which indicated that aspects of motor performance which post hoc may be considered to involve nonsequential, spatial control of hand and finger movements yielded left-hand superiority and, by inference, right-hemisphere specialization in children as young as 3 years of age. There is obvious need for further work with children younger than age 6 with various right-hemisphere type cognitive tasks. Finally, it appears that there is a sex difference in right-hemisphere specialization, in contrast to the lack of sex difference observed for left hemisphere specialization.

The Case of Braille Reading

One other issue concerning right hemisphere specialization in children is relevant here. Several studies have more recently used the reading of Braille as another method to study specialization of the right hemisphere for spatial processing. The rationale is that Braille stimuli must require spatial processing of the dot arrangements and therefore that the observation of a left-hand superiority must reflect right-hemisphere specialization for spatial processing. Most of the studies have found left-hand superiority on some performance measures of Braille reading for various groups of individuals (Critchley, 1953; Harris, Wagner, & Wilkinson, 1976; Hermelin & O'Conner, 1971; Rudel, Denckla, & Spalten, 1974). However, others have found no difference or even right-hand superiority in some instances (Fertsch, 1947; Hermelin & O'Connor, 1971; Lowenfeld, Abel, & Hatlin, 1969; Rudel, Denckla, & Spalten, 1974).

The use of hand asymmetry in Braille reading as an index of hemisphere specialization of cognitive functions assumes that the cognitive processes involved in reading Braille are known: in other words, that Braille reading is the independent variable and lateralization of function is the dependent variable. Yet it is not that clear a priori what cognitive processes are involved in Braille reading. Obviously some spatial and holistic processing must be involved. But Braille is also a language, and it is mainly a phonetically-coded language, with different dot patterns representing different phonemes or speech sounds. Sequential processing is also an important factor in Braille, at the level of both the word and the sentence. Therefore, left-hemisphere processing must also be involved. Thus the cognitive processes, or more precisely, the balance between the different cognitive processes involved in the reading of Braille are not obvious.

Within this framework, the inconsistent results of hand asymmetry in reading Braille may seem more understandable. The reports varied in type of subjects studied, that is, sighted or blind, and, in the latter case, whether of early or late origin. Accordingly, the subjects read different Grade levels of Braille, Grade I Braille (a one-to-one correlation between alphabetical letters and Braille symbols) or Grade II Braille (a contracted form), which may vary in the balance of the cognitive processes they require; they differed in the extent of their experience with Braille and with visual language; and, accordingly, varied in the ability to translate the haptic perceptions into a visual code, which, as is discussed later, may provide more direct access to phonemic associations. They also varied in sex. All these variables may affect the cognitive strategies used in reading Braille. It is suggested, therefore, that until the cognitive processes involved in Braille reading are better elucidated, hand asymmetry in Braille reading should not be used as an index of hemisphere specialization. Our knowledge of hemisphere specialization should be the independent variable, and this information should be used to elucidate the cognitive processes involved in Braille reading.

In the context of behavioral asymmetry on tasks involving dual or both types of cognitive processing, performance on a task of dichhaptic stimulation with letters (Witelson, 1974) may be relevant to the discussion of the cognitive processes involved in Braille. On this particular task, the letters had to be spatially perceived by haptic perception, but also named, and therefore at least some linguistic processing was required. Yet a significant right-hand superiority was not obtained in normal right-handed children. Braille is a language that involves phonetic processing of symbols that require spatial perception via the somesthetic modality, just as ink-writing of English is a language that involves phonetic processing of symbols that require spatial perception via the visual system. Right visual-field superiority is consistently observed for ink words (e.g., M. White, 1969), although left-field superiority has been elicited when the spatial demands of the task are sufficiently increased, as with the use of various forms of typeface such as script (Brooks, 1973; Bryden & Allard, 1976a). In contrast, right-hand superiority is usually not observed for Braille reading; more often left-hand superiority is observed. These results suggest greater left-hemisphere processing for visual language than for Braille and greater right-hemisphere processing for Braille than for visual language. By inference, then, spatial processing may play a greater role in the processing of linguistic stimuli perceived via the tactile modality than via the visual modality (Witelson,

1976b). Moreover, visual symbols may have more direct access to phonemic or auditory representations than do tactile symbols. These speculations suggest that Braille reading may depend on spatial processing more than does visual reading.

A POSSIBLE THEORY OF EARLY CEREBRAL ORGANIZATION INVOLVING LATERALIZATION OF FUNCTION AT BIRTH COEXISTENT WITH INTERHEMISPHERE PLASTICITY

Left Hemisphere Specialization

Potential for Left Lateralization of Language

On the basis of the evidence reviewed above, the following theoretical framework for early cerebral organization is postulated. There is a preprogrammed asymmetrical neural substrate for specific cognitive functions such as rapid, sequential processing of discrete items. Language functions are based on such processes. The genetic neural asymmetry provides the potential for language functions to be lateralized to the left hemisphere in most individuals. This potential is neither immutable nor all-determining. It does not prevent the right hemisphere from assuming a role in speech and language functions in instances in which the normal biological substrate is interfered with, as in the case of sufficiently large or crucially located early damage to left-hemisphere speech areas (B. Milner, 1974), or in instances in which the normal neural system is not present, as in cases of agenesis of the corpus callosum (Selnes, 1974). However, the anatomical bias favoring the left hemisphere may be a limiting factor in the mediation of language by the right hemisphere, with the latter never being able to deal as effectively with language as the former. The postulated focal versus diffuse neural organization of the left and right hemispheres, respectively (Semmes, 1968) is another possibly limiting factor in hemisphere equipotentiality.

Environmental Influences on Lateralization

This potential for a particular pattern of cerebral organization does not rule out the possibility that various environmental factors may play a role in actualizing this neural potential, as is the case, for example, in the visual system (Hirsch & Spinelli, 1970; Wiesel & Hubel, 1965). Evidence that environmental factors, particularly those related to language experience, do play some role comes from the observations that aphasia has been noted to occur equally often in association with left- or right-hemisphere lesions in illiterate adults (Cameron, Currier, & Haerer, 1971; Wechsler, 1976); that illiterate preadolescent children may not show right-ear superiority on verbal dichotic tasks comparable to matched literate children (Khadem, 1976); that right visual-field superiority on tasks involving linguistic processing was not obtained in deaf individuals (McKeever, Hoemann, Florian, & VanDeventer, 1976; Phippard, 1976); that extreme deprivation of exposure to and use of language until puberty as in the case of Genie (Fromkin, Krashen, Curtiss, D. Rigler, & M. Rigler, 1974) is associated with a lack of right-ear superiority on verbal dichotic listening tests; and that children of lower socioeconomic backgrounds, typified by less experience in using language both quantitatively and conceptually (Hunt, 1964), may have less marked right-ear superiority than their middle-class peers. All these results suggest the possibility that less marked left-hemisphere specialization is associated with some decreased experience with language.

Early Functioning of the Asymmetry

Not only is there a built-in potential for left-hemisphere specialization for particular cognitive functions, but there is also functioning asymmetry between the hemispheres right from the start. The left hemisphere has a greater role than the right for some functions in infancy. It is noted that these are two different states, potential asymmetry versus actual asymmetrical functioning.

The phonemic discriminations and sequential movements observed in neonates are likely only part of the behavior that is asymmetrically mediated early in life. With more documentation of the infant's capacity for perception and behavior, more instances of asymmetrically represented functions will likely be elucidated.

Developmental Course of Hemisphere Specialization

Left hemisphere specialization may be functional at birth, similar to Kinsbourne's (1975) suggestion, but this does not necessarily mean that it remains unchanged from infancy to senescence. The present view is that as a cognitive function develops which requires the type of processing for which the left hemisphere is specialized, then that cognitive function and any tasks dependent on such functions will be processed more by the left than the right hemisphere. In this view, what develops primarily is the extent of the child's cognitive repertoire, and as more functions are available to be processed predominantly by the left hemisphere, they are. Thus, with development, left-hemisphere specialization comes to encompass a broader scope of skills for which its particular cognitive mode of sequential, analytic, linguistic processing is particularly suited. In some sense, then, left-hemisphere specialization does increase, but only indirectly, as a secondary manifestation of cognitive development.

Is the age of 5 years a crucial point for hemisphere specialization as Krashen (1972) suggests? Krashen supports his hypothesis with data from several sources, such as the decreased incidence of speech loss associated with right-hemisphere lesions sustained after age 5 and the reduced plasticity in transfer of speech functions to the right hemisphere apparently after age 5. Recent work by Zaidel (1976a,b) provides further support for the importance of age 5 in the neural representation of language. Zaidel has been able to further explore the extent of language capacity of the disconnected right hemisphere with the use of a new stabilized visual image technique. The results indicate that the lowest level of language ability evidenced by the right hemisphere in commissurotomized individuals appears to be around the 4-to-5-year level, but it also may be no higher than the 12-year level—puberty age—an age which will be mentioned again below.

However, functioning specialization of the left hemisphere certainly exists before age 5. And some interhemisphere plasticity does seem to occur well after age 5. Therefore, it is unlikely that age 5 is either the beginning or the end stage of hemisphere specialization. Within the present theoretical framework of the relationship between hemisphere specialization and cognitive development, age 5, however, may be important as a critical age at which some cognitive skills are developed—as Krashen suggests, those skills underlying primary language learning. This speculation is supported by a report, based on behavioral studies (S. White, 1965), that indicates that numerous linguistic and cognitive abilities reach full development between the ages of 5 and 7 years. Thus, perhaps age 5 is one developmental landmark in the lateralization of cognitive skills to the left hemisphere. This implies however, in contrast to Krashen's (1972) hypothesis, that other cognitive skills are still to be learned and to be lateralized to the left hemisphere, and that interhemisphere plasticity is still possible, although perhaps never as completely as before age 5.

At what point in development is there no longer any acquisition of new mental abilities? Many theorists concerned with intellectual development (e.g., Hebb, 1942; Piaget & Inhelder, 1969; Terman & Merrill, 1937) have suggested that the end of adolescence is associated with the termination of increasing development of qualitatively new intellectual or cognitive functions. Obviously, learning occurs during adult life, but this hypothesis suggests that adult learning is more a matter of change in quantity than quality, and that it involves further learning based on already acquired cognitive skills or mental abilities. If this is so, then puberty may well be the age, as Lenneberg (1967) suggested, when left-hemisphere specialization stops developing, albeit indirectly—as a result of no further increase in the acquisition of relevant new skills. And perhaps it is at this stage of final acquisition of such species-specific cognitive skills, that neural localization of functions becomes firmly established. Specifically, it may be that it is at this time that left-hemisphere cognitive functions can no longer be assumed by other neural areas, such as the right hemisphere.

The association of the completion of the acquisition of complex species-specific behavior and lack of lateral neural plasticity may have an analogous situation in the neural control of bird song in the chaffinch. In the adult, sectioning of the left hypoglossal nerve results in loss of bird song, with little recovery, whereas right hypoglossectomy does not affect bird song. In contrast, early lesions of either nerve do not interfere with song learning, which suggests that plasticity may still be present and that either nerve may develop the dominant control for song (Nottebohm, 1970). However, as various stages of song are learned, neural plasticity decreases, and, once full song has developed, plasticity is no longer evident (Nottebohm, 1971, 1972).

It is unlikely, however, that it is only factors concerning the left hemisphere which are relevant in determining whether interhemisphere functional plasticity is possible. Also important, and perhaps even more so, is the neural and functional state of the right hemisphere. It appears that the right hemisphere plays a considerable role in language mediation in the early years, much greater than at maturity. It is also known that the right hemisphere has a predominant role in nonlinguistic, holistic, spatial processing at least as early as age 6, and possibly even in infancy. But there are insufficient data to reveal whether marked changes in the right hemisphere are occuring at particular ages, such as age 5 or puberty. What is known however is that the major part of the myelination of the corpus callosum is complete by about 6 years of age and that complete myelination of these tracts occur around age 10 (Yakovlev & Lecours, 1967). To the extent that interhemisphere inhibition and facilitation affect the lateralization of particular functions to each hemisphere and the possibility of interhemisphere transfer of functions, these data support the importance of both age 5 and puberty.

The view presented here is quite consistent with aspects of Lenneberg's theory (1967, pp. 178, 374). He suggested that all behavior including language is "the outward manifestation of physiological and anatomical interactions, under the impact of environmental stimulation;" that "language is the manifestation of species-specific cognitive propensities;" and that "cerebral lateralization becomes firmly established" at the termination of the critical period for language acquisition. It is also consistent with Chomsky's (1976) view of language. He suggests a genetic competence, a biological "organ for language," for specific skills, which allows for the development of language. What is added in the present theory is that there is functioning left-hemisphere dominance in the first few years of life. It is also explicitly stated that such early specialization is not incompatible with early equipotentiality and interhemisphere plasticity.

The recent demonstrations that chimpanzees can be taught various forms of gestural and visual language (e.g., R. Gardner & B. Gardner, 1969; Premack, 1971; Rumbaugh, Gill, & von Glasersfeld, 1972) are not incompatible with the present views. The ultimate level of the chimpanzee's conceptual information processing and, accordingly, ability to use a symbol system is certainly less than that of man. But studies have shown that these animals do have some ability to make phonemic discriminations (e.g., Morse and Snowdon, 1975) and to respond differentially to sequenced stimuli that differ only in the order of elements, which is indicative of the ability to execute sequential processing. Therefore, that they should be able to learn some behavior that is similar to human receptive and expressive language is not inconsistent with the present speculations concerning human language. In this context, the finding in monkeys of a greater role of the left hemisphere in mediating complex auditory tasks involving discrimintion of critical temporal factors (Dewson, 1976), and the observation of anatomical asymmetry in the region of the temporal lobes in chimpanzees, similar to although less in degree than that in man (Yeni-Komshian & Benson, 1976) are not inexplicable and may have important significance for the evolution of language.

Bilateral Substrate for Language

As indicated, the right hemisphere also has some role in the mediation of language in the early years. This means that to some degree there is early bilateral representation of language. Bilateral involvement, however, does not necessarily mean equal involvement. The situation appears to be that the right hemisphere has some role in processing speech and language, but less than that of the left even in the early years. Therefore, particularly in the early years, right-hemisphere mediation of language may coexist with left-hemisphere predominance in linguistic processing. The fact, however, that the right hemisphere has some role in mediating language early in life, and under some circumstances also at maturity, suggests the existence of a neural substrate for language in the right hemisphere, albeit, less developed or less efficient.

The extent of linguistic processing by the right hemisphere in adults is still not certain. However, it does appear to be less than in children. In this respect, there may be a bona fide increase in the degree of left-hemisphere predominance or specialization for language. To date we have little direct evidence of such a change from the study of either normal or brain-damaged children. But the crucial years of this change may be within the first few years of life and our present methods of studying lateralization of function in those years may still be too limited and insensitive to assess the change. It might be fruitful to extend studies such as that of Berlin *et al.* (1973) to children aged 2 to 5 years, to ascertain whether the magnitude of ear asymmetry changes in this age range. The decrease of the right hemisphere's role in language may result from an increase in inhibitory influences from the left hemisphere via the corpus callosum (Moscovitch, 1976). Such a role of the corpus callosum may be one factor underlying the observation of less lateralization of functions, particularly of language functions, in patients with agenesis of the corpus callosum (Selnes, 1974). The decrease of the right hemisphere's role in mediating language may be related also to an increased commitment to its role in mediating its own cognitive processes.

Right Hemisphere Specialization

Potential and Functioning Specialization

There are many large lacunae in our knowledge concerning right-hemisphere specialization. The little available evidence from individuals with early unilateral lesions and from hemispherectomy patients indicates that the laterality of early lesions is associated with the adult-like pattern of cognitive deficits. This suggests that there must be a genetic potential for the right hemisphere to mediate nonlinguistic spatial functions.

Actual functioning of right-hemisphere specialization appears to be present by at least 6 years of age and possibly in infancy. It is possible that right-hemisphere specialization develops in a sense similar to that of the left hemisphere: namely, that with age more cognitive skills are learned which are best processed by the specific cognitive mode of the right hemisphere and, accordingly, are then processed predominantly by the right hemisphere.

We have almost no evidence to indicate whether the left hemisphere plays an early role in spatial processing analogous to the right hemisphere's early role for language functions. In addition, there is little evidence concerning the possibility, extent, and age limits of transfer of spatial functions to the left hemisphere following early right-sided damage. From the study of cases with hemispherectomy, it is clear that the left hemisphere does have some potential to mediate at least some spatial functions after early extensive damage to the right hemisphere. To this extent, then, there may be some potential substrate for nonlinguistic, spatial processing in the left hemisphere. However, the potential of the left hemisphere to mediate spatial processing appears to be limited. It appears that each hemisphere has limitations in mediating its nonnative functions and when it is forced to process two cognitive modes, its "native" specific functions suffer least.

Sex Differences in Lateralization

There appears to be a sexual dimorphism in the neural representation of nonlinguistic spatial processing. Although not all studies have shown a sex difference, those that do consistently indicate greater specialization of the right hemisphere in males than females and this may be more marked in children than adults (for review, see Witelson, 1976a).

Interdependence of Left and Right Hemisphere Specialization

There is little evidence concerning the neural representation of spatial processing when language functions shift to the right hemisphere in individuals other than those with hemispherectomy. Does the right hemisphere then mediate both cognitive functions? If so, does this affect the level of either or both cognitive functions? There is even less information concerning the reverse situation.

Lansdell's (1969) study of individuals known to have speech functions represented in the right hemisphere (via the Wada test) subsequent to left hemisphere damage indicates that spatial functions are more impaired than verbal functions if the damage occurred before age 5. The impairment is greater the earlier the lesion occurred. In contrast, after age 5, verbal skills are more impaired. These results may suggest that right-hemisphere specialization may be more firmly established earlier than is left-hemisphere specialization. This hypothesis is not identical, but is similar to the suggestion that the right hemisphere is functionally more active or more mature than the left in the first few years of life, with the reverse situation occurring after the onset of speech (Brown & Jaffe, 1975; Carmon, Harishanu, Lowinger, & Lavy, 1972; D. Taylor & Ounsted, 1972). This hypothesis is in contrast to the more popular belief that if there is any primacy in hemisphere specialization, it must be for the left hemisphere.

The apparent sex difference in right-hemisphere specialization is relevant here. If the right hemisphere does mature earlier than the left, this may be so particularly for boys. This may be a factor in why developmental language disorders occur consistently more frequently in boys than in girls (Witelson, 1976a). The right hemisphere may be less plastic earlier in development in boys than in girls and, accordingly, less able to assume linguistic functions in the case of dysfunction in the left hemisphere. It may also be a contributing factor as to why the right hemisphere appears to have a greater role in linguistic processing in women than in men. The less-specialized right hemisphere in females may be able to assume more linguistic functions.

There is another consideration relevant to equipotentiality and interhemisphere transfer of function. The hemispheres differ not so much in what stimuli they process but in the cognitive modes with which they process information. The same task may be processed by each hemisphere, but with a different cognitive strategy (e.g., Bogen, 1969; Geffen *et al.,* 1972). It is not known to what extent right-hemisphere representation of language may be processed in a parallel–holistic fashion or to what extent left-hemisphere processing of spatial tasks employs verbal encoding and sequential strategies. Luria, several decades before the present English translation (Luria, 1970), indicated that recovery of function involved not only other cortical areas but also different cognitive approaches to the same task. A recent specific example is that of an adult who suffered dyslexia as a result of a left-hemisphere injury and who was subsequently deliberately taught to read with a spatial, holistic or "look-say" approach. It appears that she now reads via right-hemisphere processing and a visual, holistic strategy, but without phonetic decoding as she previously used (Carmon, personal communication, 1976).

Individual Differences

Although there is a typical pattern of hemisphere specialization for the majority of individuals, there are individual differences. Left-handed individuals—perhaps only a subgroup, such as those with a familial history of sinistrality (e.g., Hécaen & Sauguet, 1971) or those with noninverted hand posture in writing (Levy & Reid, 1976a)—may have different patterns of cerebral organization, particularly in respect to speech representation. This may lead to differential patterns of cognitive abilities (Levy, 1969; McGlone & Davidson, 1973).

The sexes also appear to have different patterns of lateralization, with males showing greater specialization in general. This, too, may lead to some of the observed cognitive differences in verbal and spatial skills between the sexes (L. Harris, 1976). However, any relationship between cerebral organization and cognitive skills must involve factors not yet elucidated. It is difficult to see how greater bihemisphere representation of language may be associated with lower spatial ability in women than in men, whereas greater bihemisphere representation of spatial functions may be associated with at least equal language functions in women and men.

What of individuals with developmental disorders, many of which involve language skills, notably developmental dyslexia? It has been a long-standing hypothesis that abnormal cerebral dominance underlies this clinical syndrome. Recent evidence suggests that dyslexic boys may, in fact, have a different pattern of hemisphere specialization than that typically observed for normal boys of comparable age (Witelson, 1976c, 1977). It appears that the problem may be due not to the left hemisphere showing a lack of specialization but, rather, to both hemispheres being involved in spatial processing, which results in overuse of the spatial, holistic cognitive mode. This neural and concomitant cognitive situation may underlie their cognitive difficulties.

Summary. There likely is a preprogrammed potential for each hemisphere to process specific cognitive functions. Environmental factors may influence the actualization of this potential. Specialization of each hemisphere is likely operative in infancy. Left-hemisphere specialization in the early years coexists with some, but relatively less, participation of the right hemisphere in linguistic processing. Interhemisphere plasticity occurs well after hemisphere specialization is manifest. Plasticity may decrease in stages, closely linked to the emergence of species-specific mental abilities at different stages of development. The right hemisphere may lose its plasticity earlier in development than the left. The possible mechanisms of a genetic, hormonal, neural, and environmental nature that determine hemisphere specialization, both in the normal and in the abnormal state remain to be explored.

ACKNOWLEDGMENTS

The writing of this chapter and the author's research were supported in part by the Ontario Mental Health Foundation Research Grant No. 322. I thank Diane Clews for her skill and devotion in executing a difficult typing task, Janice Swallow for her careful editing of parts of this chapter, and Susan Denburg for many thoughtful comments on earlier versions of the manuscript. And I am indebted to Henry C. Witelson for his help and generous acceptance of my absence . . . and my presence during the preparation of the manuscript.

REFERENCES

Alajouanine, Th., & Lhermitte, F. (1965) Acquired aphasia in children. *Brain, 88,* 653–662.
Anderson, A., & Barry, W. (1976) The development of cerebral dominance in children attending regular school classes, special classes for the mentally retarded and special schools for the mentally retarded. Manuscript submitted for publication.
Annett, M. (1970) The growth of manual preference and speed. *British Journal of Psychology, 61,* 545–558.
Annett, M. (1973) Laterality of childhood hemiplegia and the growth of speech and intelligence. *Cortex, 9,* 4–33.
Bakker, D.J. (1967) Left-right differences in auditory perception of verbal and non-verbal material by children. *Quarterly Journal of Experimental Psychology, 19,* 334–336.

Bakker, D.J. (1969) Ear-asymmetry with monaural stimulation: Task influences. *Cortex, 5,* 36–42.

Barnet, A.B., Vicentini, M., & Campos, M. (1974) EEG sensory evoked responses (E.Rs) in early infancy malnutrition. *Neuroscience Abstracts.* Fourth Annual Meeting of the Society for Neuroscience, St. Louis, Miss., Oct. 20–24. (Abstract) No. 43, p. 130.

Basser, L.S. (1962) Hemiplegia of early onset and the faculty of speech with special reference to the effects of hemispherectomy. *Brain, 85,* 427–460.

Bayley, N. (1969) *The Bayley Scales of infant development. Manual.* New York: Psychological Corporation.

Belmont, L., & Birch, H.G. (1963) Lateral dominance and right-left awareness in normal children. *Child Development, 34,* 257–270.

Benton, A.L., Levin, H.S., & Varney, N.R. (1973) Tactile perception of direction in normal subjects. Implications for hemispheric cerebral dominance. *Neurology, 23,* 1248–1250.

Berlin, C.I., Hughes, L.F., Lowe-Bell, S.S., & Berlin, H.L. (1973) Dichotic right ear advantage in children 5 to 13. *Cortex, 9,* 394–402.

Berlin, C.I., & McNeil, M.R. (1976) Dichotic listening. In N.J. Lass (Ed.), *Contemporary issues in experimental phonetics.* New York: Academic Press.

Bever, T.G. (1971) The nature of cerebral dominance in speech behaviour of the child and adult. In R. Huxley & E. Ingram (Eds.), *Language acquisition: Models and methods.* New York: Academic Press. Pp. 231–261.

Bever, T.G. (1975) Cerebral asymmetries in humans are due to the differentiation of two incompatible processes: Holistic and analytic. In D. Aaronson & R.W. Rieber (Eds.), Developmental psycholinguistics and communication disorders. *Annals of the New York Academy of Sciences, 263,* 251–262.

Bever, T.G., & Chiarello, R.J. (1974) Cerebral dominance in musicians and nonmusicians. *Science, 185,* 537–539.

Bogen, J.E. (1969) The other side of the brain I: Dysgraphia and dyscopia following cerebral commissurotomy. *Bulletin of the Los Angeles Neurological Society, 34,* 73–105.

Borowy, T.D., & Satz, P. (1973) Developmental parameters of the ear asymmetry phenomenon: The effects of sex, race, and socioeconomic class. Unpublished doctoral dissertation, Univ. of Florida. See Satz *et al.,* 1975.

Branch, C., Milner, B., & Rasmussen, T. (1964) Intracarotid sodium amytal for the lateralization of cerebral speech dominance. *Journal of Neurosurgery, 21,* 399–405.

Brinkman, J., & Kuypers, H.G.J.M. (1972) Splitbrain monkeys: cerebral control of ipsilateral and contralateral arm, hand and finger movements. *Science, 176,* 536–539.

Broadbent, D.E., & Gregory, M. (1969) Accuracy of recognition for speech presented to the right and left ears. *The Quarterly Journal of Experimental Psychology, 16,* 359–360.

Brooks, L.R. (1973) Treating novel stimuli in a verbal manner. Paper presented as part of a symposium, M.P. Bryden (Chm.), Recent work on perceptual asymmetry and its relation to hemispheric organization, at the 44th Annual Meeting of the Eastern Psychological Association, Washington, D.C., May 3–5.

Brown, J.W., & Jaffe, J. (1975) Hypothesis on cerebral dominance. *Neuropsychologia, 13,* 107–110.

Brown, J.W., & Wilson, F.R. (1973) Crossed aphasia in a dextral. A case report. *Neurology, 23,* 907–911.

Bryden, M.P. (1962) Order of report in dichotic listening. *Canadian Journal of Psychology, 16,* 291–299.

Bryden, M.P. (1970) Laterality effects in dichotic listening: Relations with handedness and reading ability in children. *Neuropsychologia, 8,* 443–450.

Bryden, M.P. (1976) Response bias and hemispheric differences in dot localization. *Perception and Psychophysics, 19,* 23–28.

Bryden, M.P., & Allard, F. (1976a) Visual hemifield differences depend on typeface. *Brain and Language, 3,* 191–200.

Bryden, M.P., & Allard, F. (1976b) Dichotic listening and the development of linguistic processes. In M. Kinsbourne (Ed.), *Hemispheric asymmetries of function.* New York: Cambridge Univ. Press. In press.

Bryden, M.P., Allard, F., & Scarpino, F. (1973) Unpublished studies. Univ. of Waterloo. See Bryden & Allard, 1976b.

Buffery, A.W.H. (1970) Sex differences in the development of hand preference, cerebral dominance for speech and cognitive skill. *Bulletin of British Psychological Society, 23,* 233.

Buffery, A.W.H. (1971) Sex differences in the development of hemispheric asymmetry of function in the human brain. *Brain Research, 31,* 364–365.

Buffery, A.W.H., & Gray, J.A. (1972) Sex differences in the development of spatial and linguistic skills. In C. Ounsted & D.C. Taylor (Eds.), *Gender differences. Their ontogeny and significance.* London: Churchill Livingstone. Pp. 123–157.

Byers, R.K., & McLean, W.T. (1962) Etiology and course of certain hemiplegias with aphasia in childhood. *Pediatrics, 29,* 376–383.

Cameron, R.F., Currier, R.D., & Haerer, A.F. (1971) Aphasia and literacy. *British Journal of Disorders of Communication, 6,* 161–163.

Caplan, P.J., & Kinsbourne, M. (1976) Baby drops the rattle: Asymmetry of duration of grasp by infants. *Child Development, 47,* 532–534.

Carlson, J., Netley, C., Hendrick, E.B., & Prichard, J.S. (1968) A reexamination of intellectual disabilities in hemispherectomized patients. *Transactions of the American Neurological Association, 93,* 198–201.

Carmon, A. (1975) The two human hemispheres acting as separate parallel and sequential processors. In G. Iubar (Ed.), *Signal analysis and pattern recognition in biomedical engineering.* New York: Wiley. Pp. 219–232.

Carmon, A. (1976) Personal communication.

Carmon, A., Bilstrom, D.E., & Benton, A.L. (1969) Thresholds for pressure and sharpness in the right and left hands. *Cortex, 5,* 27–35.

Carmon, A., Harishanu, Y., Lowinger, E., & Lavy, S. (1972) Asymmetries in hemispheric blood volume and cerebral dominance. *Behavioral Biology, 7,* 853–859.

Carmon, A., Kleiner, M., & Nachshon, I. (1975) Visual hemifield effects in dichoptic presentation of digits. *Neuropsychologia, 13,* 289–295.

Cattell, P. (1950) *The measurement of intelligence of infants and young children.* New York: Psychological Corporation.

Černáček, J., & Podivinský, F. (1971) Ontogenesis of handedness and somatosensory cortical response. *Neuropsychologia, 9,* 219–232.

Chomsky, N. (1976) On the nature of language. In S. Harnad, H. Steklis, & J. Lancaster (Eds.), Origins and evolution of language and speech. *Annals of the New York Academy of Sciences, 280,* 46–57.

Churchill, J.A., Igna, E., & Senf, R. (1962) The association of position at birth and handedness. *Pediatrics, 29,* 307–309.

Clifton, C. Jr., & Bogartz, R.S. (1968) Selective attention during dichotic listening by preschool children. *Journal of Experimental Child Psychology, 6,* 483–491.

Clyma, E.A., & Clarke, P.R.F. (1973) Which hand draws a better square? *Bulletin of the British Psychological Society, 26,* 141.

Cohen, A.I. (1966) Hand preference and developmental status of infants. *The Journal of Genetic Psychology, 108,* 337–345.

Cohen, G. (1972) Hemispheric differences in a letter classification task. *Perception and Psychophysics, 11,* 139–142.

Condon, W.S., & Sander, L.W. (1974) Neonate movement is synchronized with adult speech: Interactional participation and language acquisition. *Science, 183,* 99–101.

Critchley, M. (1953) Tactile thought with special reference to the blind. *Brain, 76,* 19–35.

Crowell, D.H., Jones, R.H., Kapuniai, L.E., & Nakagawa, J.K. (1973) Unilateral cortical activity in newborn humans: An early index of cerebral dominance? *Science, 180,* 205–208.

Curry, F.K.W. (1967) A comparison of left-handed and right-handed subjects on verbal and non-verbal dichotic listening tasks. *Cortex, 3,* 343–352.

Dalby, M. (1975) Air studies of speech-retarded children, evidence of early lateralization of language-function. *Abstracts.* First International Congress of Child Neurology, Toronto, Ont., Oct. 6–10. (Abstract) No. 46, p. 23.

Darby, R., & Satz, P. (1973) Developmental dyslexia: a possible lag mechanism. Unpublished Master's thesis, University of Florida. (see Satz et al., 1975)

Denckla, M.B. (1973) Development of speech in repetitive and successive finger-movements in normal children. *Developmental Medicine and Child Neurology, 15,* 635–645.

Denckla, M.B. (1974) Development of motor co-ordination in normal children. *Developmental Medicine and Child Neurology, 16,* 729–741.

Dennis, M., & Kohn, B. (1975) Comprehension of syntax in infantile hemiplegics after cerebral hemidecortication: Left-hemisphere superiority. *Brain and Language, 2,* 472–482.

Dennis, M., & Whitaker, H.A. (1976) Language acquisition following hemidecortication: Linguistic superiority of the left over the right hemisphere. *Brain and Language, 3,* 404–433.

Dewson, J.H., III. (1976) Preliminary evidence of hemispheric asymmetry of auditory function in monkeys. In S. Harnad, R.W. Doty, L. Goldstein, J. Jaynes, & G. Krauthamer (Eds.), *Lateralization in the nervous system.* New York: Academic Press. Pp. 63–74.

Dimond, S.J., & Beaumont, J.G. (Eds.) (1974) *Hemisphere function in the human brain.* London: Paul Elek.

Donchin, E., Kutas, M., & McCarthy, G. (1976) Electrocortical indices of hemispheric utilization. In S. Harnad, R.W. Doty, L. Goldstein, J. Jaynes, & G. Krauthamer (Eds.), *Lateralization in the nervous system.* New York: Academic Press. Pp. 339–384.

Dorman, M.F., & Geffner, D.S. (1974) Hemispheric specialization for speech perception in six-year-old black and white children from low and middle socioeconomic classes. *Cortex, 10,* 171–176.

Dunsdon, M.I. (1952) *The educability of cerebral palsied children.* London: Newnes.

Eimas, P.D., Siqueland, E.R., Jusczyk, P., & Vigorito, J. (1971) Speech perception in infants. *Science, 171,* 303–306.

Fedio, P., & Van Buren, J.M. (1974) Memory deficits during electrical stimulation of the speech cortex in conscious man. *Brain and Language, 1,* 29–42.

Fedio, P., & Weinberg, L.K. (1971) Dysnomia and impairment of verbal memory following intracarotid injection of sodium amytal. *Brain Research, 31,* 159–168.

Fertsch, P. (1947) Hand dominance in reading Braille. *American Journal of Psychology, 60,* 335–349.

Fitzhugh, K.B., Fitzhugh, L.C., & Reitan, R.M. (1962) Wechsler-Bellevue comparisons in groups with "chronic" and "current" lateralized and diffuse brain lesions. *Journal of Consulting Psychology, 26,* 306–310.

Forgays, D.G. (1953) The development of differential word recognition. *Journal of Experimental Psychology, 45,* 165–168.

Freud, S. (1968) *Infantile cerebral paralysis.* Translated by L.A. Russin. Coral Gables, Florida: Univ. of Miami Press.

Fromkin, V.A., Krashen, S., Curtiss, S., Rigler, D., & Rigler, M. (1974) The development of language in Genie: A case of language acquisition beyond the "Critical Period". *Brain and Language, 1,* 81–107.

Gardiner, M.F., Schulman, C., & Walter, D.O. (1974) Facultative EEG asymmetries in infants and adults. In Cerebral dominance, *Brain Information Service Conference Report,* No. *34,* Los Angeles, Univ. of California. Pp. 37–39.

Gardiner, M.F., & Walter, D.O. (1976) Evidence of hemispheric specialization from infant EEG.

In S. Harnad, R.W. Doty, L. Goldstein, J. Jaynes, & G. Krauthamer (Eds.), *Lateralization in the nervous system*. New York: Academic Press. Pp. 481–502.

Gardiner, W., Karnosh, L., McClure, C., & Gardiner, A. (1955) Residual function following hemispherectomy for tumor and infantile hemiplegia. *Brain, 78*, 487–502.

Gardner, R.A., & Gardner, B.T. (1969) Teaching sign language to a chimpanzee. *Science, 165*, 664–672.

Gazzaniga, M.S. (1970) *The bisected brain*. New York: Appleton.

Gazzaniga, M.S., & Hillyard, S.A. (1971) Language and speech capacity of the right hemisphere. *Neuropsychologia, 9*, 273–280.

Gazzaniga, M.S., & Sperry, R.W. (1967) Language after section of the cerebral commissures, *Brain, 90*, 131–148.

Geffen, G., Bradshaw, J.L., & Nettleton, N.C. (1972) Hemispheric asymmetry: Verbal and spatial encoding of visual stimuli. *Journal of Experimental Psychology, 95*, 25–31.

Geffner, D.S., & Dorman, M.F. (1976) Hemispheric specialization for speech perception in four-year-old children from low and middle socio-economic classes. *Cortex, 12*, 71–73.

Geffner, D.S., & Hochberg, I. (1971) Ear laterality performance of children from low and middle socioeconomic levels on a verbal dichotic listening task. *Cortex, 7*, 193–203.

Geschwind, N., & Levitsky, W. (1968) Human brain: Left-right asymmetries in temporal speech region. *Science, 161*, 186–187.

Gesell, A., & Amatruda, C.S. (1940) *The first five years of life, a guide to the study of the preschool child*. Part Three. New York: Harper.

Gesell, A., & Ames, L.B. (1947) The development of handedness. *The Journal of Genetic Psychology, 70*, 155–175.

Ghent, L. (1961) Developmental changes in tactual thresholds on dominant and nondominant sides. *Journal of Comparative and Physiological Psychology, 54*, 670–673.

Gilbert, J.H.V. (1976) Dichotic listening in children 2 to 3 CA: A note. *Neuropsychologia*, in press.

Goldman, P.S., Crawford, H.T., Stokes, L.P., Galkin, T.W., & Rosvold, H.E. (1974) Sex-dependent behavioral effects of cerebral cortical lesions in the developing rhesus monkey. *Science, 186*, 540–542.

Goodglass, H. (1967) Binaural digit presentation and early lateral brain damage. *Cortex, 3*, 295–306.

Goodglass, H. (1973) Developmental comparison of vowels and consonants in dichotic listening. *Journal of Speech and Hearing Research, 16*, 744–752.

Gordon, H.W. (1970) Hemispheric asymmetries in the perception of musical chords. *Cortex, 6*, 387–398.

Gordon, H.W. (1974a) Auditory specialization of the right and left hemispheres. In M. Kinsbourne & W.L. Smith (Eds.), *Hemispheric disconnection and cerebral function*. Springfield, Illinois: Charles C. Thomas. Pp. 126–136.

Gordon, H.W. (1974b) Olfaction and cerebral separation. In M. Kinsbourne & W.L. Smith (Eds.), *Hemispheric disconnection and cerebral function*. Springfield, Illinois: Charles C. Thomas. Pp. 137–154.

Gordon, H.W. (1976) Hemisphere asymmetry for dichotically presented chords in musicians and non-musicians, males and females. Manuscript submitted for publication.

Guttman, E. (1942) Aphasia in children. *Brain, 65*, 205–219.

Harris, A.J. (1958) *Harris Tests of lateral dominance*. (3rd ed.) New York: Psychological Corporation.

Harris, L.J. (1976) Sex differences in spatial ability: Possible environmental, genetic, and neurological factors. In M. Kinsbourne, (Ed.), *Hemispheric asymmetries of function*. New York: Cambridge Univ. Press. In press.

Harris, L., Wagner, N., & Wilkinson, J. (1976) Hand difference in Braille discrimination by blind and sighted subjects. Paper presented at the Fourth Annual Meeting of the International Neuropsychology Society, February 5–7.

Hayashi, T., & Bryden, M.P. (1967) Ocular dominance and perceptual asymmetry. *Perceptual and Motor Skills, 25*, 605–612.

Hebb, D.O. (1942) The effect of early and late brain injury upon test scores, and the nature of normal adult intelligence. *Proceedings of the American Philosophical Society, 85*, 275–292.

Hécaen, H. (1976) Acquired aphasia in children and the ontogenesis of hemispheric functional specialization. *Brain and Language, 3*, 114–134.

Hécaen, H., & Sauguet, J. (1971) Cerebral dominance in left-handed subjects. *Cortex, 7*, 19–48.

Hermelin, B., & O'Connor, N. (1971) Functional asymmetry in the reading of Braille. *Neuropsychologia, 9*, 431–435.

Heron, W. (1957) Perception as a function of retinal locus and attention. *American Journal of Psychology, 70*, 38–48.

Hicks, R.E., Provenzano, F.J., & Rybstein, E.D. (1975) Generalized and lateralized effects of concurrent verbal rehearsal upon performance of sequential movements of the fingers by the left and right hands. *Acta Psychologia, 39*, 119–130.

Hillier, W. (1954) Total left hemispherectomy for malignant glioma. *Neurology, 4*, 718–721.

Hirsch, H.V.B., & Spinelli, D.N. (1970) Visual experience modifies distribution of horizontally and vertically oriented receptive fields in cats. *Science, 168*, 869–887.

Hiscock, M., & Kinsbourne, M. (1976) Perceptual and motor measures of cerebral lateralization in children. Paper presented at the 37th Annual Meeting of the Canadian Psychological Association, Toronto, Ont., June 9–11.

Hochberg, F.H., & LeMay, M. (1975) Arteriographic correlates of handedness. *Neurology, 25*, 218–222.

Hunt, J. McV. (1964) The psychological basis for using pre-school enrichment as an antidote for cultural deprivation. *Merrill-Palmer Quarterly of Behavior and Development, 10*, 209–248.

Inglis, J., & Sykes, D.H. (1967) Some sources of variation in dichotic listening performance in children. *Journal of Experimental Child Psychology, 5*, 480–488.

Ingram, D. (1975a) Motor asymmetries in young children. *Neuropsychologia, 13*, 95–102.

Ingram, D. (1975b) Cerebral speech lateralization in young children. *Neuropsychologia, 13*, 103–105.

Ingram, T.T.S. (1964) *Paediatric aspects of cerebral palsy.* Edinburgh: Livingstone.

Jarvella, R.J., Herman, S.J., & Pisoni, D.B. (1970) Laterality factors in the recall of sentences varying in semantic constraint. *Journal of the Acoustical Society of America, 47*, 76(A).

Jasper, H.H. (1932) A laboratory study of diagnostic indices of bilateral neuromuscular organization in stutterers and normal speakers. *Psychological Monographs, 43*, (Whole No. 194) 72–174.

Kennard, M.A. (1942) Cortical reorganization of motor function: Studies on series of monkeys of various ages from infancy to maturity. *Archives of Neurological Psychiatry, 48*, 227–240.

Khadem, F. (1976) Unpublished studies on illiteracy and cerebral dominance. McGill Univ.

Kimura, D. (1961a) Some effects of temporal lobe damage on auditory perception. *Canadian Journal of Psychology, 15*, 156–165.

Kimura, D. (1961b) Cerebral dominance and the perception of verbal stimuli. *Canadian Journal of Psychology, 15*, 166–171.

Kimura, D. (1963) Speech lateralization in young children as determined by an auditory test. *Journal of Comparative and Physiological Psychology, 56*, 899–902.

Kimura D. (1966) Dual functional asymmetry of the brain in visual perception. *Neuropsychologia, 4*, 275–285.

Kimura D. (1967) Functional asymmetry of the brain in dichotic listening. *Cortex, 3*, 163–178.

Kimura, D. (1969) Spatial localization in left and right visual fields. *Canadian Journal of Psychology, 23,* 445–457.

Kimura, D. (1973) Manual activity during speaking–1. Right-handers. *Neuropsychologia, 11,* 45–50.

Kimura, D. (1976) The neural basis of language qua gesture. In H. Avakian-Whitaker & H.A. Whitaker (Eds.), *Studies in neurolinguistics.* Vol. 2. New York: Academic Press. Pp. 145–156.

Kimura, D., & Durnford, M. (1974) Normal studies on the function of the right hemisphere in vision. In S.J. Dimond & J.G. Beaumont (Eds.), *Hemisphere function in the human brain.* London: Elek Science. Pp. 25–47.

Kimura, D., & Vanderwolf, C.H. (1970) The relation between hand preference and the performance of individual finger movements by left and right hands. *Brain, 93,* 769–774.

Kinsbourne, M. (1971) The minor cerebral hemisphere. *Archives of Neurology, 25,* 302–306.

Kinsbourne, M. (1972) Eye and head turning indicates cerebral lateralization. *Science 176,* 539–541.

Kinsbourne, M. (1973) The control of attention by interaction between the cerebral hemispheres. In S. Kornblum, (Ed.), *Attention and performance IV.* New York: Academic Press. Pp. 239–256.

Kinsbourne, M. (1975) The ontogeny of cerebral dominance. In D. Aaronson & R.W. Rieber (Eds.), Developmental psycholinguistics and communication disorders. *Annals of the New York Academy of Sciences, 263,* 244–250.

Kinsbourne, M., & Cook, J. (1971) Generalized and lateralized effects of concurrent verbalization on a unimanual skill. *Quarterly Journal of Experimental Psychology, 23,* 341–345.

Kinsbourne, M., Hotch, D., & Sessions, T. (1976) Unpublished studies. Univ. of Toronto. See Kinsbourne and Hiscock, this volume, Chapter 14.

Kinsbourne, M., & McMurray, J. (1975) The effect of cerebral dominance on time sharing between speaking and tapping by preschool children. *Child Development, 46,* 240–242.

Kinsbourne, M., & Smith, W.L. (Eds.) (1974) *Hemispheric disconnection and cerebral function.* Springfield, Illinois: Charles C. Thomas.

Kling, A., & Tucker, T.J. (1968) Sparing of function following localized brain lesions in neonatal monkeys. In R.L. Isaacson (Ed.), *The neuropsychology of development.* New York: Wiley. Pp. 121–145.

Knights, R.M., & Moule, A.D. (1967) Normative and reliability data on finger and foot tapping in children. *Perceptual and Motor Skills, 25,* 717–720.

Knox, C., & Kimura, D. (1970) Cerebral processing of nonverbal sounds in boys and girls. *Neuropsychologia, 8,* 227–237.

Kohn, B., & Dennis, M. (1974a) Patterns of hemispheric specialization after hemidecortication for infantile hemiplegia. In M. Kinsbourne & W.L. Smith (Eds.), *Hemispheric disconnection and cerebral function.* Springfield, Illinois: Charles C. Thomas. Pp. 34–47.

Kohn, B., & Dennis, M. (1974b) Selective impairments of visuo-spatial abilities in infantile hemiplegics after right cerebral hemidecortication. *Neuropsychologia, 12,* 505–512.

Krashen, S.D. (1972) Language and the left hemisphere. *UCLA Working Papers in Phonetics, 24,* 1–72.

Krashen, S.D. (1975) The critical period for language acquisition and its possible bases. In D. Aaronson & R.W. Rieber (Eds.), Developmental psycholinguistics and communication disorders. *Annals of the New York Academy of Sciences, 263,* 211–224.

Lake, D.A., & Bryden, M.P. (1976) Handedness and sex differences in hemispheric asymmetry. *Brain and Language, 3,* 266–282.

Lansdell, H. (1962) A sex difference in effect of temporal-lobe neurosurgery on design preference. *Nature, 194,* 852–854.

Lansdell, H. (1969) Verbal and nonverbal factors in right-hemisphere speech: Relation to early neurological history. *Journal of Comparative and Physiological Psychology, 69,* 734–735.

Lashley, K.S. (1937) Functional determinants of cerebral localization. *Archives of Neurological Psychiatry, 38,* 371–387.

Lechelt, E.C., & Tanne, G. (1976) Laterality in the perception of successive tactile pulses. *Bulletin of the Psychonomic Society, 7,* 452–454.

LeMay, M. (1976) Morphological cerebral asymmetries of modern man, fossil man and nonhuman primate. In S. Harnad, H. Steklis, & J. Lancaster (Eds.), Origins and evolution of language and speech. *Annals of the New York Academy of Sciences, 280,* 349–366.

Lenneberg, E. (1967) *Biological foundations of language.* New York: Wiley.

Leong, C.L. (1976) Lateralization in severely disabled readers in relation to functional cerebral development and synthesis of information. In R. Knights & D. Bakker, (Eds.), *The neuropsychology of learning disorders: theoretical approaches.* Baltimore, Maryland: University Park Press. Pp. 221–231.

Levy, J. (1969) Possible basis for the evolution of lateral specialization of the human brain. *Nature, 224,* 614–615.

Levy, J., Nebes, R.D., & Sperry, R.W. (1971) Expressive language in the surgically separated minor hemisphere. *Cortex, 7,* 49–58.

Levy, J., & Reid, M. (1976a) Variations in writing posture and cerebral organization. *Science, 194,* 337–339.

Levy, J., & Reid, M. (1976b) Unpublished studies. Univ. of Pennsylvania.

Liepmann, H. (1908) Drei aufsätze aus dem apraxiegebiet. Berlin: Karger.

Ling, A.H. (1971) Dichotic listening in hearing-impaired children. *Journal of Speech and Hearing Research, 14,* 793–803.

Lomas, J., & Kimura, D. (1976) Intrahemispheric interaction between speaking and sequential manual activity. *Neuropsychologia, 14,* 23–33.

Lowenfeld, B, Abel, G., & Hatlen, P. (1969) *Blind children learn to read.* Springfield, Illinois: Charles C. Thomas.

Luria, A.R. (1970) *Traumatic aphasia. Its syndromes, psychology and treatment.* Translated by D. Bowden. Paris: Mouton. Pp 49–76.

Maccoby, E.E., & Konrad, K.W. (1966) Age trends in selective listening. *Journal of Experimental Child Psychology, 3,* 113–122.

MacFarlane, R., & Witelson, S.F. (1976) Verbal and nonverbal dichotic listening in boys and girls. Unpublished studies.

Marcel, T., Katz, L., & Smith, M. (1974) Laterality and reading proficiency. *Neuropsychologia, 12,* 131–139.

Marcel, T., & Rajan, P. (1975) Lateral specialization for recognition of words and faces in good and poor readers. *Neuropsychologia, 13,* 489–497.

McCarthy, J.J. (1963) Referred to in Pribram, K.H., Neurological Theory and Research on Aphasia. In C. E. Osgood & M.S. Miron (Eds.), *Approaches to the study of aphasia.* Urbana, Illinois: Univ. of Illinois, Press. P. 50.

McFie, J. (1961a) The effects of hemispherectomy on intellectual functioning in cases of infantile hemiplegia. *Journal of Neurology, Neurosurgery and Psychiatry, 24,* 240–249.

McFie, J. (1961b) Intellectual impairment in children with localized post-infantile cerebral lesions. *Journal of Neurology, Neurosurgery and Psychiatry, 24,* 361–365.

McGlone, J., & Davidson, W. (1973) The relation between cerebral speech laterality and spatial ability with special reference to sex and hand preference. *Neuropsychologia, 11,* 105–113.

McKeever, W.F., Hoemann, H.W., Florian, V.A., & VanDeventer, A.D. (1976) Evidence of minimal cerebral asymmetries for the processing of English words and American sign language in the congenitally deaf. *Neuropsychologia, 14,* 413–423.

McKeever, W.F., & Huling, M.D. (1970) Lateral dominance in tachistoscopic word recognitions of children at two levels of ability. *Quarterly Journal of Experimental Psychology, 22,* 600–604.

McKeever, W.F., and Huling, M.D. (1971) Lateral dominance in tachistoscopic word recognition performances obtained with simultaneous bilateral input. *Neuropsychologia, 9,* 15–20.

McKinney, J.P. (1967) Handedness, eyedness and perceptual stability of the left and right visual fields. *Neuropsychologia, 5,* 339–344.

McRae, D.L., Branch, C.L., & Milner, B. (1968) The occipital horns and cerebral dominance. *Neurology, 18,* 95–98.

Miller, E.A., Goldman, P.S., & Rosvold, H.E. (1973) Delayed recovery of function following orbital prefrontal lesions in infant monkeys. *Science, 182,* 304–306.

Miller, L.K., & Turner, S. (1973) Development of hemifield differences in word recognition. *Journal of Eductional Psychology, 65,* 172–176.

Milner, B. (1962) Laterality effects in audition. In V.B. Mountcastle (Ed.), *Interhemispheric relations and cerebral dominance.* Baltimore: Johns Hopkins Univ. Press. Pp. 177–195.

Milner, B. (1974) Hemispheric specialization: Scope and limits. In F.O. Schmitt & F.G. Worden (Eds.), *The neurosciences, third study program.* Cambridge, Massachusetts: MIT Press. Pp. 75–89.

Milner, B., Branch, C., & Rasmussen, T. (1964) Observations on cerebral dominance. In A.V.S. De Reuck & M. O'Connor (Eds.), *Disorders of language (Ciba Foundation Symposium).* London: Churchill, Pp. 200–241.

Milner, B., Branch, C., & Rasmussen, T. (1964) Observations on cerebral dominance. In A. V. S. some non-right-handers. *Transactions of the American Neurological Association, 91,* 306–308.

Milner, P.M. (1970) *Physiological psychology.* New York: Holt. Pp. 171–174.

Molfese, D.L. (1976) The ontogeny of cerebral asymmetry in man: Auditory evoked potentials to linguistic and non-linguistic stimuli. In J.E. Desmedt (Ed.), *Recent developments in the psychobiology of language: The cerebral evoked potential approach.* London: Oxford Univ. Press. In press.

Molfese, D.L., Freeman, R.B., Jr., & Palermo, D.S. (1975) The ontogeny of brain lateralization for speech and nonspeech stimuli. *Brain and Language, 2,* 356–368.

Molfese, D.L., Nunez, V., Seibert, S.M., & Ramanaiah, N.V. (1976) Cerebral asymmetry: Changes in factors affecting its development. In S. Harnad, H. Steklis, & J. Lancaster (Eds.), Origins and evolution of language and speech. *Annals of the New York Academy of Sciences, 280,* 821–833.

Morse, P.A. & Snowdon, C.T. (1975) An investigation of categorical speech perception by rhesus monkeys. *Perception and Psychophysics, 17,* 9–16.

Moscovitch, M. (1976) On the representation of language in the right hemisphere of right-handed people. *Brain and Language, 3,* 47–71.

Mountcastle, V.B. (Ed.) (1962) *Interhemispheric relations and cerebral dominance.* Baltimore: Johns Hopkins Univ. Press.

Nachshon, I., & Carmon, A. (1975) Hand preference in sequential and spatial discrimination tasks. *Cortex, 11,* 123–131.

Nagafuchi, M. (1970) Development of dichotic and monaural hearing abilities in young children. *Acta Otolaryngology, 69,* 409–414.

National Institute of Health (1973) Information Centre for Hearing, Speech, and Disorders of Human Communication, Bibliography, 1-1078, *Childhood Aphasia.* The Johns Hopkins Medical Institutions, Baltimore, Maryland.

Neville, H. (1975) The development of cerebral specialization in normal and congenitally deaf children: An evoked potential and behaviorial study. Paper presented at the Third Annual Meeting of the International Neuropsychology Society, Tampa, Florida, Feb. 5–7.

Nottebohm, F. (1970) Ontogeny of bird song. *Science, 167,* 950–956.

Nottebohm, F. (1971) Neural lateralization of vocal control in a Passerine bird. I. Song. *The Journal of Experimental Zoology, 177,* 229–261.

Nottebohm, F. (1972) Neural lateralization of vocal control in a Passerine bird. II. Subsong, calls, and a theory of vocal learning. *The Journal of Experimental Zoology, 179,* 35–49.

Obrador, S. (1964) Nervous integration after hemispherectomy in man. In G. Schaltenbrand & C.N. Woolsey (Eds.), *Cerebral localization and organization.* Madison: Univ. of Wisconsin Press. Pp. 133–154.

Olson, M.E. (1973) Laterality differences in tachistoscopic word recognition in normal and delayed readers in elementary school. *Neuropsychologia, 11,* 343–350.

Orton, S.T. (1928) A physiological theory of reading disability and stuttering in children. *New England Journal of Medicine, 199,* 1046–1052.

Papçun, G., Krashen, S., Terbeek, D., Remington, R., & Harshman, R. (1974) Is the left hemisphere specialized for speech, language and/or something else? *Journal of the Acoustical Society of America, 55,* 319–327.

Pearlman, A.L. (1975) Anatomy and physiology of central visual pathways. In R.A. Moses (Ed.), *Adler's Physiology of the eye. Clinical application. (6th Ed.).* St. Louis: Mosby. Pp. 420–452.

Penfield, W., & Roberts, L. (1959) *Speech and brain-mechanisms.* Princeton, New Jersey: Princeton Univ. Press.

Phippard, D. (1976) Hemifield differences in visual perception in deaf and hearing subjects. Manuscript submitted for publication.

Piaget, J., & Inhelder, B. (1969) *The psychology of the child.* New York: Basic Books.

Pizzamiglio, L., & Cecchini, M. (1971) Development of the hemispheric dominance in children from 5 to 10 years of age and their relations with the development of cognitive processes. Abstract. *Brain Research, 31,* 363–364.

Polyak, S. (1957) *The vertebrate visual system.* Chicago: Univ. of Chicago Press.

Porter, R.J., Jr., & Berlin, C.I. (1975) On interpreting developmental changes in the dichotic right-ear advantage. *Brain and Language, 2,* 186–200.

Posner, M.I., & Mitchell, R.F. (1967) Chronometric analysis of classification. *Psychological Review, 74,* 392–409.

Premack, D. (1971) Language in chimpanzee? *Science, 172,* 808–822.

Rasmussen, T. (1964) In discussion following O.L. Zangwill. The current status of cerebral dominance. In *Disorders of communication, Association for Research in Nervous and Mental Disease, 42,* 113–115.

Reitan, R.M. (1971) Sensorimotor functions in brain-damaged and normal children of early school age. *Perceptual and Motor Skills, 33,* 655–664.

Reitsma, P. (1975) Visual asymmetry in children. In *Lateralization of brain functions.* Boerhaave Committee for Postgraduate Education. The Netherlands: Univ. of Leiden Press. Pp. 85–98.

Riese, W., & Collison, J. (1964) Aphasia in childhood reconsidered. *Journal of Nervous and Mental Diseases, 138,* 293–295.

Risberg, J., Halsey, J.H., Wills, E.L., & Wilson, E.M. (1975) Hemispheric specialization in normal man studied by bilateral measurements of the regional cerebral blood flow—A study with the 133 Xe inhalation technique. *Brain, 98,* 511–524.

Rudel, R., Denckla, M., & Spalten, E. (1974) The functional asymmetry of Braille letter learning in normal sighted children. *Neurology, 24,* 733–738.

Rudel, R.G., Teuber, H.-L., & Twitchell, T.E. (1974) Levels of impairment of sensori-motor functions in children with early brain damage. *Neuropsychologia, 12,* 95–108.

Rumbaugh, D.M., Gill, T.V., & von Glasersfeld, E.C. (1972) Reading and sentence completion by a chimpanzee (Pan). *Science, 183,* 731–733.

Satz, P. (1976) Laterality tests: An inferential problem. *Cortex,* in press.

Satz, P., Bakker, D.J., Teunissen, J., Goebel, R., & Van der Vlugt, H. (1975) Developmental parameters of the ear asymmetry: A multivariate approach. *Brain and Language, 2,* 171–185.

Satz, P., Rardin, D., & Ross, J. (1971) An evaluation of a theory of specific developmental dyslexia. *Child Development, 42,* 2009–2021.

Schulman-Galambos, C. (1976) Hemispheric specialization in school children: Response to dichotically presented words. Manuscript submitted for publication.

Selnes, O.A. (1974) The corpus callosum: Some anatomical and functional considerations with reference to language. *Brain and Language, 1,* 111–139.

Semmes, J. (1968) Hemispheric specialization: A possible clue to mechanisms. *Neuropsychologia, 6,* 11–26.

Seth, G. (1973) Eye-hand co-ordination and 'handedness': A developmental study of visuomotor behaviour in infancy. *The British Journal of Educational Psychology, 43,* 35–49.

Shankweiler, D., & Studdert-Kennedy, M. (1975) A continuum of lateralization for speech perception? *Brain and Language, 2,* 212–225.

Slorach, N., & Noehr, B. (1973) Dichotic listening in stuttering and dyslalic children. *Cortex, 9,* 295–300.

Smith, A., & Burklund, C.W. (1966) Dominant hemispherectomy: Preliminary report on neuropsychological sequelae. *Science, 153,* 1280–1282.

Sobotka, K.R. (1974) Neuropsychological and neurophysiological correlates of developmental dyslexia. Unpublished master's thesis, Univ. of New Orleans, New Orleans, Louisiana.

Sommers, R.K., & Taylor, M.L. (1972) Cerebral speech dominance in language-disordered and normal children. *Cortex, 8,* 224–232.

Sparrow, S., & Satz, P. (1970) Dyslexia, laterality and neuropsychological development. In D.J. Bakker & P. Satz (Eds.), *Specific reading disability: Advances in theory and method.* Rotterdam, The Netherlands: Rotterdam Univ. Press. Pp. 41–60.

Sperry, R.W. (1971) How a developing brain gets itself properly wired for adaptive function. In E. Tobach, L.R. Aronson, & E. Shaw (Eds.), *The biopsychology of development.* New York: Academic Press. Pp. 27–42.

Sperry, R.W., Gazzaniga, M.S., & Bogen, J.H. (1969) Interhemispheric relationships: The neocortical commissures; syndromes of hemisphere disconnection. In P.J. Vinken & G.W. Bruyn (Eds.), *Handbook of clinical neurology. Disorders of speech, perception, and symbolic behavior,* Vol. 4. New York: Wiley. Pp. 273–290.

Spreen, O., Miller, C.G., & Benton, A.L. (1966) The phi-test and measures of laterality in children and adults. *Cortex, 2,* 308–321.

Studdert-Kennedy, M., & Shankweiler, D. (1970) Hemispheric specialization for speech perception. *Journal of the Acoustical Society of America, 48,* 579–594.

Taylor, D.C., & Ounsted, C. (1972) The nature of gender differences explored through ontogenetic analyses of sex ratios in disease. In C. Ounsted & D.C. Taylor (Eds.), *Gender differences: Their ontogeny and significance.* London: Churchill Livingstone. Pp. 215–240.

Taylor, L.B. (1962) Perception of digits presented to right and left ears in children with reading difficulties. Paper presented at Canadian Psychological Association meeting, Hamilton, Ontario.

Terman, L.M., & Merrill, M.A. (1937) *Measuring intelligence.* Boston: Houghton Mifflin.

Teszner, D., Tzavaras, A., Gruner, J., & Hécaen, H. (1972) L'asymétrie droite-gauche du *planum temporale:* Á propos de l'étude anatomique de 100 cerveaux. *Revue Neurologique, 126,* 444–449.

Teuber, H.-L., & Rudel, R.G. (1962) Behavior after cerebral lesions in children and adults. *Developmental Medicine and Child Neurology, 4,* 3–20.

Towbin, A. (1960) *The pathology of cerebral palsy.* Springfield, Illinois: Charles C. Thomas.

Trehub, S.E., & Rabinovitch, M.S. (1972) Auditory-linguistic sensitivity in early infancy. *Developmental Psychology, 6,* 74–77.

Trevarthen, C. (1974a) Conversations with a two month-old. *New Scientist, 64,* 230–235.

Trevarthen, C. (1974b) The psychobiology of speech development. In E.H. Lenneberg, (Ed.),

Language and brain: Developmental aspects. *Neurosciences Research Program Bulletin,* *12,* 570–585.

Turkewitz, G., & Creighton, S. (1974) Changes in lateral differentiation of head posture in the human neonate. *Developmental Psychobiology, 8,* 85–89.

Turkewitz, G., Gordon, E.W., & Birch, H.G. (1965a) Head turning in the human neonate: Spontaneous patterns. *Journal of Genetic Psychology, 107,* 143–158.

Turkewitz, G., Gordon, E.W., & Birch, H.G. (1965b) Head turning in the human neonate: Effect of prandial condition and lateral preference. *Journal of Comparative and Physiological Psychology, 59,* 189–192.

Ulatowska, H.K., & Baker, T. (1974) *Linguistic deficits in right hemisphere lesions.* Paper presented at the Fourth Annual Meeting of the Society for Neuroscience, St. Louis, Missouri, October 20–24, (Abstract) No. *695,* 456.

Van der Vlugt, H. (1975) Dichotic listening. In *Lateralization of brain functions.* Boerhaave Committee for Postgraduate Education. The Netherlands: Univ. of Leiden Press. Pp. 183–200.

Wada, J.A. (1976) Cerebral anatomical asymmetry in infant brains. Paper presented as part of a symposium, D. Kimura (Chm.), *Sex differences in brain asymmetry,* at the 4th Annual Meeting of the International Neuropsychology Society, Toronto, Ontario, February 4–7.

Wada, J.A., Clarke, R., & Hamm, A. (1975) Cerebral hemispheric asymmetry in humans. *Archives of Neurology, 32,* 239–246.

Wada, J.A., & Rasmussen, T. (1960) Intracarotid injection of sodium amytal for the lateralization of cerebral speech dominance: Experimental and clinical observations. *Journal of Neurosurgery, 17,* 266–282.

Walls, G.L. (1951) A theory of ocular dominance. *Archives of Ophthalmology, 45,* 387–412.

Warrington, E.K. (1969) Constructional apraxia. In P.J. Vinken and G.W. Bruyn (Eds.), *Handbook of clinical neurology: Disorders of speech perception, and symbolic behavior.* Vol. 4. New York: Wiley. Pp. 67–83.

Wechsler, A.F. (1976) Crossed aphasia in an illiterate dextral. *Brain and Language, 3,* 164–172.

Weinstein, S. (1968) Intensive and extensive aspects of tactile sensitivity as a function of body part, sex, and laterality. In D.R. Kenshalo (Ed.), *The skin senses.* Springfield, Illinois: Charles C. Thomas. Pp. 195–222.

White, H. (1961) Cerebral hemispherectomy in the treatment of infantile hemiplegia. *Confinie Neurologicia, 21,* 1–50.

White M.J. (1969) Laterality differences in perception: A review. *Psychological Bulletin, 72,* 387–405.

White, M.J. (1973) Does cerebral dominance offer a sufficient explanation for laterality differences in tachistoscopic recognition? *Perceptual and Motor Skills, 36,* 479–485.

White, S. (1965) Evidence for a hierarchical arrangement of learning processes. In L.P. Lipsett & C. Spiker (Eds.), *Advances in child development and behavior.* Vol. 2. New York: Academic Press.

Wiesel, T.N., & Hubel, D.H. (1965) Extent of recovery from the effects of visual deprivation in kittens. *Journal of Neurophysiology, 28,* 1060–1072.

Witelson, S.F. (1962) Perception of auditory stimuli in children with learning problems. Unpublished master's thesis, McGill Univ.

Witelson, S.F. (1966) Learning as a function of cortical damage at different ages. Unpublished doctoral dissertation, McGill Univ.

Witelson, S.F. (1974) Hemispheric specialization for linguistic and nonlinguistic tactual perception using a dichotomous stimulation technique. *Cortex, 10,* 3–17.

Witelson, S.F. (1975) Brain lateralization in children: normal and dyslexic. In *Lateralization of brain functions.* Boerhaave Commission. Leiden, Netherlands. Pp. 122–146.

Witelson, S.F. (1976a) Sex and the single hemisphere: Right hemisphere specialization for spatial processing. *Science, 193,* 425–427.

Witelson, S.F. (1976b) Lateralization issues in haptics. Paper presented as part of a symposium,

J. Kennedy, (Chm), Haptics as a perceptual system, at the 4th Annual Meeting of the Canadian Psychological Association, Toronto, Ontario, June 9–11.

Witelson, S.F. (1976c) Abnormal right hemisphere specialization in developmental dyslexia. In R. Knights & D. Bakker, (Eds.), *The neuropsychology of learning disorders: Theoretical approaches.* Baltimore, Maryland: University Park Press. Pp. 233–255.

Witelson, S.F. (1976d) Verbal dichotic stimulation in 3 to 5 year olds. Unpublished studies.

Witelson, S.F. (1976e) Lateral tachistoscopic studies in children. Unpublished studies.

Witelson, S.F. (1977) Neural and cognitive correlates of developmental dyslexia: age and sex differences. In C. Shagass, S. Gershon, and A. Friedhoff (Eds.) *Psychopathology and brain dysfunction.* New York: Raven, in press.

Witelson, S.F., & Gibson, T. (1976) Right hemisphere specialization in 3 to 5 year olds. Unpublished studies.

Witelson, S.F., & Pallie, W. (1973) Left hemisphere specialization for language in the newborn: Neuroanatomical evidence of asymmetry. *Brain, 96,* 641–647.

Witelson, S.F., & Rabinovitch, M.S. (1971) Children's recall strategies in dichotic listening. *Journal of Experimental Child Psychology, 12,* 106–113.

Witelson, S.F., & Rabinovitch, M.S. (1972) Hemispheric speech lateralization in children with auditory-linguistic deficits. *Cortex, 8,* 412–426.

Wolff, P.H., & Hurwitz, I. (1976) Sex differences in finger tapping: A developmental study. *Neuropsychologia, 14,* 35–41.

Woods, B.T., & Teuber, H.-L. (1973) Early onset of complementary specialization of cerebral hemispheres in man. *Transactions of the American Neurological Association, 98,* 113–117.

Yakovlev, P.I., & Lecours, A.-R. (1967) The myelogenetic cycles of regional maturation in the brain. In A. Minkowski (Ed.), *Regional development of the brain in early life.* Oxford: Blackwell. Pp. 3–70.

Yeni-Komshian, G. (1973) Dichotic listening studies. Unpublished studies.

Yeni-Komshian, G.H., & Benson, D.A. (1976) Anatomical study of cerebral asymmetry in temporal lobe of humans, chimpanzees, and rhesus monkeys. *Science, 192,* 387–389.

Yeni-Komshian, G.H., Isenberg, S., & Goldberg, H. (1975) Cerebral dominance and reading disability: Left visual field deficit in poor readers. *Neuropsychologia, 13,* 83–94.

Zaidel, E. (1976a) Unilateral auditory language comprehension on the token test following cerebral commissurotomy and hemispherectomy. *Neuropsychologia, 15,* 1–17.

Zaidel, E. (1976b) Auditory vocabulary of the right hemisphere following brain bisection or hemidecortication. *Cortex, 12,* 191–211.

Zangwill, O.L. (1964) The current status of cerebral dominance. In Disorders of communication. *Association for Research in Nervous and Mental Disease, 42,* 103–118.

Zangwill, O.L. (1967) Speech and the minor hemisphere. *Acta Neurologica et Psychiatrica Belgica, 67,* 1013–1020.

Zurif, E.B., & Carson, G. (1970) Dyslexia in relation to cerebral dominance and temporal analysis. *Neuropsychologia, 8,* 351–361.

17

Manual Specialization in Infancy: Implications for Lateralization of Brain Function

GERALD YOUNG

The traditional index of handedness is manual preference which involves consistent unilateral usage on daily highly practised tasks. In this sense, most adults are right-handed. However, by manual specialization we mean the differential use of the hands in terms of strategies or processes in dealing with complex tasks in the environment. Picking up the phone with the right hand or performing other common tasks with the right hand tells us nothing about differential skill, since presumably the left hand is capable of doing all these tasks as well. Consequently, it is important to look at specific behaviors on specific tasks that the hands perform when the demand characteristics of the tasks predispose the individual to optimal performance if asymmetric response strategies are employed. Tasks should cover a range so that constraints include both *limitations* on using both hands and *demands* to use both hands but in different ways. In the first case, we measure if the individual adapts to his environment more efficiently with, for example, unilateral as opposed to bimanual reaching. In the second case we determine whether the two hands can coordinate and assume different roles to optimize performance.

Pertinent to this is the need to devise tasks that are relatively more serial or spatial in nature, relatively more or less demanding of fine motor sequencing. Increasingly, research is pointing to *left*-hand superiority in *right*-handers on a variety of tasks involving spatial discrimination and localization (e.g., Nachson & Carmon, 1975, with adults; and Witelson, 1975, with children). Nachson & Carmon (1975) gave right-handed normal adults sequential or spatial sensorimotor discrimination tasks. In the bimanual response mode the right hand performed better on sequential tasks but the left hand excelled on spatial tasks. Findings such as these can only lead us to heed Denckla (1974) who writes that "the age-specific distribution of right–left differences in various motor performances may be a more important aspect of 'lateralization' . . . than are distributions of preference [p. 729] ." This is why the present review speaks more of manual specialization than of handedness.

There is a series of issues involving the development of lateralization of manual behavior and brain functioning in infancy, and the absence of careful longitudinal research precludes their resolution. These issues are now reviewed.

DEVELOPMENT OF LATERALIZATION OF MANUAL BEHAVIOR

Early Studies

The development of manual skills in infancy has been extensively investigated (Touwen, 1971; White, 1969; etc.) and has been related to the development of sensorimotor intelligence (Piaget in particular, e.g., 1963). Nevertheless, the development of differential behavior by the left and right hands has been relatively ignored in the modern era. Studies prior to 1945 tend to have poor methodologies, which minimizes the validity of their results. Samples are small and drawn from institutions. No interobserver reliability is calculated for the behaviors observed. Observation systems are generally limited in size. Task selection is limited as well. Care is not taken in administering the tasks—such as ensuring that objects are presented equally to the left, right, and midline in a randomly determined order by an experimenter holding the object with two hands or suspending it on a string. Statistics are entirely lacking, and data analysis often lumps data across individuals, obscuring individual differences.

Given this cautionary note, a review of the early studies involving more than one or two infants follows, for infants up to 1 year of age. Surprisingly, the right hand seems spontaneously more active than the left hand in the neonatal period (Giesecke, 1936; Stubbs & Irwin, 1933; Valentine & Wagner, 1934; cf. Watson, 1919), although no strength differences are evident (Sherman, Sherman, & Flory, 1936; Watson, 1919). In the first half year of life, on reaching tasks, most studies find either no lateral preference or equal left and right lateral preference (Giesecke, 1936; Halverson, 1931; Lesné & Peycelon, 1934; Lippman, 1927; Shirley, 1931; Voelckel, 1913; Watson, 1919).

Contrary to these findings for reaching, Halverson (1937a, b) found that young infants grasped with the right hand more and clung with the left hand more. Halverson (1937a) pressed rods against the palms of supine infants aged 1 to 24 weeks, scoring closing and grasping (involving a tighter grip than close). I regrouped Halverson's complex data analysis in an effort to find clearer trends than his tables gave. The reanalysis showed that when the infant grasped with one hand, irrespective of whether the other one closed or did nothing, the right hand proved more active throughout except at 12 and 20 weeks. At 12 and 20 weeks, the infant closed more with his right than his left hand when grasping with the left hand was not involved. Clearly, a right-hand preference seems evident. In another study, Halverson (1937b) tested the clinging strength of infants in the first year of life with a rod and spring which he used to lift the infant. Infants seemed stronger with the left hand throughout the first year, according to Halverson. However, closer scrutiny of his data shows that the left hand of girls was clearly stronger only in the first week and that the right hand dominated after the first month. The left hand of boys proved stronger for the first 2 months and at times thereafter.

For the second half year of life, the early studies on the development of differential manual behavior show that right-hand preference for reaching begins to appear, although the trend is not marked and is sometimes entirely absent (Halverson, 1931; Lesné & Peycelon, 1934; Lippman, 1927; Shirley, 1931; Valentine & Wagner, 1934; Voelckel, 1913; cf. Giesecke, 1936; Lederer, 1939). Several studies emphasized the long-term instability of hand preference in the first year of life (Lederer, 1939; Valentine & Wagner, 1934; cf. Giesecke, 1936).

More Recent Studies

The studies done since 1945 are an improvement over earlier ones but still suffer in part from some of the limitations referred to. The modern studies are not numerous; they are described here in greater detail to give a flavor of their methodological approaches.

Studies of Reaching in Early Infancy

Gesell and Ames (1947) examined sitting and supine infants presented objects to the midline. Infants were observed longitudinally and eventually emerged right-handed. The authors coded contacts of objects. No detail is offered of how they determined lateralized scores for contacting. No hand preference was evident for infants of 8 and 12 weeks. However, at 16 to 20 weeks preference was more left-handed; it then oscillated throughout infancy, from left to right to neither. Until 28 weeks, the left hand predominated in most cases when laterality was evident.

Seth's (1973) research supports Gesell and Ames's (1947) view that the left hand is preferred for reaching in early infancy. Seth (1973) examined the development of reaching and manipulation of objects placed on a table before 20- to 52-week-old infants, some of whom were observed longitudinally. The presentation of his data is confusing and individual differences are essentially neglected. Seth noted a clear left-hand preference in the younger subjects and a right-hand preference in the older ones, but there was no one age period where this shift occurred, as it varied with task and type of data analysis. In terms of both relative amounts of visual–motor coordination during activity and success in contacting (grasping, manipulating), the left hand seemed preferred up to 28 weeks when confronted with a cube, up to 32 weeks with a pellet, and sometimes as late as 44 to 52 weeks with a bell, depending upon the particular data analysis examined. In terms of quantity of movements, initial approaches, and the percentage of individuals showing left- or right-hand preference, the left hand was preferred up to 28 weeks for the cube and bell and up to 40 weeks for the pellet. In conclusion, the 28- to 32-week period seems the critical transition point, although Seth did not try to specify a particular period when left-hand reaching transforms into right-hand reaching.

This apparent finding of an initial left-hand reaching in infancy has important implications for the ontogenesis of lateralization of brain functioning. However, it should be noted that in neither Seth's (1973) nor Gesell and Ames's (1947) data were statistics used. When this is done for the one set of data in each study that account for individual differences, all supposed left-hand preferring trends wash out (the binomial test was applied to Table 4, p. 46, in Seth, 1973; and to Figure 1, p. 158, in Gesell & Ames, 1947).

Studies of Grasping in Early Infancy

White (1969) and White, Castle, and Held (1964) observed institution-reared infants longitudinally from 1 to 6 months of age on two tasks: (a) putting an object in the hand (method unspecified), and (b) holding an object before the infant to the left (45°), right, and midline. No mention is made of hand preference for the second task. As for the first one, a preferred hand could be specified for most infants although the scoring procedure for making such a judgment was not described. White (1969) found that infants would watch their preferred hand if it had an object in it during the third month of life; several weeks later, they would stare at an object in their preferred hand, but bring the preferred hand over to explore an object if it was in the nonpreferred hand. Although White did not specify which hand was predominantly preferred, he later revealed it was the right hand (personal communication).

More recently Caplan and Kinsbourne (1976) observed young infants on two task sequences, one where a rattle was placed in one hand on alternate trials and one where identical rattles were placed, one in each hand. The right hand was preferred, both in grasp duration and in trial scores per hand per subject, in the first part of the study but not in the second. However, the result for the first part of the study may be explained in two conflicting ways, as Caplan and Kinsbourne themselves point out. Although they support the idea that the right hand grasped longer because it was attended to more, reflecting a right-hand preference, it may very well be that the left hand dropped the rattle sooner to be free for some other purpose, reflecting a left-hand preference. As for the second part of the study, although no one hand consistently maintained contact longer when each hand held a rattle, it could be that each hand was performing differently. For example, consistent right-hand manipulating and left-hand holding would imply a right-hand preference despite equal contact duration. Nevertheless, taken together, the Halverson (1937a), White (1969), and Caplan and Kinsbourne (1976) studies suggest an early right-hand preference for grasping.

Studies of Reaching in Older Infants

Cohen (1966) observed normal, family-reared 8-month-olds in a hospital setting. Hand preference, shown by reaching for and grasping objects at the midline with the same hand in 9 of 12 trials, was associated with higher Bayley test performance, whereas poorer test performance was related to no hand preference. In addition, in individuals showing hand preference, the right hand was preferred more than the left. Grapin and Perpère (1968) held toys at the midline before seated infants 3 to 15 months of age. Without specifying their criterion of establishing unilateral preference, they report that out of 75 infants with left- or right-hand preference for object contact, 57 were right-hand preferring. However, from their data it is impossible to determine the age when this trend begins, although the mean age for one particular subgroup of right-hand preferring infants was 7 months. Černáček and Podivinský (1971, 1972) examined infants from 3½ months onward when they were trying to seize a small doll presented to the left, right, or midline. Preference was considered manifested if the percentage of left minus right hand seizures exceeded ±10. Of eight infants 7 to 12 months old, three seemed to show a hand preference, all to the right. No differences were found in younger infants. Flament (1973) examined 3- to 12-month-olds in a partly longitudinal study on reaching tasks and tests of possible bimanual coordination (using a cube in a cup, for example). She noted that once the object is reached for and contacted in the reaching tasks there is an adjustment phase of the hand on the object preceding manipulation. This adjusted phase evidenced the first signs of asymmetry in the population studied (5 months), but the direction of asymmetry was not specified. In the second half of the first year, three successive signs of right-hand preference developed. The right hand was used first and more quickly to reach and grasp. Next, it was preferred in terms of precise adjustment movements on objects. Then, more precise movements in fine prehension during bimanual coordination was performed more by the right hand, while the left hand performed more subordinate behaviors. In informal observations, Sherick, Greenman, and Legg (1976) noticed a shift from bilaterality to unilaterality, in reaching at 28 weeks of age. However, they did not specify whether the left or right side was preferred.

The trends across all studies seem to be that the young infant grasps more with the right hand yet may reach more with the left, if a preference is shown. Muir (1976; personal communication, Queen's U., Kingston, Ont.) has found that the left hand is preferred when infants prereach in the first few weeks of life and Chorazyna (1976) describes a shift in the preference from the left to the right hand in a longitudinal study of a baby chimpanzee. By the end of the first year of life and perhaps as early as 7 or 8 months, the right hand is preferred for reaching and begins to show ascendancy in bimanual coordination tasks as well. However, only careful, controlled observations can confirm or disconfirm this global impression and the surprising suggestion that infants may begin life with an initial left-hand preference for reaching.

Author's Investigation

Pilot research (Young & Wolff, 1976) has produced results counter to the trends described in the past research. Normal 15-week-olds were observed in the home, primarily while seated, while trying to reach at distant objects and when objects were in or near the hands. Rather than obtaining overall handedness scores, greater right- or left-hand frequency for a variety of behaviors on each task was calculated for each infant. The main thrust of the results is that, given appropriate tasks and an observation system maximizing possible laterality differences, young infants manifested a right-hand preference for directed swiping and a left-hand preference for nondirected finger—hand movements with no arm activity, especially when a large rattle was held before the infant. The various types of behaviors (manipulating, touching, pinching, holding) performed when objects were in or near the hands were preferred by neither hand. Consistency or stability from task to task and even trial to trial was quite rare, except for directed swiping. Patterns of behavior coordination, that is, either the same or opposite hand being preferred for a pair of behaviors, was especially evident on tasks where objects were held in the infant's hands. Holding was preferred by the opposite hand preferred for manipulating and pinching, whether this hand was the left or the right one. This kind of precursor complementary hand usage both in the reaching and grasping tasks illustrates the importance of taking into account the concept of manual specialization in observing the development of lateralized manual behavior. Since the study concerned a specific age group, it is hard to compare unequivocally with past research. Previous findings of left-handed reaching and right-handed grasping may still be found in early infancy using other ages. Hopefully future studies will be aware of the methodological problems noted earlier in reviewing the past research.

IMPLICATIONS FOR HEMISPHERIC SPECIALIZATION

Contrary to what has previously been thought (Lenneberg, 1967; Zangwill, 1960) the neonate or very young infant is already manifesting a pattern of hemispheric specialization analogous to the adult model (Kinsbourne and Hiscock, Chapter 14, this volume; *per contra*, Bay, 1975; Lenneberg, 1975; Sherick, Greenman, & Legg, 1976). Studies of subtle behavior deficits in hemidecorticates (Dennis, 1975; Dennis & Whitaker, Chapter 8, this volume) and of other patients with early unilateral brain insult (Milner, 1974), as well as anatomical (Wada, Clark, & Hamm, 1975; Witelson & Pallie, 1973) behavioral, and electrophysiological studies of normal infants (Molfese, Freeman, & Palermo, 1975; Chapters 2 and 6, this volume) all suggest an early templating of the hemispheres along adult lines. However, the exact nature of early hemispheric specialization has not been fully elucidated and its developmental course is still subject to debate. The present section details some of these issues about the development of lateralization of brain function and how knowledge of the longitudinal development of manual specialization may help resolve them in part.

Rate of Lateralization of Hemispheric Specialization

Beyond the issue of early hemispheric equipotentiality is the question of the rate of lateralization of brain function. Gazzaniga (1974) argued that such structural–genetic factors as the enlarged temporal planum on the left side of the brain are important antecedents that predispose relatively more right-hand exploration of the environment although the left hand is also extensively used. This slight right bias leads to slightly more engram formation of learning in the left hemisphere, which in turn feeds back to encourage more right- than left-hand exploration. Thus, although the hemispheres are not equipotential at birth, the left hemisphere lead for its typical functions is only slight. Kinsbourne (1975a; and Kinsbourne and Hiscock, Chapter 14) have presented an alternative view to Gazzaniga's; they suggest that the left hemisphere may be very dominant for language functions from early in life onward (*per contra*, Kinsbourne, 1975b). To be more cautious, the left hemisphere may be extensively specialized to deal with linguistic precursors from early in life onward. Then, the described trends of age changes in the effects of left-brain insult on behavioral (especially language) output (Hécaen, 1976) may not be the result of an increasing lateralization of brain function with development but may be because of a progressive loss of plasticity of the right hemisphere as its own fully templated primary functions become increasingly active. Right hemisphere plasticity is lost due to increasing commitment to its own different potentialities (Goldman, 1974), its relative lack of language function experience, and possible inhibition—interference via the corpus callosum from the left hemisphere (Kinsbourne, 1974). There seems to be a scale in the ontogenesis of cerebral functional reorganization (Hécaen, 1976). A similar explanation applies to why the right hemisphere may be functionally active for its particular specialization from early in life onward while the left hemisphere is presumably plastic enough to undertake right-hemisphere functioning early in life, if necessary, with decreasing facility thereafter.

This argument implies either of two possibilities: First, it may be that each hemisphere is dually templated for its own (primary) and the other (secondary) specialization from birth or soon thereafter. The left and right hemispheres become differentially active functionally along the adult (primary) model from early in life onward and gradually realize this direction more while losing the plasticity of their secondary templates. The second possible implication is that each hemisphere is templated early in life only in accord with the adult model—the left hemisphere for language-related phenomena and the right one for space-related phenomena. There is enough lack of commitment of these templated areas and of other zones not preformed which can account for early plasticity. With commitment and opposite hemisphere inhibition, plasticity gradually decreases as described. Both models differ from Gazzaniga's, where lateralization of cerebral functioning is seen as a gradual, continuing process. In the present two models the differences in specialization of the two hemispheres are inherently present in full from early in life onward and await experiential or maturational activation processes to consolidate or commit the different templates, rendering them functional. Kinsbourne (1975b) feels innate congenital lateral-orienting synergisms (e.g., head turning) is involved in this activation. Kinsbourne and Hiscock (Chapter 14) postulate that the innate hemispheric differences described lie in clerical midbrain activity, not in differential hemispheric neuronal organization. Research is needed to verify those conjectures.

Support for either of the two models I have proposed would be that, in early life, aspects of peripheral (especially manual) behavior exhibit scores for novel and practiced tasks comparable in distribution to older children and adults (Annett, 1970; Kinsbourne & Hiscock, Chapter 14, this volume). That is, it should be determined whether distributions of asymmetric manual behavior in infancy follow a normal distribution of relative manual efficiency skewed slightly to the right hand for novel tasks and an inverted U-curve skewed heavily to the right hand (J-curve) for practiced tasks. Along these lines, Caplan and Kinsbourne (1976) argued that, in their study of 3-month-olds' contact duration with rattles, the score distribution complied to a normal curve skewed to the right, as Annett (1970) would predict, fitting with the novelty of this task for the age range concerned. However, the clarity of Caplan and Kinsbourne's data and interpretations can be questioned (see earlier). Other possibly relevant data are that both spontaneous head turning (Turkewitz, Gordon, & Birch, 1965) and tonic neck reflex activity (Gesell & Ames, 1947) in neonates exhibit bimodal J-shaped distributions heavily skewed to the right, analogous to hand-preference distributions for highly practised tasks in older children and adults. However, the relationship between head turning, the tonic neck reflex, manual lateralization of function, and hemispheric specialization is hard to determine specifically. Consequently, to date there seems to be no corroborated direct support in terms of lateralized score distributions of peripheral (especially manual) behavior for or against the concept of a gradual course in the lateralization of brain functioning activation.

A qualification of the nature of the relevant data needed to answer the question of the rate of lateralization follows. Any one behavior need not necessarily show the same distribution throughout the life cycle; such an inference ignores relevant motor, perceptual, and cognitive advancement with age. Rather, it may be that, especially early in life, different behaviors in different tasks will show the relevant distribution at different ages. This hypothesis is consistent with Satz's (Satz, Rardin, & Ross, 1971) conjecture that reading disability may simply reflect a lag in left-hemisphere maturation in the normal hierachical order of acquisition of motor, somatosensory, and, finally, speech lateralization. Moreover, in a further refinement of the problem, Porter and Berlin (1975) have concluded that different aspects of language or language-related skills manifest left-hemisphere lateralization at different ages, depending on their complexity. Reviewing dichotic listening studies in children, they noted that auditory and phonetic processes may exhibit right-ear (left-hemisphere) advantage in younger children to the same extent as older children, whereas more slowly acquired or maturing mnemonic processes may become evidently lateralized only in older children. Different outputs come to reflect the asymmetrically specialized left hemisphere at different ages. The conclusion to this section can only be that careful longitudinal study of central and peripheral lateralization of function is needed.

Left or Right Hemisphere Ascendency

Do left- and right-hemispheric specialization follow the same developmental course or does one or the other lateralize or activate more quickly, or influence behavior more directly? For example, Moscovitch (1976) presents several hypotheses on the development of lateralization of brain function including the following. He predicts that specialization of language-related phenomena in the left hemisphere precedes right-hemisphere specialization for nonlinguistic functions. Research with infants is needed to establish if the assumption is indeed valid. Related to this issue is whether it is the left or the right hemisphere that is generally more mature or functionally active in early infancy (e.g., controls motor output such as manipulation), irrespective of whether it is slower in being fully lateralized for its specialized functions than the other hemisphere is for its own. Based on very little direct observation of normal infant behavior, some investigators support an earlier left-hemisphere maturation (e.g., Corballis & Beale, 1976; Moscovitch, 1976; Steffen, 1975), some an earlier right-hemisphere maturation (Brown & Jaffe, 1975; Carmon, Harishanu, Lowinger, & Lavy, 1972; Fromkin, Krashen, Curtiss, Rigler, & Rigler, 1974; etc.).

Brown and Jaffe (1975) carry this argument one step further. They argue that Gesell and Ames's (1947) and Seth's (1973) findings of an initial preference in infancy for the left hand in reaching lends support to their point of view of an initial right-hemisphere *dominance* in infancy. However, as has been pointed out, Seth's and Gesell and Ames's data do not show a left-hand preference in the reaching of young infants when the data are more carefully analyzed. Brown and Jaffe (1975) offer a variety of other types of arguments, based largely on research with infants, supporting their point of view, but the infant data are not conclusive. For example, they argue that the infant hears mostly nonlinguistic sounds. However, it has been shown that the linguistic processing capacities of infants are well developed early in life (Eimas, 1974; Trehub & Rabinovitch, 1972). Brown and Jaffe (1975) cite Aronson and Rosenbloom (1971), who found visual–auditory spatial integration (a right hemisphere function) in young infants. However, studies by Lyons-Ruth (1975) and McGurk and Lewis (1974) using more careful methodology could not replicate Aronson and Rosenbloom's (1971) results. Brown and Jaffe (1975) point out that the infant turns his head spontaneously to the right (Turkewitz & Creighton, 1975), exposing the left ear and left visual field and leading to right-hemisphere processing of visual and auditory stimuli. However, right head turning may be analogous to right hand usage, that is, due to left-hemisphere motor control. Another aspect considered by Brown and Jaffe (1975) is that the neonate is sensitive to photic driving in the right hemisphere before the left, while in the adult no sensitivity differences are found (Crowell, Jones, Kapuniai, & Nakagawa, 1973). However, assumptions about longitudinal development cannot be drawn from Crowell *et al.*'s study, since only neonates were examined.

Despite these comments on Brown and Jaffe's (1975) data sources, important evidence for their hypothesis can be found in the work of Taylor (1969). Taylor examined the distribution of age at time of onset of first fit in temporal lobe epilepsy where onset was before the tenth year. The left hemisphere was most at risk in the first year, while the right hemisphere was most at risk in the second and third years. In that functional inactivity and seizure activity are correlated, this suggests that the right hemisphere may be dominant early in life. Annett (1970) presented similar findings. However, until differences in the performance of the hands in the longitudinal development of manual behavior in early infancy are studied, an important set of data that may help to confirm or disconfirm Brown and Jaffe's (1975) hypothesis is lacking.

Sex Differences in Lateralization

Hemispheric specialization is often referred to in terms of language- or space-related skills, and it appears that girl infants are in advance of boy infants on a variety of language-related variables; but few investigators (Witelson, 1976) consider possible neurological substrate differences between the sexes in infancy, despite several models that do so for adults and children (Buffery & Gray, 1972; Harris, 1975). Girl infants vocalize the full range of phonemes earlier, speak the first word earlier, and develop vocabularies earlier (Harris, 1975). In contrast, despite later-developing superior spatial skills and the supposed genetic base for such superiority, boy infants do not have an early superiority in such skills compared to girl infants (Maccoby & Jacklin, 1974).

In may be that early hormonal (Reinisch, 1974) or information-processing strategy differences (Bryden, 1976) account for these behavior differences across the sexes in infancy, either in whole or in part. It is also conceivable that some aspect of bilateral brain maturation may help explain these differences. For example, Goldman, Crawford, Stokes, Galkin, and Rosvold (1974) observed the effects of bilateral orbital prefontal lesions in very young or older juvenile male and female rhesus monkeys. On object discrimination reversal tasks or spatial delayed-response problems, males were impaired at 2½ months, whereas females showed similar impairment only at 15 and 18 months. The orbital cortex may thus functionally manifest earlier in male monkeys; this may be a model to explain the sex differences in behavior observed in man, although this speculation needs research and refinement.

Another possible explanation of the described developmental shifts in sex differences in behavior may lie in sex differences in differential left–right brain organization or maturation (Lake & Bryden, 1976; Kimura, 1976). In this regard, Denckla (1973) suggests that girls may be in advance of boys in left-hemisphere skills whereas boys show better but not earlier right-hemisphere dependent skills. There are several possible ways of explaining this advance in left-hemisphere skills in girls. It could be that the left hemisphere matures more quickly in girls (Taylor, 1969), or is more relied on in girls due to greater sensitivity in the auditory channel from early in life (J. Sherman, 1971), or develops cerebral connections with the right hemisphere more quickly (Denckla, 1973). There is no evidence for the last suggestion in terms of differential rates of corpus callosum myelinization (Yakovlev & Lecours, 1967). The supposed greater auditory sensitivity in girls has not been corroborated by research findings (Maccoby & Jacklin, 1974), nor do there seem to be any data showing advanced physical maturation of the left hemisphere in girls (Wada et al., 1975; Witelson & Pallie, 1973). Taylor (1969) analyzed sex differences in maturation across both hemispheres in one set of data and left—right differences in another. Despite how some have interpreted his results, nowhere is the question of sex differences in left- versus right-hemisphere maturation specifically addressed.

Even if some data could be found supporting these explanations for early sex differences in behavior, they present two problems. (a) They look for gross physical differences instead of looking at more fruitful possible explanations, such as differential cerebral organization or templates in one or the other or both hemispheres. (b) They would be hard pressed to explain the developmental shifts in sex differences described earlier. Developmental models can only be formulated after careful longitudinal study of the ontogenesis of central and peripheral lateralization of function in boys and girls (in coordination with language-related and space-related observation).

Early Determinants of Lateralization of Function

Genetic and environmental—enculturation theories (Annett, 1975; Levy & Nagylaki, 1972) and their rebuttals (Collins, 1974; Corballis & Beale, 1976; Hudson, 1975) are numerous, but a review of this topic is beyond the scope of the present article. Instead, early determinants or mechanisms that may mediate in genetic or environmental models of lateralization of function are discussed. Gesell and Ames (1947) thought that handedness is largely influenced by the spontaneous tonic neck reflex (TNR) exhibited in the first few months of life. They found that even most (87%) prematures as young as 26 weeks gestational age exhibit the TNR and that most infants (77%) exhibit the reflex largely to the right. Of 19 cases of infants showing asymmetric TNRs, 10 right-side preferring infants became right-handed at 10 years of age, 4 left-side preferring infants became left-handed, and 5 cases showed no correlation. Gesell's thesis is plausible, since in the TNR an arm is extended outward on the side to which the head turns. Consequently, a majority of infants show more right- than left-arm extension. Such constant predispositions may very well lead to the extended arm being favored later on. However, one could argue that the extended arm, which is flexed toward the body, may have more material (skin, clothes) to manipulate and thus lead to later preference for that limb. That is, the TNR might favor left-hand preference and may account for the data showing early reversal of the typical right-hand preference, if this trend is replicated. Caplan and Kinsbourne (1976) further differentiated Gesell's thesis; they argued that a visual orienting component induces the TNR, and that a right-space (left-hemisphere) attentional bias leads to right-arm extension in the TNR and an eventual right-hand preference. However, there are no data to support or refute the presence of a visual component to the TNR.

Both Churchill, Igna, and Senf (1962) and Grapin and Perpère (1968) related the way in which the head is turned in delivery at birth to later hand preference. They found that left head turning is associated with later right-handedness, whereas the head turned to the right correlated with later left-handedness. In both studies handedness was determined by a gross motor act such as reaching. The apparent extent of variance that the association between birth position and handedness accounts for is minimal and there are many exceptions to the rule in their data. At best they are showing that differential head position during delivery may affect later handedness, due to possible differential cerebral injury or blood flow. Oettlinger (1975) discussed a possible relationship between eye, hand, and cortical dominance. He argued that the TNR is associated with eye preference and that eye preference precedes hand preference in development. Consequently, eye preference may be a good measure of cortical dominance and a causal relationship may be involved. However, this hypothesis is presented without any data. The low percentage of right-eye sighting dominance in adults (60 to 65%, Coren, 1974) compared to the high percentage of left-hemisphere dominance and right-handedness argues against Oettlinger's hypothesis.

Turkewitz et al., (1965) had shown that 85% of 3-day-old normal neonates spontaneously turn their heads only to the right. Further research suggested an association between right head turning and greater right-side sensitivity to perioral stimulation (Turkewitz, Moreau, Davis, & Birch, 1969). Turkewitz and Creighton (1975) then showed that by maintaining the head in position at the midline, thereby reducing or eliminating lateral differences in sensitivity, right turning of the head was eliminated only in infants younger than 12 hours. Presumably then, in the first 12 hours of life lateral differences in sensitivity reinforce an initial head turning bias to the right, interrelating the two phenomena. After 12 hours of age, however, head turning can become independent of lateral sensitivity. Given the possible association of head turning and handedness, lateral differences in sensitivity may explain much about why we are generally right-handed. However, only longitudinal research involving such measures as lateral sensitivity, eye sighting dominance, manual behavior, head turning, and measures of hemispheric specialization can fully test Turkewitz and Creighton's (1975) hypothesis and the others presented in this section.

Evolution of Lateralization

The young infant possesses linguistic competency (Eimas, 1974; Trehub & Rabinovitch, 1972) but his typical vocal performance is not speech. Thus hemi-

spheric specialization, which seems present at birth, may precede speech in development. If this progression in ontogenesis could be confirmed, it would add power to
the argument (Trevarthen, 1974a) that hemispheric specialization preceded language acquisition in evolution. Others argue that if language was not the evolutionary pressure for hemispheric specialization then it may have derived from pressures
either for bimanual coordination (e.g., in tool using and making, Steklis & Harnad,
in press) or for gestural speech (Hewes, in press) in our protohominid ancestors.
Changes in peripheral behavior in the course of evolution is implied to have led
exclusively to corresponding central hemispheric accommodation. However, the
evolutionary pressure that favored asymmetry of function may have been related
centrally to the brain itself, rather than peripherally to behavior. This idea is
supported in the work of Levy (1969, 1972) who argues that the left hemisphere is
an analytic serial information processor and output director while the right hemisphere is more gestalt, holistic and parallel in its functioning. On the basis of studies
of split-brain patients, she concluded that the specialized functions of the two
hemispheres are mutually antagonistic or competitive, so that their segregation in
different hemispheres is advantageous.

It could very well be that the environmental aspect needing more acute information processing in our early ancestors was terrain recognition, especially for men
involved in hunting and women involved in gathering. Both the analytic–sequential
and the holistic–parallel information-processing demands in achieving these goals
may have become so complex that a brain organization favoring their segregation
and lack of competition evolved. Equally plausible is that conspecific social
behavior became so complex that information processing of the sequential stream
of intricate gestalt displays demanded the segregation we are talking about. In
conclusion, this section describes several possible evolutionary origins of hemisphere specialization which do not directly involve language, and longitudinal
research on the ontogenetic course of hemispheric specialization, linguistic competency, and manual specialization may shed some light by analogy on the problem.

Applied Implications

Two studies suggest that deficits in either fine motor skills or lateral differences
in behavior in the neonate and young infant may be associated with at-risk factors
or prematurity. Turkewitz, Moreau, and Birch (1968) demonstrated a direct relationship between laterality of behavior and condition of birth in term neonates.
Infants of variable 1-min Apgar scores who seemed normal at age 1 to 3 days were
tested for head turning directed to perioral stimulation. Normal (Apgar 9–10)
infants showed clear right preferences, whereas poor birth condition infants (Apgar
1–6) showed no lateral preferences. Infants with Apgar scores 7–8 showed intermediate patterns. The authors concluded that early disturbances in lateral differentiation may be related to similar later disturbances and disabilities in older children.
Kopp (1974) examined term and preterm infants at 8 months of age on sensorimotor tasks. Infants were classified as coordinated or clumsy when they reached

and grasped on the first task. On the following tasks, coordinated infants explored more with their mouths, while clumsy infants, who were mostly preterm, tended to watch objects more. These have been the only two studies of such a nature; neither considered manual specialization and neither was longitudinal. Yet the two studies point to the need for longitudinal research of manual specialization, beginning at birth, because of possible practical applications.

The most relevant application of results deriving from the proposed longitudinal studies of manual specialization concerns possible early diagnostic criteria of later developmental or neurological problems. If manual behavior reflects both under-lying neurological organization and intelligent adaptation from early life onward, it is conceivable that altered patterns of manual specialization in the developing infant may help in the diagnosis and prognosis of individual cases where *subtle* detection techniques are needed. The relationship between early perinatal problems and later learning disabilities is pertinent in this regard. It may even be possible to diagnose different types of risk on the basis of different alterations of the normal develop-mental pattern of manual specialization.

The criticisms of Orton's (1937) theory that mixed or crossed cerebral *dominance* is a cause of learning (reading) disabilities (Kinsbourne, 1973) might seem to militate against the suggested applied relevance of longitudinal study of manual specialization. However, researchers who not only look at hand and eye preference but also use more refined means and examine manual specialization and lateraliza-tion of brain function in detail are beginning to support revised versions of Orton's position phrased in terms of lateralization of manual behavior and hemispheric specialization (Beaumont, 1974; Benton, 1975; Guyer & Friedman, 1975; Thompson, 1976; etc.).

CONCLUSIONS

Careful longitudinal study of manual specialization and of differential hemi-spheric functioning in infancy is needed and it should give results that will help to clarify the issues of which hand is initially preferred in early infancy, which hemisphere is initially dominant, when sex differences and individual differences in lateralization of function begin to emerge, as well as what is the origin of manual specialization and lateralization of hemispheric function and what is their presumed interrelationship. Other issues not dealt with in this review (e.g., a critical period for lateralization of brain function and first language acquisition, Fromkin *et al.,* 1974; Lenneberg, 1967; Krashen, 1975; Wechsler, 1976) may also profit from such longitudinal studies. Until these longitudinal studies are undertaken a comment by Trevarthen (1977) will stand as a worthy conclusion. He notes that

We must concede that the connection between lateralization of manipulative practice and lateralization of language remains obscure. Both are undoubtedly consequences of an inborn asymmetry in cerebral organization of the mechanisms which effect orientation to complex tasks and there may or may not be a close functional between them [p. 53 of galley proof].

APPENDIX

Is There Contralateral Left Hemisphere Control of Arm Movement?

Ipsilateral Arm Movement Control

The question of what manual behaviors are relevant in relation to hemispheric specialization is discussed, since early manual behavior is dominated by reaching and such gross motor movements may not be as relevant as more fine motor movements (Trevarthen, 1974b). The novelty of this review is that it places emphasis on logic and research showing possible hemispheric control of gross motor movements, often neglected in favor of analyses with respect to fine motor movements. Selected more recent evidence is dealt with, rather than giving a historical perspective. Split-brain monkeys were observed performing a visual—motor task with one eye covered, restricting visual input to one half of the brain (Brinkman & Kuypers, 1972, 1973). When tactile guidance of movement was limited by placing small food morsels in deep wells, the contralateral hand reached and manipulated accurately but the ipsilateral hand could only reach accurately, its manipulatory search resembling the behavior of blindfolded animals. Without tactile guidance masking, manipulatory exploration was accurate. The studies suggest that there is ipsilateral as well as contralateral cerebral control of independent arm movements involving axial and proximal musculature. However, independent hand or finger movements (involving distal musculature) with or without arm movements seem to be only under contralateral control.

These results suggest that gross motor arm movements may be less relevant than fine motor and finger movements for the determination both of lateral differences in behavior and of the relationship between cerebral hemispheric specialization and contralateral manual behavior. Some developmental data obtained by Denckla (1974) fits with Brinkman and Kuyper's hypothesis. Denckla administered 5- to 11-year-old normal right-handed children a battery of motor coordination tasks. She found greater right-hand superiority only on tasks involving distal muscle movements. Also, just after surgery, chiasm-sectioned split-brain monkeys can use ipsilateral eye—hand combinations to grab a rapidly moving object, but discriminatory visual attention to stimuli is impaired even on tasks for which the monkeys were highly trained preoperatively (Trevarthen, 1977).

Contralateral Arm Movement Control

One cannot totally exclude gross arm movements, such as reaching, from consideration as behaviors possibly amenable to contralateral hemispheric control, for the following two sets of reasons. The first set concerns the corticomotoneu-ronal connections described by Brinkman and Kuypers (1972). Despite both contra- and ipsilateral pathways controlling arm movements, contralateral pathways may somehow occlude or dominate ipsilateral ones for gross motor arm movements in daily activity, creating an analogous contralateral cerebral control in organization found for distal fine motor movements. Furthermore, there may be differential efficacy in left and right ipsilateral pathways, allowing for the left or the right hemisphere leading for arm movements.

The second set of reasons pointing to the possibility that gross motor arm movements may be under contralateral hemispheric control concerns associated confounding factors. Three aspects are considered. First, whole arm movements may be visually guided or not, and differing opinions exist as to whether this possible guidance inhibits bilateral control fo the behavior. Lomas and Kimura (1976) argue that their studies of intrahemispheric interaction between speaking and sequential motor (including whole arm) activity support the idea that, with minimal visual guidance involved, lateralized (to the left) control of rapid limb or limb part placement occurs. In contrast, Van Der Staak (1975) insists that regula-tion of movement by visual information facilitates finding intrahemispheric or interhemispheric control (or both) for various arm movements. The two studies were aimed at different problems, so that their differing emphases on visual–motor control are not entirely opposing, yet they highlight a possible secondary variable related to the question of contralateral hemispheric control of whole arm move-ments.

A second possibly confounding factor in considering the relationship of whole arm movements and cortical control is illustrated by Preilowski's (1972, in Sperry, 1974) distinction between new and old motor activities. Commissurotomy patients were severely impaired in novel bimanual coordinations but not in old habits like tying shoelaces. One explanation offered was that central control for old habits shifted from the cortex to lower, undivided subcortical centers such as the cerebel-lum. The same shift might occur for well-learned whole arm movements; that is, the initial learning of such a movement as reaching in the infant may be cerebrally mediated and liable to lateralization. It may even be that, once initiated, a whole arm movement is subcortically controlled but the decision to perform that move-ment requires higher cortical involvement and possible lateralization.

The final distinction made about whole arm gross motor movements that is relevant to the question of their contralateral hemispheric control is derived from Van Der Staak (1975). He found a distinction between abductive (e.g., reaching) movements away from the body and adductive movements toward the body when right-handed students were fixating a midpoint in two tasks. In terms of speed and accuracy in moving from a target to a start button, and in reciprocal tapping, abductive movements were controlled by the contralateral hemisphere while adduc-tive movements were controlled bilaterally. This seems to be the general case for humans according to Van Der Staak, unlike the special case of split-brain monkeys used by Brinkman and Kuypers (1972), where all arm movements seem to be bilaterally controlled.

Left-Hemisphere Arm Movement Control

Up to this point, reasons why gross motor arm movements such as reaching may be contralaterally controlled in the hemispheres was discussed without emphasizing left- or right-side differences. Evidence and lines of reasoning are now offered that the left rather than the right hemisphere may be more in control of motor output, including whole arm movements. Hemisphere impairment for control of sensori-motor functioning differs with the complexity and demand characteristics of the task at hand, so that generalizations about cerebral versus subcortical, bilateral versus unilateral, contralateral versus ipsilateral, and left- versus right-hemispheric control are premature; but contralateral cerebral control by the left hemisphere is more often implied than are other explanations. For example, Haaland and Clee-land (1976) administered a battery of simple and complex motor tasks to patients with unilateral cerebral insult and found no group differences on less complex tasks but differential motor performance for more complex tasks. For maze coordination (involving whole arm movements in particular) and a grooved pegboard test, left-hemisphere patients manifested bilateral deficits whereas right hemisphere patients were deficient only with the left hand. It is not simply a question of whether a behavior is lateralized or not but rather of whether the functions to which a movement or behavior is applied—that is, the task's characteristics and demands—induce lateralization or not.

Another relevant task-demand characteristic is the extent of associated or prior factors inducing left- or right-hemisphere priming or activation of attention (Bowers & Heilman, 1976; Kinsbourne & Hiscock, Chapter 14, this volume; Klein, Mosco-vitch, & Vigna, 1976; Lomas & Kimura, 1976, including whole arm movement tapping). Interference with motor performance of the right hand or arm may or may not occur depending on whether left-hemisphere language-related processing or output direction is concurrently going on. These data imply that some aspect of left-hemisphere control for the arm as well as the hand overlaps with left-hemi-sphere control of speech.

This close association between motor and language control in the left hemi-sphere (Wolff & Hurwitz, 1976) has been supported in studies of apraxics (Heil-man, 1975; Heilman, Schwartz, & Geschwind, 1975), aphasics (Duffy, Duffy, & Pearson, 1975), and brain-injured patients (Kimura & Archibald, 1974). For example, Kimura and Archibald (1974) observed that right-handers who incurred left unilateral cerebral insult were more impaired, relative to right-hemisphere damaged patients, in copying unfamiliar, meaningless movement sequences of the arm as well as the hand. This was not found for isolated finger flexion or copying static hand postures. These findings support the hypothesis that the left may be the hemisphere controlling motor sequencing of the whole arm, finger and hand.

However, the exact nature of left-hemisphere control of activity of the whole arm is still open to debate. There may be greater ipsilateral representation of the left than of the right hand in the motor cortex (Kimura & Vanderwolf, 1970), which also may lead to greater left-hemisphere control of arm movements. Another possibility is that the left-hemisphere control for fine motor finger movements may generalize to gross motor arm movements (e.g., reaching in order to manipulate), resulting in the same contralateral (right) limb preference found for manipulation itself. Lomas and Kimura (1976) present evidence against Wyke (1967) who argues that control of speed of movement per se is involved. Both Lomas and Kimura (1976) and Flowers (1975) emphasize feel or sensory feedback control being crucial in dominant- (left-) hemisphere control of motor activity. This latter idea goes beyond the hypothesis that the left hemisphere leads for control of sequential movement, as it differentiates a sensory feedback loop that may be involved in serial activity. Only further research can help to qualify the exact nature of left-hemisphere control of motor activity and how this may differ for fine motor and gross motor movements. However, despite the argument that reaching may not be contralaterally controlled in the hemispheres, it appears that control of motor activity, including gross motor arm movements in general and reaching in particular, may very well be controlled in the left hemisphere, depending on the task characteristics involved in eliciting the behavior. How true this may be in the infant still needs to be established, but there are no *a priori* reasons for excluding the study of reaching and arm movements in infancy as possible indices of the development of lateralization of brain function.

ACKNOWLEDGMENTS

This chapter was written while the author was supported by a National Research Council of Canada postdoctoral fellowship. Thanks are due to Peter H. Wolff, Deborah Waber, and A. Roch Lecours for reading an earlier draft of this chapter.

REFERENCES

Annett, M. (1970) The growth of manual preference and speed. *British Journal of Psychology, 61,* 545–558.

Annett, M. (1975) Hand preference and the laterality of cerebral speech. *Cortex, 11,* 305–328.

Aronson, E., & Rosenbloom, S. (1971) Space perception in early infancy: Perception within a common auditory-visual space. *Science, 172,* 1161–1163.

Beaumont, J. (1974) Handedness and hemisphere function. In S. Dimond & J. Beaumont (Eds.), *Hemisphere function in the human brain.* New York: Wiley.

Benton, A. (1975) Developmental dyslexia: Neurological aspects. In W. Friedlander (Ed.), *Advances in neurology.* Vol. 7. New York: Raven.

Bowers, D., & Heilman, K. (1976) Material specific hemispheric arousal. *Neuropsychologia, 14,* 123–127.

Brinkman, J., & Kuypers, H. (1972) Splitbrain monkeys: Cerebral control of ipsilateral and contralateral arm, hand and finger movements. *Science, 176,* 536–539.

Brinkman, J., & Kuypers, H. (1973) Cerebral control of contralateral and ipsalateral arm, hand, and finger movements in the splitbrain rhesus monkey. *Brain, 96,* 653–674.

Brown, J., & Jaffe, J. (1975) Hypothesis on cerebral dominance. *Neuropsychologia, 13,* 107–110.

Bryden, M. (1976) Sex differences in cerebral organization. In D. Kimura (Chair), Sex differences in brain asymmetry. Symposium presented at the meeting of the International Neuropsychology Society, Toronto, Feb.

Buffery, A., & Gray, J. (1972) Sex differences in development of spatial and linguistic skills. In C. Ounsted & D. Taylor (Eds.), *Gender differences: Their ontogeny and significance.* London: Churchill.

Caplan, P., & Kinsbourne, M. (1976) Baby drops the rattle: Asymmetry of duration of grasp by infants. *Child Development, 47,* 532–534.

Carmon, A., Harishanu, Y., Lowinger, E., & Lavy, S. (1972) Asymmetries in hemispheric blood volume and cerebral dominance. *Behavioral Biology, 7,* 853–859.

Černáček, J., & Podivinský, F. (1971) Ontogenesis of handedness and somatosensory cortical response. *Neuropsychologia, 9,* 219–232.

Černáček, J., & Podivinský, F. (1972) Changes of contralateral and ipsalateral somatosensory cortical responses during infancy. In J. Černáček & F. Podivinský, (Eds.), *Cerebral interhemispheric relation.* Bratislava: Publishing House of the Slovak Academy of Sciences.

Chorazyna, H. (1976) Shifts in laterality in a baby chimpanzee. *Neuropsychologia, 14,* 381–384.

Churchill, J., Igna, E., & Senf, R. (1962) The association of position at birth and handedness. *Pediatrics, 29,* 307–309.

Cohen, A. (1966) Hand preference and developmental status of infants. *Journal of Genetic Psychology, 108,* 337–345.

Collins, R. (1974) When left-handed mice live in right-handed worlds. *Science, 187,* 181–184.

Corballis, M., & Beale, I. (1976) *Psychology of left and right.* Hillsdale, New Jersey: Lawrence Erlbaum.

Coren, S. (1974) Development of ocular dominance. *Developmental Psychology, 10,* 304.

Crowell, D., Jones, R., Kapuniai, L., & Nakagawa, J. (1973) Unilateral cortical activity in newborn humans: An early index of cerebral dominance? *Science, 180,* 205–208.

Denckla, M. (1973) Development of speed in repetitive and successive finger movements in normal children. *Developmental Medicine and Child Neurology, 15,* 635–645.

Denckla, M. (1974) Development of motor coordination in normal children. *Developmental Medicine and Child Neurology, 16,* 729–741.

Dennis, M. (1975) Hemispheric specialization in adulthood after hemidecortication for infantile cerebral disease. In L. Harris (Chair), Functional specialization of the cerebral hemispheres in infants and children: New experimental and clinical evidence. Symposium presented at the meeting of the Society for Research in Child Development, Denver.

Duffy, R., Duffy, J., & Pearson, K. (1975) Pantomime recognition in aphasics. *Journal of Speech and Hearing Research, 18,* 115–132.

Eimas, P. (1974) Auditory and linguistic processing of cues for place of articulation by infants *Perception and Psychophysics, 16,* 513–521.

Flament, F. (1973) Intelligence pratique et lateralité: Etude genétique de la synergie et de la prevalence manuelle chez le nourrisson. *Bulletin de Psychologie, 27,* 681–684.

Flowers, K. (1975) Handedness and controlled movements. *British Journal of Psychology, 66,* 39–52.

Fromkin, V., Krashen, S., Curtiss, S., Rigler, D., & Rigler, M. (1974) The development of language in Genie: A case of language acquisition beyond the critical period. *Brain and Language, 1,* 81–107.

Gazzaniga, M. (1974) Cerebral dominance viewed as a decision system. In S. Dimond & J. Beaumont (Eds.), *Hemisphere function in the human brain.* New York: Wiley.

Gesell, A., & Ames, L. (1947) The development of handedness. *Journal of Genetic Psychology, 70,* 155–175.

Giesecke, M. (1936) The genesis of hand preference. *Monograph of the Society for Research in Child Development, 1* (5, Serial No. 5).

Goldman, P. (1974) Recovery of function after CNS lesions in infant monkeys. In E. Eidelberg & D. Stein (Eds.), Functional recovery after lesions of the nervous system. *Neurosciences Research Progress Bulletin, 12,* 217–222.

Goldman, P., Crawford, H., Stokes, L., Galkin, T., & Rosvold, H. (1974) Sex-dependent behavioral effects of cerebral cortical lesions in the developing rhesus monkey. *Science, 186,* 540–542.

Grapin, P., & Perpère, C. (1968) Symmetrie et lateralization du nourrisson. In R. Kourilsky & P. Grapin (Eds.), *Main droite et main gauche.* Paris: Presses Universitaire de France.

Guyer, B., & Friedman, M. (1975) Hemispheric processing and cognitive styles in learning-disabled and normal children. *Child Development, 46,* 658–668.

Haaland, K., & Cleeland, C. (1976) *Motor performance after unilateral hemisphere damage.* Paper presented at the meeting of the International Neuropsychology Society, Toronto, Feb.

Halverson, H. (1931) An experimental study of prehension in infants by means of systematic cinema records. *Genetic Psychology Monographs, 10,* 107–286.

Halverson, H. (1937a) Studies of the grasping responses of early infancy, I. *Journal of Genetic Psychology, 51,* 371–392.

Halverson, H. (1937b) Studies of the grasping responses of early infancy, II. *Journal of Genetic Psychology, 51,* 393–424.

Harris, L. (1975) Interaction of experiential and neurological factors in the patterning of human abilities: The question of sex differences in right hemisphere skills. In L. Harris (Chair) Functional specialization of the cerebral hemispheres in infants and children: New experimental and clinical evidence. Symposium presented at the meeting of the Society for Research in Child Development, Denver, April.

Hécaen, H. (1976) Acquired aphasia in children and the ontogenesis of hemispheric functional specialization. *Brain and Language, 3,* 114–134.

Heilman, K. (1975) A tapping test in apraxia. *Cortex, 11,* 25–263.

Heilman, K., Schwartz, H., & Geschwind, N. (1975) Defective motor learning in ideomotor apraxia. *Neurology, 25,* 1018–1020.

Hewes, G. (in press) The current status of the gestural theory of language origin. *Annals of the New York Academy of Sciences.*

Hudson, P. (1975) The genetics of handedness—a reply to Levy and Nagylaki. *Neuropsychologia, 13,* 331–339.

Kimura, D. (Chair). (1976) Sex differences in brain asymmetry. Symposium presented at the meeting of the International Neuropsychology Society, Toronto, Feb. (Abstract of symposium in meeting programme)

Kimura, D., & Archibald, Y. (1974) Motor functions of the left hemisphere. *Brain, 97,* 337–350.

Kimura, D., & Vanderwolf, C. (1970) The relation between hand preference and the performance of individual finger movement by left and right hands. *Brain, 93,* 769–774.

Kinsbourne, M. (1973) Minimal brain dysfunction as a neurodevelopmental lag. *Annals of the New York Academy of Sciences, 205,* 268–273.

Kinsbourne, M. (1974) Mechanisms of hemispheric interaction in man. In M. Kinsbourne & W. Smith (Eds.), *Hemisphere disconnection and cerebral function.* Springfield, Illinois: Thomas.

Kinsbourne, M. (1975a) The ontogeny of cerebral dominance. *Annals of the New York Academy of Sciences, 263,* 244–250.
Kinsbourne, M. (1975b) Minor hemisphere language and cerebral maturation. In E. Lenneberg & E. Lenneberg (Eds.), *Foundations of language development: A multidisciplinary approach.* Vol. 2. New York: Academic.
Klein, D., Moscovitch, M., & Vigna, C. (1976) Attentional mechanisms and perceptual asymmetries on tachistoscopic recognition of words and faces. *Neuropsychologia, 14,* 55–66.
Kopp, C. (1974) Fine motor abilities of infants. *Developmental Medicine and Child Neurology, 16,* 629–636.
Krashen, S. (1975) The critical period for language acquisition and its possible bases. *Annals of the New York Academy of Sciences, 263,* 211–224.
Lake, D., & Bryden, P. (1976) Handedness and sex differences in hemispheric asymmetry. *Brain and Language, 3,* 266–282.
Lederer, R. (1939) An exploratory investigation of handed status in the first two years of life. In R. Lederer & J. Redfield (Eds.), Studies in infant behavior. Vol. 5. *University of Iowa Studies: Studies in Child Welfare, 16,* 1–103.
Lenneberg, E. (1967) *Biological foundations of language.* New York: Wiley.
Lenneberg, E. (1975) In search of a dynamic theory of aphasia. In E. Lenneberg & E. Lenneberg (Eds.), *Foundations of language development: A multidisciplinary approach.* Vol. 2. New York: Academic.
Lesné, & Peycelon (1934) A quel age un enfant cesse-t-il d'être ambidextre pour devenir droitier? *Bulletin de la Societé de la Pédiatrie, 32,* 436–439.
Levy, J. (1969) Possible basis for lateral specialization of the human brain. *Nature, 224,* 614–615.
Levy, J. (1972) Lateral specialization of the human brain: Behavioral manifestations and possible evolutionary basis. In J. Kiger, Jr. (Ed.), *The biology of behavior.* Corvallis: Oregon State Univ. Press.
Levy, J., & Nagylaki, T. (1972) A model for the genetics of handedness. *Genetics, 72,* 117–128.
Lippman, H. (1927) Certain behaviour responses in early infancy. *Journal of Genetic Psychology, 34,* 424–440.
Lomas, J., & Kimura, D. (1976) Intrahemispheric interaction between speaking and sequential manual activity. *Neuropsychologia, 14,* 23–33.
Lyons-Ruth, K. (1975) Integration of auditory and visual spatial information during early infancy. Paper presented at the meeting of the Society for Research in Child Development, Denver, April.
Maccoby, E., & Jacklin, C. (1974) *The psychology of sex differences.* Stanford, California: Stanford Univ. Press.
McGurk, H., & Lewis, M. (1974) Space perception in early infancy: Perception within a common auditory-visual space? *Science, 186,* 649–650.
Milner, B. (1974) Hemispheric specialization: Scope and limits. In F. Schmitt & F. Worden (Eds.), *The neurosciences: Third study program.* Cambridge, Mass.: M.I.T. Press.
Molfese, D., Freeman, R., Jr., & Palermo, D. (1975) The ontogeny of brain lateralization for speech and nonspeech stimuli. *Brain and Language, 2,* 356–368.
Moscovitch, M. (1976) On the representation of language in the right hemisphere of right-handed people. *Brain and Language, 3,* 47–71.
Nachson, L., & Carmon, A. (1975) Hand preference in sequential and spatial discrimination tasks. *Cortex, 11,* 123–131.
Oettlinger, L., Jr. (1975) The asymmetrical tonic neck reflex. *Developmental Medicine and Child Neurology, 17,* 119.
Orton, S. (1937) *Reading, writing and speech problems in children.* New York: Norton.
Piaget, J. (1963) *The origins of intelligence in children.* New York: Norton.
Porter, R., & Berlin, C. (1975) On interpreting developmental changes in the dichotic right-ear advantage. *Brain and Language, 2,* 186–200.

Preilowski, B. (1972) Interference between limbs during independent bilateral movements. Paper presented at the 80th Annual Convention of the American Psychological Association, Washington. (Cited in Sperry, 1974).

Reinisch, J. (1974) Fetal hormones, the brain and human sex differences: A heuristic, integrative review of the recent literature. *Archives of Sexual Behavior, 3,* 51–90.

Satz, P., Rardin, D., & Ross, J. (1971) An evaluation of a theory of specific developmental dyslexia. *Child Development, 42,* 2009–2021.

Seth, G. (1973) Eye-hand co-ordination and "handedness": A developmental study of visuomotor behaviour in infancy. *British Journal of Educational Psychology, 43,* 35–49.

Sherick, I., Greenman, G., & Legg, C. (1976) Some comments on the significance and development of midline behavior during infancy. *Child Psychiatry and Human Development, 6,* 170–183.

Sherman, J. (1971) *On the psychology of women.* Springfield, Illinois: Thomas.

Sherman, M., Sherman, I., & Flory, C. (1936) Infant behavior. *Comparative Psychology Monographs, 12* (4, Serial No. 59).

Shirley, M. (1931) *The first two years: A study of twenty-five babies.* Vol. 1, *Postural and locomotor development.* Minneapolis: Univ. of Minnesota Press.

Sperry, R. (1974) Lateral specialization in the surgically separated hemispheres. In F. Schmitt & F. Worden (Eds.), *The neurosciences: Third study program.* Cambridge, Massachusetts: M.I.T. Press.

Steffen, H. (1975) Cerebral dominance: The development of handedness and speech. *Acta Psychopediatrica, 41,* 223–235.

Steklis, H., & Harnad, S. (in press) From hand to mouth: Some critical stages in the evolution of language. *Annals of the New York Academy of Sciences.*

Stubbs, E., & Irwin, O. (1933) Laterality of limb movements of four newborn infants. *Child Development, 4,* 358–359.

Taylor, D. (1969) Differential rates of cerebral maturation between sexes and between hemispheres. *Lancet, 2,* 140–142.

Thompson, M. (1976) A comparison of laterality effects in dyslexics and controls using verbal dichotic listening tasks. *Neuropsychologia, 14,* 243–246.

Touwen, B. (1971) A study on the development of some motor phenomena in infancy. *Developmental Medicine and Child Neurology, 13,* 435–446.

Trehub, S., & Rabinovitch, M. (1972) Auditory linguistic sensitivity in early infancy. *Developmental Psychology, 6,* 74–77.

Trevarthen, C. (1974a) The psychobiology of speech development. In E. Lenneberg (Ed.), Language and brain: Developmental aspects. *Neurosciences Research Progress Bulletin, 12,* 570–585.

Trevarthen, C. (1974b) Functional relations of disconnected hemispheres with the brainstem and with each other: Monkey and man. In M. Kinsbourne & W. Smith (Eds.), *Hemispheric disconnection and cerebral function.* Springfield, Illinois: Thomas.

Trevarthen, C. (1977) Manipulative strategies of baboons and the origins of cerebral asymmetry. In M. Kinsbourne (Ed.), *Hemispheric asymmetry of Function.* New York: Cambridge Univ. Press.

Turkewitz, G., & Creighton, S. (1975) Changes in lateral differentiation of head posture in the human neonate. *Developmental Psychobiology, 8,* 85–90.

Turkewitz, G., Gordon, E., & Birch, H. (1965) Head turning in the human neonate: Spontaneous patterns. *Journal of Genetic Psychology, 107,* 143–158.

Turkewitz, G., Moreau, T., & Birch, H. (1968) Relation between birth condition and neurobehavioral organization in the neonate. *Pediatric Research, 2,* 243–249.

Turkewitz, G., Moreau, T., Davis, L., & Birch, H. (1969) Factors affecting lateral differentiation in the human newborn. *Journal of Experimental Child Psychology, 8,* 483–493.

Valentine, W., & Wagner, I. (1934) Relative arm motility in the newborn infant. *Ohio University Studies, 12,* 53–68.

Van Der Staak, C. (1975) Intra- and interhemispheric visual-motor control of human arm movements. *Neuropsychologia, 13,* 439–448.

Voelckel, E. (1913) Untersuchungen über die Rechtshändigkeit beim Säugling. *Zeitschrift für Kinderheilk, 8,* 351–358.

Wada, J., Clarke, R., & Hamm, A. (1975) Cerebral hemispheric asymmetry in humans: Cortical speech zones in 100 adult and 100 infant brains. *Archives of Neurology, 32,* 239–246.

Watson, J. (1919) *Psychology from the standpoint of a behaviorist.* Philadelphia: Lippincott.

Wechsler, A. (1976) Crossed aphasia in an illiterate dextral. *Brain and Language, 3,* 164–172.

White, B. (1969) The initial coordination of sensorimotor schemas in human infants—Piaget's ideas and the role of experience. In D. Elkind & J. Flavell (Eds.), *Studies in cognitive development: Essays in honor of Jean Piaget.* New York: Oxford Univ. Press.

White, B., Castle, P., & Held, R. (1964) Observations on the development of visually-directed reaching. *Child Development, 35,* 349–364.

Witelson, S. (1975) Age and sex differences in the development of right hemisphere specialization for spatial processing as reflected in a dichotomous tactual stimulation task. In L. Harris (Chair), Functional specialization of the cerebral hemispheres in infants and children: New experimental and clinical evidence. Symposium presented at the meeting of the Society for Research in Child Development, Denver, April.

Witelson, S. (1976) Sex and the single hemisphere: Right hemisphere specialization for spatial processing. *Science, 193,* 425–427.

Witelson, S., & Pallie, W. (1973) Left hemisphere specialization for language in the newborn: Neuroanatomical evidence of asymmetry. *Brain, 96,* 641–646.

Wolff, P., & Hurwitz, I. (1976) Sex differences in finger tapping: A developmental study. *Neuropsychologia, 14,* 35–41.

Wyke, M. (1967) The effect of brain lesions on the rapidity of arm movement. *Neurology, 17,* 1113–1120.

Yakovlev, P., & Lecours, A. (1967) The myelogenetic cycles of regional maturation of the brain. In A. Minkowski (Ed.), *Regional development of the brain in early life.* Oxford: Blackwell.

Young, G., & Wolff, P. (1976) *Lateralization of manual behavior in 15-week-olds.* Manuscript submitted for publication.

Zangwill, O. (1960) *Cerebral dominance and its relation to psychological function.* Edinburgh: Oliver and Boyd.

Part IV

Speech Perception

SPEECH PERCEPTION AND LANGUAGE MODELS

How do we gather discrete language experiences from a continuous, complex sound wave? Speech perception study can be seen as a special case of the general psychological pattern recognition problem (Corcoran, 1971; Uhr, 1973).

Few research topics have stimulated people in as many disciplines. Psychologists, linguists, neurologists, philosophers, speech pathologists, audiologists, electrical engineers, computer scientists, and biologists are among the diverse interests active in this field. A consequence of this multidisciplinary interest has been a proliferation of terms and techniques as well as a large body of literature (for reviews, see Lindgren, 1965; Flanagan, 1972; Paap, 1975. Collections of germinal papers are found in Lehiste, 1900; Flanagan & Rabiner, 1973; Small, in press). It is not surprising that a number of integrative conferences have been held (see, Nagy, 1966; Wathen-Dunn, 1967).

Yet, only two essential research strategies appear to dominate speech perception work. As in psychology and linguistics, these approaches have their historical and philosophical roots in the rationalism—empiricism dichotomy (see Chapter 1).

Empiricists employ an analysis-by-analysis technique, which reduces the perceptual language experience to some "basic" perceptual unit and then seeks to relate (by correlation, association, etc.) tokens of the perceptual unit to real or theoretical invariants in the speech wave-form (e.g., Chapter 18).

Perceptual Units

Theories of speech and language are expressed in discrete categories. But, speech wave-forms, even though they exhibit stops and starts, transitions, and a variety of features, are essentially continuous across many linguistic boundaries. Consequently, researchers often feel compelled to assign a particular linguistic category the status of a "basic" or "minimal" perceptual unit. (For a review of some of these choices, see Lehiste, 1972.) The choices have not been generally agreed upon, and they include distinctive features (Jakobson, Fant, & Halle, 1969), context-sensitive allophones (Wickelgren, 1969a, b), phonemes (Cole, Chapter 18, this volume), and syllables (Savin & Bever, 1970; Liberman, Cooper, Shankweiler, & Studdert-Kennedy, 1967), as well as "word" or "morpheme-like" strings (Morton & Broadbent, 1967).

As in linguistics, rationalist-oriented approaches attempt to duplicate important aspects of the language experience by generating or synthesizing crucial surface elements of the experience from explicitly expressed, more abstract, and deeper theoretical elements (Chomsky, 1957, 1965; Liberman, 1970; Stevens, 1960, 1970; Stevens & Halle, 1962, 1967). In speech perception research, the surface elements generated are aspects of the acoustic signal. This is accomplished with the assistance of electrical and mechanical speech synthesizers, which are generally computer driven (see, Flanagan & Rabiner, 1973).

Empirical analysis-by-analysis techniques initially focus on surface aspects of the speech signal (and the linguistic analysis, e.g., the phone and spectrographic plosive "bursts"), claiming that the data base rests in the more observable facets of the speech stream.

Rationalist analysis-by-synthesis techniques, by contrast, focus on hypothesized underlying rule structures and conditions whose necessity is mandated by various configurations assumed to be encoded in the speech signal or by combinatorial properties of the linguistic system. In general, this latter approach requires a complex hierarchy of equally significant units which are related by well-defined rules (Chomsky & Halle, 1968; Jakobson *et al.,* 1969).

Cole (Chapter 18) defends the analysis-by-analysis approach and maintains that an adequate description of speech perception is possible by a sophisticated concatenation of surface units with real speech, although it may not be as successful with "degraded," synthetically produced speechlike sounds. He maintains that a fundamental invariance by which we can recognize the linguistic elements in speech are contained in the acoustic signal at the phonetic level. By contrast, a number of investigators (Katz & Postal, 1964; Liberman, 1970; Stevens & Halle, 1967) claim that important aspects of the speech signal do not appear on the surface at all. They maintain that, depending on the linguistic context, the same acoustic signal can result in two different perceptual experiences; or, that the converse can be true: that two very different patterns of sound wave can result in the same linguistic experience. This is a strong case for the significance of linguistic context; it does not, however, necessarily mean that the crucial contextual elements are not represented in the acoustic signal. It suggests rather that the speech signal is very highly encoded (Liberman, 1957). In fact, a classical synthesis experiment by Delattre, Liberman, and Cooper (1955) on transitional surface cues in the perception of /b/, /d/, and /g/ stop consonants in CV contexts for English-speaking listeners demonstrates that the rate of change of the second formant—concentration of acoustical energy in the speech spectrum—is at least partly responsible for the identification of these sounds. However, the actual cue itself is absent from an immediate surface representation. Delattre *et al.* (1955) argue that it is *the direction (frequency) to which the transition points* that is responsible for distinguishing these three phonemes.

An essential difference between authors who seek surface cues and those who argue for deeper cues would appear to be in the amount and type of processing required for the recognition and identification of speech sounds. There is no serious argument that many cues must be coded into the acoustic stream of speech. The question is open, though, as to what kind of machinery will be required to recover those cues. That is, how deeply encoded is the linguistic material woven into the speech stream.

Strategies used to scan the speech signal, for example, may be serial or parallel. Arbitrary elements A,B,C, . . . , may be processed sequentially according to some predetermined order or they may be processed simultaneously. Both scanning methods, and probably mixtures of the two, appear to be formally feasible, and there is some evidence that, at least in visual perception, newly learned recognition strategies may first be serial and later, with practice, become parallel (Corcoran, 1971).

Although the speech stream enters the ear serially, there is some impetus for claiming that a parallel processing capacity is required for the extraction of linguistic information, due to the speed with which humans communicate. In speech at rates of 200 to 300 words per minute—which is easily understood by most people—we are handling some 10 to 30 phonemes per second, or, in information-processing terms, about 50 bits per second (Liberman *et al.,* 1967; Stetson, 1951). This is clearly too high a rate to resolve auditorily for a nonspeech stream, as over a half century of experience in attempting to devise reading machines for the blind has demonstrated (Liberman, 1970; Liberman *et al.,* 1967).

This does not mean that parallel processing is necessitated. It does appear to indicate one of the following: that parallel processing is required; that the speech signal is highly encoded; or that the fundamental units of perception are larger than the phoneme—or some combination of these alternatives.

A decoding strategy may also be considered "active" or "passive." That is, does the nervous system have to generate and synthesize some kind of neural impulse to match the ones received from lower auditory pathways? Or does the nervous system analyze input signals on the basis of some "selective tuning"? In short, do we accept a generative model or a filtering model? As with the other positions discussed, rationalist-oriented researchers lean toward the active synthesis model, whereas empirical-oriented scientists prefer the passive analysis model.

An influential active model, the "motor theories" type, proposes the matching or mapping process on a neurological level using articulatory—motor reference as the necessary comparator (Chistovich, 1962; Liberman, 1957; Liberman, Cooper, Harris, & MacNeilage, 1962).

It is generally recognized, however, that, to achieve an adequate match, the signals or neural patterns must occur at the same level; that is, the signals require auditory and motor transformations such that adequate linguistic comparisons can be possible.

Passive theories, on the other hand, require some "generalizing filter" (Corcoran, 1971; Morton & Broadbent, 1967; Treisman, 1960). A central requirement of this type of model is some initial store of features or units to which the filter can respond and some "tuning" or "learning" mechanism which can refine and expand the range of inputs recognized as the speech it receives warrants (Morton & Broadbent, 1967; Chapters 18 and 20.).

In this regard, the discovery of neural acoustic feature detectors (see Chapter 18), which appear to be present in the squirrel monkey (Funkenstein, Nelson, Winter, Wollberg, & Newman, 1972) provides some possible mechanism. In addition, the finding that chinchillas are able to perceive the voice—voiceless distinction in English speech for initial plosives in CV pairs suggests that at least certain speech perception abilities are also possessed by other mammals, although we cannot be certain the same mechanism is responsible for this cross-species ability (Kuhl & Miller, 1975).

Alternatively, some verification of a three-dimensional, lingual muscle-spindle network in man that can mediate dynamic space—time information is apparent (Sussman, 1972). Such a network and finely tuned feedback apparatus in the tongue can be interpreted as lending credence to motor theory speculations.

These and other bits of neurological and behavioral evidence, however, do not yet weigh the arguments for or against active versus passive or parallel versus sequential proposals. They can readily be incorporated without serious modification into existing theories. Further, a variety of theories are proposed that utilize a mixture of these positions.

Fant (1962, 1963, 1967), for example, proposes a model that suggests an acoustic feature recognition device at the subphonemic level and a synthesis device at higher linguistic levels. Morton and Broadbent (1967) admit that some motor information input is possible in accounting for the recognition of dialect variations. The positions are not, in principle, exclusive and, at least at this stage of investigation, tend to be matters of emphasis.

The abilities of some nonhuman mammals to perceive aspects of English (and presumably all human) speech, and proposals that suggest innate mechanisms for speech perception, direct the researcher's attention to the acquisition of speech perception abilities. Experience in listening to foreign languages clearly illustrates for most of us that certain of the discrimination abilities we apply in daily life are learned. The natural questions are, which ones, and when? With some factual knowledge in these areas we are able to speculate on possible mechanisms.

Gilbert and Cooper (Chapters 19 and 20) review and provide speculation regarding production evidence. Cole (Chapter 18) reports on work in this area from receptive evidence. All three researchers concur on an innate component or at least an extremely early-developing component in speech perception abilities, coupled with a later-maturing production capacity. Each also appears to be representative of the more empirical school of thought, at least with respect to the problems presented here.

REFERENCES

Chistovich, L.A. (1962) Continuous recognition of speech by man. *Mashinnyi Perevod i Prikladnaia Lingvistika*, (Machine Translation and Applied Linguistics), 7, 3–44.

Chomsky, Noam (1957) *Syntactic structures*. The Hague: Mouton.

Chomsky, Noam (1965) *Aspects of the theory of syntax*. Cambridge, Massachusetts: MIT Press.

Chomsky, Noam, & Halle, M. (1968) *The sound pattern of English*. New York: Harper.

Corcoran, D.W.J. (1971) *Pattern recognition*. Baltimore: Penguin Books.

Delattre, P.C., Liberman, A.M., & Cooper, F.S. (1955) Acoustic loci and transitional cues for consonants. *Journal of the Acoustical Society of America, 27*, 769–773.

Fant, C.G.M. (1962) Descriptive analysis of the acoustic aspects of speech. *Logos, 5*, 3–17.

Fant, C.G.M. (1963) Comments by G. Fant to paper D3, a motor theory of speech perception. In *Proceedings of the speech communication seminar. Vol. 3* Stockholm: Royal Institute of Technology.

Fant, C.G.M. (1967) Auditory patterns of speech. In W. Wathen-Dunn (Ed.), *Models for the perception of speech and visual form*. Cambridge, Massachusetts: MIT Press.

Flanagan, J.L. (1972) *Speech analysis, synthesis and perception*. (2nd ed.) New York: Springer-Verlag.

Flanagan, J.L., & Rabiner, L.R. (Eds.) (1973) *Speech synthesis*. Stroudsburg, Pennsylvania: Dowden, Hutchinson & Ross.

Funkenstein, H.H., Nelson, P.G., Winter, P., Wollberg, Z., & Newman, J.D. (1972) Unit responses in auditory cortex of awake squirrel monkeys to vocal stimulation. in M.B. Sachs (Ed.), *Physiology of the auditory system*. Baltimore: National Educational Consultants.

Jakobson, R., Fant, C.G.M., & Halle, M. (1969) *Preliminaries to speech analysis: The distinctive features and their correlates*. Cambridge, Massachusetts: MIT Press.

Katz, J.J., & Postal, P.M. (1964) *An integrated theory of linguistic descriptions*. Cambridge, Massachusetts: MIT Press.

Kozhevnikov, J.A., & Chistovich, L. (1965) *Rech: Articulyatsiai vospriyatiye* (Speech, Articulation and Perception). Moscow-Lenningrad: Nanka. (Translated by U.S. Dept. of Commerce, Joint Publications Research Service (JPRS) Washington, D.C., No. 30)

Kuhl, P.K., & Miller, J.D. (1975) Speech perception by the chinchilla: Voiced-voiceless distinction in alveolar plosive consonants. *Science, 190,* 69–72.

Lehiste, I. (Ed.) (1967) *Readings in acoustic phonetics.* Cambridge, Massachusetts: MIT Press.

Lehiste, I. (1972) The units of speech perception. In. J.H. Gilbert (Ed.), *Speech and cortical functioning.* New York: Academic Press. Pp. 187–235.

Liberman, A.M. (1957) Some results of research on speech perception. *Journal of the Acoustical Society of America, 29,* 117–123.

Liberman, A.M. (1970) The grammars of speech and language. *Cognitive Psychology, 1,* 301–323.

Liberman, A.M., Cooper, F.S., Harris, K.S., & MacNeilage, P.F. (1962) A motor theory of speech perception. *Proceedings of the Speech Communication Seminar,* Session D3, Stockholm, Royal Institute of Technology, 1–10.

Liberman, A.M., Cooper, F.S., Shankweiler, D.P., & Studdert-Kennedy, M. (1967) Perception of the speech code. *Psychological Review, 74,* 431–461.

Lindgren, N. (1965) Machine recognition of human language. *IEEE Spectrum, 2,* 114–136.

Morton, J., & Broadbent, D.E. (1967) Passive versus active recognition models or is your homunculus really necessary? In W. Wathen-Dunn (Ed.), *Models for the perception of speech and visual form.* Cambridge, Massachusetts: MIT Press. Pp. 103–110.

Nagy, G. (1966) Pattern recognition 1966 IEEE Workshop Special Conference Report. *IEEE Spectrum,* February.

Savin, H.B., & T.G. Bever (1970) The nonperceptual reality of the phoneme. *Journal of Verbal Learning and Verbal Behavior, 9,* 295–302.

Small, A. (Ed.) (in press) *Psychological acoustics.* Stroudsburg, Pennsylvania: Dowden, Hutchinson & Ross.

Stetson, R.H. (1951) *Motor phonetics.* (2nd ed.) Amsterdam: N. Holland.

Stevens, K.N. (1960) Towards a model for speech recognition. *Journal of the Acoustical Society of America, 32,* 47–55.

Stevens, K.N. (1970) Segments features and analysis-by-synthesis. In J.F. Kavanagh & I.G. Mattingly (Eds.), *Language by eye and ear.* Cambridge, Massachusetts: MIT Press. Pp. 41–52.

Stevens, K.N., & Halle, M. (1962) Speech recognition: A model and a program for research. *IRE Trans. IT-8,* 155–159.

Stevens, K.N. & Halle, M. (1967) Remarks on analysis by synthesis and distinctive features. In W. Wathen-Dunn (Ed.), *Models for the perception of speech and visual form.* Cambridge, Massachusetts: MIT Press.

Sussman, H.M. (1972) What the tongue tells the brain. *Psychological Bulletin, 77,* 262–272.

Treisman, A.M. (1960) Contextual cues in selective listening. *Quarterly Journal of Experimental Psychology, 12,* 242–248.

Uhr, L. (1973) *Pattern Recognition, Learning and Thought.* Prentice-Hall.

Wathen-Dunn, W. (Ed.) (1967) *Models for the perception of speech and visual form.* Cambridge, Massachusetts: MIT Press.

Wickelgren, W.A. (1969a) Context-sensitive coding, associative memory, and serial order in (speech) behavior. *Psychological Review, 1,* 1–15.

Wickelgren, W.A. (1969b) Context-sensitive coding in speech recognition, articulation and development. In K.N. Leibovic (Ed.), *Information processing in the nervous system.* Berlin: Springer-Verlag. Pp. 85–95.

18

Invariant Features and Feature Detectors: Some Developmental Implications

RONALD A. COLE

Developmental psychology, perhaps more than any other area in psychology, is goal directed. While the developmental psychologist may concern himself with the qualitative nature of the child's world at a particular stage of functioning, he must eventually explain the transition to the adult mode of function. Thus, any widely accepted theory of adult behavior is bound to have a profound influence on the conceptions and research strategies of the developmental psychologist. Compare, for example, developmental accounts of language acquisition during the reign of behaviorism and following the basic acceptance of Chomsky's views on linguistic competence.

In the present chapter, I would like to describe briefly the currently popular view of speech perception. I hope to show that this view, which is based on experiments with synthetic speech, does not offer much hope for research to the developmental psychologist and, in fact, is not supported by experiments with real speech. Finally, I will describe an alternative model of speech perception, and outline its relevance to the development of speech perception in humans.

The study of speech perception has dealt mainly with the perception of phonemes. A phoneme, as I use the term, is a perceptual segment used to discriminate among the words of a language. Phonemes are the basic building blocks of speech—the consonant and vowel segments that make up syllables. A word such as BIT is composed of three phonemes; the words PIT, BET, and BID hold each of these phonemes in minimal contrast and demonstrate their perceptual importance.

A point of major agreement among students of speech perception is that a spoken utterance can be adequately described as an ordered series of phonetic segments[1] and that speech perception involves, at some level of analysis, the identification of an ordered series of phonemes. A fundamental problem in speech perception, then, is to specify the acoustic cues for phonemes and the process by which they are identified from the physical stimulus—the sounds of speech.

The present chapter follows, and is in some part a reaction to, over 20 years of research directed to the understanding and specification of the acoustic cues for phoneme perception. Most of this research has used synthetically produced speech, and the great majority of experiments have investigated the perception of stop consonants. The general view that has emerged from this research, a view which dominates the contemporary psychological literature, is that phonemes do not exist as physical entities in the speech wave (Liberman, Cooper, Shankweiler, & Studdert-Kennedy, 1967; Liberman, 1970). This is not a simple statement that there is lack of a general one-to-one correspondence between sound and perceived phoneme, but rather, that there is a complete and total lack of correspondence between any given segment of the speech wave and any particular phoneme.

This general statement about phoneme perception is based on the results of experiments with synthetic speech conducted at Haskins Laboratories. Figure 1 displays hand-painted speech spectrograms which, when converted to sound on a speech synthesizer, are heard as [di] (dee) and [du] (do). The two steady-state bars of energy in each syllable are called formants, and the relative frequency of the first two formants of a vowel are sufficient for its perception. The frequencies of the (lower) first formant and the (upper) second formant in real speech are determined mainly by the position of the tongue in the mouth. The relative height of the tongue determines the frequency of the first formant, while the relative front—backness of the raised portion of the tongue determines the frequency of the second formant. The tongue is raised toward the roof of the mouth for both /i/ and /u/, so that both vowels have a similar first formant. For /i/ the tongue is raised and pushed forward, which results in a second formant near 3000 Hz. For /u/ the tongue is also raised but is further back in the mouth, resulting in a second formant centered at about 600 Hz.

The acoustic feature *in these stimuli* responsible for perception of the stop consonant /d/ (as opposed to /b/ or /g/) is the frequency glide or *transition* to the upper or second formant. Note that the second formant transition in Figure 1 points to the same frequency for /di/ and /du/. This is because the starting frequency or locus of the second formant transition is determined by the place of articulation of the consonant, and the place of articulation just prior to the release of /d/ is approximately the same before all vowels. Soon after /d/ is released the vocal cords start vibrating while the vocal apparatus is gliding to the position assumed for the vowel. It is this movement of the articulators as the vocal tract is in

---

[1] In fluent speech, a phrase such as "Did you want to?" may be realized phonetically as /ʃawana/. The present chapter is concerned with how listeners recognize the series of phones in /ʃawana/ from the acoustic signal. The question of how listeners decode the (intended) words in an utterance from a partial phonetic representation is not considered in the present chapter, although my current research is directed to precisely this problem.

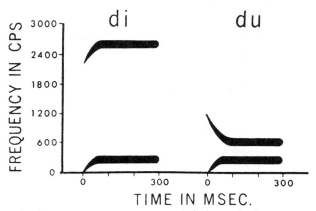

Figure 1. Hand-painted speech spectrograms of /di/ and /du/. (From Liberman, A.M., Cooper, F.S., Shankweiler, D.P., & Studdert-Kennedy, M., Perception of the speech code, *Psychological Review, 74,* 1967, 431–461. Copyright 1967 by the American Psychological Association. Reprinted by permission.)

transition from one target position to another that produces the formant transitions. Since the articulators must glide to different positions for /i/ and /u/, the second formant transition is quite different before the two vowels.

The important point is that the acoustic feature that determines perception of /d/, the second formant transition, is radically different before /i/ and /u/. There is, as shown in Figure 1, a lack of correspondence between sound and perceived phoneme.

The consonant /d/ is said to be highly *encoded* into the syllable (Liberman *et al.,* 1967), since the transition that determines its perception is an integral part of the vowel. It is not possible to articulate a transition without producing a vowel. The transitions only exist in relation to the vowel, so there is no specific segment of sound in the speechwave corresponding to the perceived phoneme /d/. It is not possible, for example, to remove the transitions from before the steady-state vowel, or to interchange the transitions between /i/ and /u/, and still perceive /d/.

The point I want to stress is that this specific property of encodedness—the lack of discrete acoustic features for individual phonemes—is currently held to be the single most essential aspect of speech. The relationship between sound and phoneme that has been observed for synthetic stop consonants has been generalized to most other phonemes, and has formed the central assumption for many current models of speech perception. This view has been stated most explicitly by Liberman *et al.* (1967):

> Acoustic cues for successive phonemes are intermixed in the sound stream to such an extent that definable segments of sound do not correspond to segments at the phoneme level. Moreover, the same phoneme is most commonly represented in different phonemic environments by sounds that are vastly different. There is, in short, a marked lack of correspondence between sound and perceived phoneme [p. 432: From Liberman, A.M., Cooper, F.S., Shankweiler, D.P., & Studdert-Kennedy, M., Perception of the speech code, *Psychological Review,* 1967, *74.* Copyright 1967 by the American Psychological Association. Reprinted by permission.].

MOTOR THEORIES OF SPEECH PERCEPTION

Given that phonemes are highly encoded into the signal, and that there are no discrete invariant cues for phonemes, we are left with two interesting questions: (a) what is the process by which listeners recover phonemes from the speechwave? and (b) how do children learn the phonemic system of their language?

Elaborate conceptual attempts have been made to describe the conversion from sound to phoneme as a "grammatical conversion" (Liberman, 1967) or "analysis by synthesis" (Stevens, 1972; Stevens & Halle, 1967). These models of speech perception assume that speech perception is mediated by the processing mechanisms involved in the *production* of speech, and are thus known as "motor theories" of speech perception. The original motor theory of speech perception, proposed by Liberman (1957) and elaborated by Liberman *et al.* (1967) and Liberman (1970), was advanced to explain how listeners could perceive segmental phonemes without reference to invariant acoustic features. The theory is based on the assumption that, whereas there is a lack of correspondence between sound and perceived phoneme, *production* of a particular phoneme involves reference to an invariant set of centrally stored motor commands. Perception of phonemes, then, is mediated by reference to these invariant commands.

> The listener uses the inconstant sound as a basis for finding his way back to the articulatory gestures that produces it and thence, as it were, to the speaker's intent [Liberman *et al.*, 1967, p. 453].

And,

> The assumption is that at some level or levels of the production process there exist neural signals standing in one-to-one correspondence with the various segments of the language—phoneme, word, phrase, etc. Perception consists in somehow running the process backward, the neural signals corresponding to the various segments being found at their respective levels. In phoneme perception—our primary concern in this paper—the invariant is found far down in the neuromotor system, at the level of the commands to the muscles [p. 454].

Although the motor theory offers an elaborate conceptualization of the perceptual process, it does not describe the information-processing routines by which listeners convert the incoming sounds to the invariant motor commands. That is, the motor theory offers a conception, but no mechanism. In fact, in a subsequent paper Liberman (1970) suggests that the conversion from sound to phoneme is actually a grammatical transformation and is therefore a part of a listener's innately determined linguistic competence.

A second problem with motor theories is that they cannot adequately account for certain recent findings about infant speech perception. Eimas and his colleagues (Cutting & Eimas, 1975; Eimas, 1974; Eimas, Sequeland, Jusczyk, & Vigorito, 1971) have shown that infants are able to perceive certain phonetic distinctions by the age of 1 month. As Eimas (1974) points out:

> Although motor theories of speech perception are possible models of adult speech perception, the application of this class of model to the speech-processing capability of the infant raises certain difficulties. Most prominent of these is the need to explain how the young, virtually inarticulate infant has come to possess the complex knowledge

required for the conversion of phonetic features to articulatory commands, and how he has come to associate particular auditory patterns with articulatory commands. Without ascribing this knowledge to the biological endowment of the infant, there would appear to be no way in which an infant could have acquired this information by traditional means during the first few weeks or months of life. However, to attribute this knowledge to the infant's biological endowment would seem to extend considerably the cognitive competencies that we are willing to impute to genetically determined factors [p. 518: From Eimas, P.D., Auditory and linguistic processing of cues for place of articulation by infants, *Perception & Psychophysics,* 1974, *16*(3).].

In summary, although elaborate conceptual attempts have been made to describe the conversion from sound to phoneme, the process may still be considered magical. The name for the magician is the "special decoder." He works in the "speech mode" and he lives in the "speech processor," which is located in the land of the left hemisphere. Research with synthetic speech has thus led to a general mystique about speech perception. Phenomena of categorical perception and results of dichotic listening experiments have all added to the speech mystique—speech is a special code, and speech perception is a special, uniquely human process.

THE INVARIANT FEATURES OF SPEECH

Thus far I have attempted to show that the general mystique about speech perception has grown out of one basic assumption—that phonemes are not generally accompanied by invariant acoustic features. Although most researchers interested in speech perception have accepted this basic assumption, it should be noted that several investigators, most notably Fant (1967), have advocated a continued search for invariant cues for phonemes.[2] Stevens (1973) has suggested that invariance is a necessary condition for the development of phoneme perception. He argues that:

In spite of this apparent lack of invariance, it is recognized that, at a stage when a child is acquiring language, he needs some basis on which to organize and classify the acoustic events in speech. Some invariant property must exist in the acoustic events associated with phonetic segments that have a particular feature in common, so that a child can identify these events as belonging to the same category or feature [p. 155: From Stevens, K.N., Potential role of property detectors in the perception of consonants, M.I.T. Research Laboratory of Electronics, 1973, QPR No. 110, July 15.].

In the next section, I will attempt to show that there is in fact a great deal of invariant information accompanying the consonant phonemes of English.

The Extent of Invariance for Consonant Phonemes

In the past four years my colleagues and I at the University of Waterloo and more recently at Carnegie-Mellon University have examined the cues for consonant phonemes in English using natural speech. We have found that the encoded portions

---

[2] An invariant cue is defined as an acoustic feature that remains constant for a given phoneme across different syllable contexts, and provides information about the identity of the phoneme.

of speech—the vowel transitions—provide important information about the place of articulation of certain phonemes. However, the major source of information about the identity of individual phonemes is signaled by invariant acoustic features (Cole & Scott, 1974b).

Our research has shown that most consonant phonemes are accompanied by invariant energy that provides sufficient information to specify the phoneme uniquely. For other phonemes, the invariant energy limits perception to a possible pair of phonemes. The remainder of this chapter briefly describes the invariant features of speech as well as some recent research that sheds new light on the response characteristics of analyzers or "feature detectors" that mediate speech perception. The final section of the chapter discusses the implications of invariant features and feature detectors for developmental theories of speech perception.

Invariant Features for Stop Consonants?

In the present chapter, discussion is restricted to the acoustic features that accompany consonant phonemes in stressed CV syllables. I assume, along with Stevens (1973) and others, that these syllables are most salient to the prelinguistic child, contain the most invariant information, and form the basis for the development of more acoustically complex phonemic discriminations.

To begin, how do we know if the initial energy in a consonant—vowel (CV) syllable is invariant? We can test for perceptual invariance by a very simple experiment. If a segment of energy is invariant across different syllable environments and uniquely specifies a particular phoneme, then it should be possible to physically remove the segment from before one vowel, splice it onto any other steady-state vowel, and still perceive the original phoneme.

Brian Scott and I performed a tape-splicing experiment of this kind with stop consonants. In English, the voiced stops /b, d, g/ in stressed CV syllables consist of a short stop burst lasting from 6 to 10 msec, followed by a 10- to 20-msec "open" interval of relative silence, followed by transitions to the steady-state vowel. For the voiceless stops /p, t, k/ the burst is followed by a breathy interval of noise, called aspiration, that lasts from 40 to 70 msec. The voiceless stops have weak vowel transitions compared to the voiced stops because the vocal tract glides to the vowel during the aspiration. The formant transitions are thus embedded within the aspirated portion of the syllable. Speech spectrograms of the stop consonants spoken before /i/ and /u/ are displayed in Figure 2.

Cole and Scott (1974a) recorded each of the stop consonants before /i/ and /u/. In control syllables, the vowel transitions were first removed from before the vowel and the entire aperiodic noise segment that preceded the vowel transitions was then spliced back onto the steady-state vowel. Listeners were essentially perfect in identifying all of the stops when vowel transitions were removed and the burst plus open interval (for voiced stops) or the burst plus aspiration (for voiceless stops) was spliced onto its original steady-state vowel. To test for invariance, the entire aperiodic portion of energy prior to the onset of the first glottal pulse was

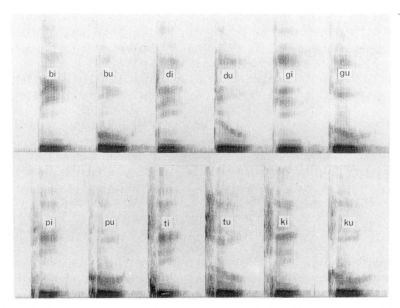

Figure 2. Speech spectrograms of the stop consonants before /i/ and /u/. (From Cole, R.A., & Scott, B., Toward a theory of speech perception, *Psychological Review,* 1974, *81,* 348–374. Copyright 1974 by the American Psychological Association. Reprinted by permission.)

transposed between steady-state tokens of /i/ and /u/. Results of the identification test revealed that the transposed energy was invariant across the /i/–/u/ environments for /b/, /d/, /p/ and /t/.[3] There was some evidence for invariance for the burst plus aspiration portion of /k/, but no evidence for invariance was found for /g/.

In a recent experiment, Just, Suslick, Michaels, and Shockey (1977) replicated and extended our results in a carefully performed experiment using a computerized tape-splicing system. Just *et al.* recorded each voiced and voiceless stop before /i/, /a/, and /u/ and determined the precise duration of the burst and open interval for

[3] The tape-splicing experiment we performed has produced a substantial amount of agitation in speech perception circles as well as a good deal of criticism. (Dorman, Raphael, & Studdert-Kennedy, 1975). The main criticism directed against this study was that the transposed segments of noise were too long, since they contained not only the stop burst but also the onset of formant transitions embedded in the aperiodic noise. This criticism is based on the naive view that there is a single acoustic feature such as the stop burst that signals the identity of a given stop consonant across different vowels. Rather, we have taken the view that both bursts and transitions are essential to perception of stop consonants; that these cues contribute differentially to perception of a stop consonant before different vowels; and, most important, that these cues interact to provide an invariant pattern. To restate our original conclusion: "The essential point demonstrated in this experiment is that the entire energy spectrum that accompanies a stop consonant prior to the vowel transitions contains invariant perceptual information [Cole & Scott, 1974a, p. 106]."

each voiced stop and of the burst and aspirated portion of each voiceless stop. This energy was then removed from before the original vowel and spliced onto a different steady-state vowel. The percentage of correct identification responses for each stop in each vowel environment are shown in Table 1. It can be seen that listeners' identification responses are well above chance (17%) for both control and transposed syllables for /b/, /d/, /p/, /t/, and also for /k/, with one exception (/i/ → /u/).

It seems that the aperiodic portion of a voiced stop consonant carries a great deal of information about the identity of the consonant and is relatively invariant across the point vowels /i/, /a/, and /u/. It should be reemphasized that the burst and transition do not contribute equally to perception of the voiced stops before different vowels, as Fischer-Jørgenson (1972) has confirmed for Danish stops. Just *et al.* found that, while the burst is a sufficient and invariant cue for /d/ before /i/ and /u/, the transition carries more information than the burst when /d/ occurs before /a/. Still, listeners identify /d/ when the burst from /da/ is transposed to /i/ or /u/.

For the voiceless stops, the burst plus aspiration carries sufficient information for listeners to identify the stop consonant whether this energy is presented in isolation (Winitz, Scheib, & Reeds, 1972) or is transposed between /i/, /a/, and /u/ (Cole & Scott, 1974a, Experiment 2; Just *et al.,* 1976). It is clear, however, that some of the information about the voiceless stop is carried by the transitions embedded within the aspiration. This fact was confirmed by Just *et al.,* who found

TABLE 1 Percentage of Correct Identifications of Stop Consonants Based on Information Prior to Vowel Transitions

	Voiced			Voiceless		
	b	d	g	p	t	k
Control						
/i/ → /i/	87	97	79	98	100	100
Transposed						
/i/ → /u/	95	74	11	91	87	18
/i/ → /a/	81	43	12	87	72	40
Control						
/a/ → /a/	74	37	13	92	86	97
Transposed						
/a/ → /i/	57	83	27	88	95	47
/a/ → /u/	92	55	32	96	61	76
Control						
/u/ → /u/	96	93	75	97	100	99
Transposed						
/u/ → /i/	65	66	51	83	87	82
/u/ → /a/	81	50	38	86	87	98

in a subsequent experiment that replacing the aspiration with silence greatly reduced the subject's ability to identify the voiceless stop. For the voiced stops, Blumstein and Stevens (1976) have shown that identification of the stop is essentially perfect if listeners are presented with the burst and the first two glottal pulses of the vowel.

I believe it is an extremely important fact of speech perception that listeners are able to identify a stop consonant when the burst and transitions are presented outside of their original syllable context. This result suggests that a stop consonant does not need to be decoded from a larger syllable unit.

Despite the evidence for a high degree of invariance for certain stop consonants, it is clear that perception of stop consonants depends not upon identification of any one particular acoustic feature but upon the interaction of various features. This statement is supported by at least two results that have emerged across studies. First, syllables that have been altered in some way, even when identified well above chance, are rarely identified as well as unaltered versions of the same syllable. Second, identification preformance based on one or more features almost always improves when the listener is presented with additional features. Thus, Sharf and Hemeyer (1972) found identification performance was well above chance for voiceless stops when listeners were presented with all of the aperiodic noise prior to the vowel, but a significant improvement was observed when listeners were provided with this energy plus the first 100 msec of vowel. These results suggest that, while certain features may be relatively invariant and carry a high information load for a given stop consonant, "normal" perception of stop consonants requires information from a variety of features that interact in complex ways before different vowels.

One possibility that has occurred to several investigators (e.g., Fant, 1967) is that the acoustic features for a given stop consonant before different vowels may combine to form an invariant pattern or "gestalt." In what may turn out to be the light at the end of the tunnel in the search for invariance, Stevens (1973) and Stevens and Blumstein (1976) have reported evidence for context-independent spectral *configurations* for stop and nasal consonants in CV syllables. Stevens notes that certain acoustic features are evident for consonants preceding stressed vowels in all phonetic environments. One such feature is a rapid frequency change in the energy spectrum following the release of the consonant. Examining spectrograms and short-time spectra for stop and nasal consonants in CV syllables, Stevens (1973) has described three general spectral patterns corresponding to the three places of articulation of the stop consonants:

Labial consonants are generally characterized by a rapid spectrum change in which the spectrum at the initial onset of energy has an energy concentration that is lower in frequency than that in the spectrum sampled a few milliseconds later.

A rapid spectrum change in which the onset of energy at high frequencies precedes the onset at lower frequencies characterizes a *coronal* consonant, i.e., a consonant produced with the tongue blade. For example, the falling second-formant transition in a syllable containing /d/ or /n/ followed by a back vowel would result in a spectrum change of this type.

Still another type of rapid spectrum change occurs for *velar* and other dorsal consonants. In this case, the major energy concentration at the onset is in the middle frequency range. Immediately following this onset there is a spreading or broadening of the spectral energy to frequency regions above and below this middle range [p. 161].

Furthermore,

All of these cues for place of articulation occur within the rapid spectrum change at the onsets of consonant–vowel syllables. They identify features of place of articulation without reference to acoustic events remote from this point in time. That is, these cues are absolute properties of the speech signal, and are context-independent. Determination of place of articulation from these properties does not require that attributes of the signal be placed in some kind of precategorical auditory store, since there is no need to interpret one portion of the signal with reference to another portion that occurs at a different time [p. 164].

It should be noted that Stevens's description of context-independent spectral patterns for place of articulation considers transitions to the third vowel formant. Thus, the synthetic [di] in Figure 1 has a rising second formant transition and would appear to violate the rule that coronals change from higher to lower frequencies. However, Stevens notes that "there may be a slightly rising F_2 transition, but this is offset by a strongly falling F_3 transition [p. 163]." It should also be noted that the frequency of the stop burst is generally high for the coronals, low for the labials, and intermediate for the velars (Halle, Hughes, & Radley, 1957), consistent with Stevens's analysis of the spectral pattern of the transitions and vowels.

To summarize, it appears that certain features carry a high information load for certain stop consonants and provide sufficient information to allow listeners to identify the consonant in most phonetic environments. Perhaps more important, preliminary evidence provided by Stevens suggests that, "for a majority of consonant–vowel syllables, the labial, coronal, and velar categories have the simple primary context-independent characteristics described above [Stevens, 1973, p. 165]."

The Invariant Structure of CV Syllables

Examination of naturally spoken CV syllables for the remaining consonant phonemes in English reveals a typical pattern—the CV syllable is composed of an initial invariant portion of energy followed by transitions to the steady-state vowel. Figure 3 displays speech spectrograms of six different CV syllables. Each of these syllables has an initial invariant portion of energy which serves to specify the consonant phoneme uniquely. The fricatives /s/, /z/, /š/ and /ž/ are characterized by a gradual onset and a particular spectral distribution of frication. For /s/ and /z/, the fricative noise is centered in a region from approximately 4000 to 7000 Hz, whereas the fricative noise for /š/ and /ž/ has a wider bandwidth extending into the lower frequencies. The distinction between /s/ and /z/ and between /š/ and /ž/, in the present example, is that the voiced fricatives /z/ and /ž/ are accompanied by

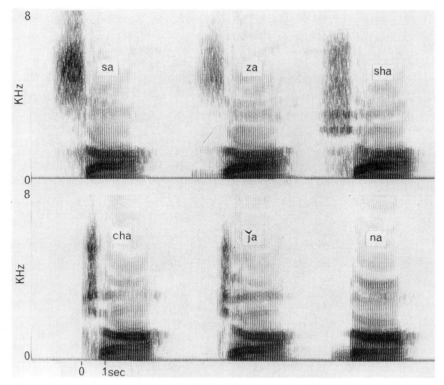

Figure 3. Speech spectrograms of selected fricatives and affricates (from Cole & Scott, 1974b).

voicing—resonant energy at the lower frequencies—while the voiceless fricatives /s/ and /š/ are never accompanied by low-frequency resonant energy. The affricates /č/ (as in "chair") and /ǰ/ (as in "job") are distinguished from the fricatives by an abrupt onset. Like the stops, the affricates are released with an explosive burst, so the /č/ and /ǰ/ are characterized by an abrupt onset. In general, the fricative portion of /č/ is longer than the fricative portion of /ǰ/.

The invariant portion of the CV syllable serves as a sufficient cue for identification of the fricatives /s/, /š/, /z/, and /ž/, and the affricates /č/ and /ǰ/. For these phonemes, the initial segment of noise can be removed from before the vowel transitions in the CV syllable and spliced onto a different steady-state vowel, and the original phoneme will still be heard.

Immediately following the invariant energy, vowel transitions may be clearly observed in each of these syllables. As mentioned earlier, the starting frequency of the second formant transition is determined by the place of articulation of the consonant. Since all of the consonants in Figure 3 have a similar place of articulation, the vowel transitions are similar. However, these vowel transition do *not* aid in perception of these consonants. The consonants /s, š, z, ž, č, and ǰ/ are perfectly

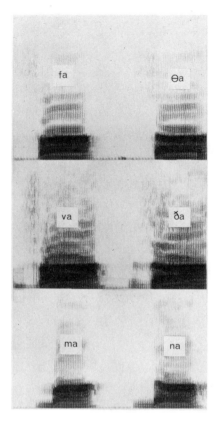

Figure 4. Speech spectrograms of selected fricatives and nasals (from Cole & Scott, 1974b).

intelligible if the initial invariant energy is removed from the syllable and spliced onto a steady-state vowel (Cole & Scott, 1973).

The remaining consonant phonemes /m/, /n/; /f/, /θ/; and /v/, /ð/ also contain invariant portions, but, for these phonemes, the invariant energy limits perception to a pair of possible phonemes, as shown in Figure 4. Thus, the low-frequency nasal resonance limits perception to /m/ or /n/, the low amplitude frication cues either /f/ or /θ/, and the frication plus voicing cues either /v/ or /ð/. In order to discriminate between the members of each pair, the vowel transitions are needed (Harris, 1958, Malécot, 1956). The first member of each pair in Figure 4 has a rising second formant transition, since it is articulated toward the front of the mouth; the second member of each pair has a falling second formant transition, since it is articulated toward the center of the mouth. Thus, perception of these phonemes requires identification of both invariant and context-conditioned cues.

To summarize, the fricatives /s/, /z/, /š/, and /ž/, the affricates /č/ and /ǰ/ are accompanied by invariant acoustic features that serve to identify the phoneme uniquely. In addition, the fricatives /f/, /θ/, /v/, and /ð/, and the nasals /m/ and [n] are also accompanied by invariant features in CV syllables, but the invariant information in the syllable limits perception to a pair of possible phonemes. Of the entire set of English consonant phonemes, only the velar stops /g/ and /k/ are signaled entirely by context-conditioned cues, and, as Stevens points out, the velar stops may be characterized in terms of a diverging spectrum in most phonetic environments. Thus, in stressed CV syllables, 16 of the 18 consonant phonemes in English (and perhaps all 18) are accompanied by invariant configurations of sound.

Given the extent of invariant information present in the speech wave, it seems highly unlikely that listeners ignore this information in order to process the highly encoded portions of speech. In fact, speech devoid of the phonemic information signaled by invariant features for consonants is completely unintelligible (Cole & Scott, 1974b, pp. 360–362). It is therefore necessary to assume that listeners attend to invariant features (in addition to the context-conditioned variations in speech) in order to perceive the phonemic message. Similarly, we may assume that the child attends to the invariant features of speech in order to master the phonemic system of his language.

FEATURES AND FEATURE DETECTORS

In the previous section I have argued that consonant phonemes are signaled by discrete acoustic features, many of them invariant, that are readily observable in real speech. One of the implications of this view is that speech perception may be mediated by a finite number of finely-tuned auditory feature detectors (Abbs & Sussman, 1971; Cole & Scott, 1972; Eimas, 1974). In the past year, W.E. Copper and I have been investigating this possibility.

Eimas and Corbit (1973) first reported evidence for the existence of phonetic feature detectors using a selective adaptation paradigm. In their experiment, subjects were randomly presented with syllables from a series in which the syllables varied in discrete acoustic steps from a voiced to voiceless stop consonant (e.g., /b/ to /p/ or /d/ to /t/). Stimuli varied in 5-msec steps in terms of their voice onset time (VOT), defined as the interval between the onset of the stop burst and the onset of vocal cord vibration (voicing). Stimuli ranged from 0 msec VOT (a distinct /b/) to 60 msec VOT (a distinct /p/). A stimulus with a VOT of 30 msec was heard equally often as /b/ and /p/, and this stimulus defined the phoneme boundary.

Eimas and Corbit found that repeated presentation of a stimulus from one end of the continuum resulted in a shift of the phoneme boundary toward the adapting stimulus. That is, repeated presentation of /b/ resulted in fewer /b/ responses for stimuli near the boundary, while repeated presentation of /p/ resulted in fewer /p/ responses. Their results cannot be easily explained in terms of response bias, since adaptation along a bilabial voiced–voiceless continuum (i.e., /b/–/p/) was produced using an apical stop (i.e., /d/ or /t/) as the adapting stimulus. Thus, adaptation with the voiced stop /d/ resulted in fewer /b/ responses to syllables near the boundary of the /b/—/p/ series, while adaptation with /t/ resulted in fewer /p/ responses. This result suggests that a phonetic feature was adapted, and not a particular consonant.

Eimas and Corbit argued that the shift in perception following adaptation was caused by fatigue of feature detectors responsive to a certain range of VOT values. According to their account, the unadapted response range of one analyzer partially overlaps the response range of an opponent analyzer. For stimuli that excite both analyzers—that is, stimuli near the phoneme boundary—the output of the analyzer with the greater response overrides the output of the other analyzer and results in a decision about the phonetic identity of the syllable. A stimulus that excites both analyzers equally is heard as ambiguous and represents the phoneme boundary. The fatigue model states that adaptation produces a decrease in the responsiveness of one analyzer across its entire range with respect to the opponent analyzer, thus producing a shift in the location of the phoneme boundary.

Selective adaptation has also been demonstrated along the place of articulation dimension by Cooper (1974). Cooper varied the starting frequency of the second and third formant transitions to produce a series of synthetic CV syllables that varied in discrete steps from /b/ to /d/ to /g/. Adaptation with /b/ shifted the /b/—/d/ boundary toward /b/ but did not significantly affect the /d/—/g/ boundary. Similarly, adaptation with /g/ shifted the /d/—/g/ boundary toward /g/ but did not affect the /b/—/d/ boundary. Finally, adaptation with /d/ shifted both boundaries toward /d/. From these results, Cooper argued for the existence of a bilabial, apical, and velar subset of feature detectors for the place of articulation dimension.

An experiment by Cooper and Blumstein (1974) suggests that finely tuned feature detectors for vowel transitions may be responsible for perception of place of articulation for synthetically produced stop consonants. Cooper and Blumstein presented subjects with five different real speech adapting stimuli—/bæ/, /mæ/, /væ/, /wæ/, and /pʰæ/, and tested for adaptation along a /bæ/—/dæ/—/gæ/ continuum. Syllables in the test series differed only in the starting frequency of the second and third formant transitions. The results showed a large and nearly identical decrease in /b/ responses following adaptation with /bæ/, /mæ/, and /væ/, but not following repeated presentation of /wæ/ and /pʰæ/. These results are interesting because the three adapting syllables that produced a large effect (/bæ/, /mæ/, and /væ/) have identical vowel transitions (see Figure 5) whereas the vowel transitions are quite different for /wæ/ and /pʰæ/.

The experiment by Cooper and Blumstein suggests the existence of finely tuned feature detectors for vowel transitions. In addition, their results provide exciting support for the feature-detector model proposed by Stevens (1973) to account for perception of the invariant spectral patterns he observed for stop and nasal consonants. Stevens speculates that:

> Detection of place of articulation of stop and nasal consonants preceding stressed vowels can be achieved if three different property detectors are available in the receiver: (i) a detector that responds when the onset of energy in one frequency region is followed by the onset of energy in an adjacent lower frequency region; (ii) a detector that responds when the onset of energy in one frequency region is followed by the onset of energy in an adjacent higher frequency region; and (iii) a detector that responds when the onset of energy in one frequency region is followed by the onset of energy in *both* an adjacent

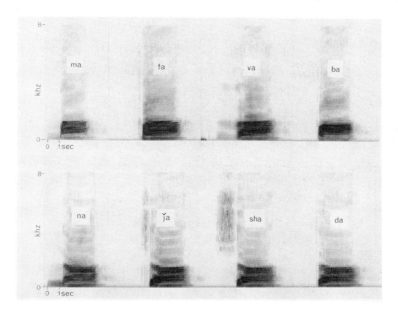

Figure 5. Speech spectrograms of consonants articulated toward the front of the mouth (top panel) and center of the mouth (bottom panel). Note the relationship between place of articulation and starting frequency of the second formant transition. (From Cole, R.A., Cooper, W.A., Allard, F., & Singer, J., Selective adaptation of English consonants using real speech, *Perception & Psycholophysics*, 1975, *18*, 227–244.)

higher frequency region *and* an adjacent lower frequency region. It is conceivable that only two such detectors are required—one responding to rising spectral energy and the other to falling spectral energy. Both detectors respond to a velar consonant in which the energy at an onset spreads both upward and downward in frequency [p. 163].

It is clear that the selective adaptation procedure provides an exciting paradigm for investigating the properties of hypothetical feature detectors. However, because the adaptation procedure requires series of stimuli that vary in precise acoustic steps, all of the experiments to date have been restricted to continua composed of synthetic stop consonants that differ along the voiced—voiceless dimension or the place of articulation dimension.

Cole, Cooper, Allard, and Singer (1975) recently performed a series of adaptation experiments in which the adapting syllable and the series of test syllables were all constructed from naturally spoken CV syllables. The construction of a variety of different test series was made possible by the fact that most English consonants have other consonants "embedded" within them (Carlson, Granstrom, & Pauli, 1972; Cole & Scott, 1974a; Gerstman, 1957; Grimm, 1966; Scott, 1971). Embedded sounds exist because the structure of a CV syllable, as previously mentioned, consists of an invarant set of features followed by a transition-vowel unit.

If we remove the invariant portion of the syllable, we are left with the embedded transition-vowel unit, and a stop consonant—vowel syllable is heard. If the original consonant is articulated toward the front of the mouth, the second formant

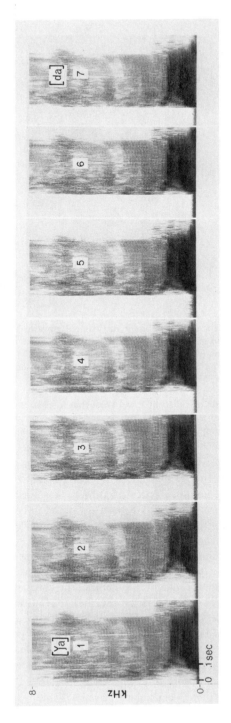

Figure 6. Speech spectrograms of a /ǰa/-/da/ continuum produced by splicing increasingly longer segments from the onset of a naturally spoken /ǰa/ (from Cole *et al.*, 1975).

transition begins at a low frequency, as shown in the upper panel of Figure 5. Thus, the vowel transitions in /ma/, /fa/, and /va/ are similar to the transitions in /ba/. When the nasal resonance is excised from /ma/, or the fricative portion from /fa/ or /va/, the syllable /ba/ is clearly perceived. Similarly, syllables in the lower panel in Figure 5 have the same vowel transitions as /da/, and the syllable /da/ is embedded in /na/, /ša/, and /ǰa/. By splicing successive segments from the onset of the original CV syllable, it is possible to construct continua that vary in discrete acoustic steps from, for example /ma/ to /ba/, /va/ to /ba/, /na/ to /da/, or /ǰa/ to /da/. Using continua constructed in this way, Cole *et al.* have demonstrated adaptation for voiced and voiceless stops, nasals, affricates and fricatives.

Let me briefly describe the procedure used to construct a natural speech continuum and present some identification data for a /ǰa/ to /da/ series. The original /ǰa/ was recorded on magnetic tape at 7-1/2 ips. The syllable contained 70 msec of fricative noise measured from burst onset to the onset of the first glottal pulse (the start of the vowel transitions). The /ǰa/ was duplicated a number of times and the onset of the consonant was marked on the recording tape for each duplicated syllable. This was done by drawing the magnetic type manually over the playback head of the tape recorder, listening for the onset of the fricative noise, and then marking the appropriate place on the magnetic tape with a grease pencil. After each syllable was marked, the desired segment of fricative noise was removed from the beginning of the syllable by tape splicing. Speech spectrograms of the seven syllables in the /ǰa/–/da/ series are shown in Figure 6. The syllable at the far left of

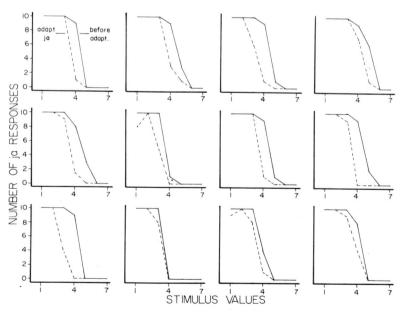

Figure 7. Individual subject's identification responses to syllables along a /ǰa/-/da/ continuum before and after repeated presentation of /ǰa/ (from Cole *et al.*, 1975).

the figure is the original /ʃa/ containing 70 msec of frication, while each successive syllable contains 10 msec less of frication.

Once we have constructed a continuum, it is possible to test for adaptation effects. Subjects in the first experiment we performed with the /ʃa/–/da/ series participated in two separate sessions at least 2 days apart (Cole *et al.,* 1975). Each session consisted of an initial identification test in which each of the seven syllables were presented 10 times each in random order. The identification test was followed, after a 5-min rest period, by seven adaptation trials. Each adaptation trial consisted of 200 repetitions of either Syllable 1 (/ʃa/) or Syllable 7 (/da/) (depending upon the session) at the rate of three repetitions every 2 sec. Following these repetitions, subjects were randomly presented with 10 stimuli from the test series for identification as /ʃa/ or /da/. Thus, in the two sessions subjects identified each of the seven stimuli 10 times as /ʃa/ or /da/, either before or after listening to either the /ʃa/ or /da/ adapter.

The results of this experiment are presented for the individual subjects, for the /ʃa/ adapter in Figure 7 and for the /da/ adapter in Figure 8. A significant change in the phoneme boundary in the predicted direction was produced by both adapters. Thus, compared to the preadaptation test series (the solid lines) there were fewer /ʃ/ responses following repeated presentation of /ʃa/, and fewer /d/ responses following repeated presentation of /da/. It is clear from Figures 7 and 8 that adaptation is selective, in that the change in the subjects' responses occurred only to those stimuli near the phoneme boundary.

A dramatic result of this experiment was that the amount of change following

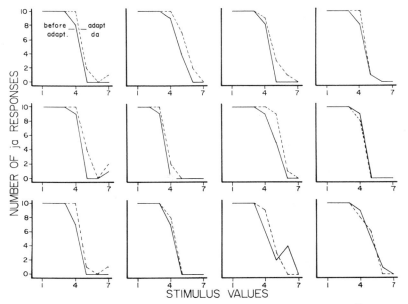

Figure 8. Individual subject's identification responses to syllables along a /ʃa/-/da/ continuum before and after repeated presentation of /da/ (from Cole *et al.,* 1975).

adaptation with /ja/ was significantly greater than that following adaptation with /da/ ($p < .01$). A comparison of the magnitude of the boundary shift for the individual subjects revealed that all 12 subjects exhibited a greater shift in the phoneme boundary following adaptation with /ja/ than /da/. This result has been termed asymmetrical adaptation, and is assumed to reflect the fact that some analyzers mediating phoneme perception are more resistant to fatigue than others.

Adaptation with Fluent Speech

All of the experiments reported to date on adaptation of speech have employed isolated syllables as the adapting stimuli. The question natuarlly arises: Is it possible to produce adaptation by presenting listeners with meaningful, connected speech?

Rudnicky and Cole (1977) performed a series of experiments that provide an affirmative answer to this question. Three experiments were performed, each examining adaptation of a different phonetic feature using ongoing speech. The test series used in the three experiments are shown in Figure 9. The stop consonant (/ti/−/di/), affricate (/ja/−/da/), and nasal (/ma/−/ba/) test series were constructed by removing the appropriate duration of energy from /ti/, /ja/, and /ma/, respectively, just prior to the onset of the vowel, and then splicing the initial consonant energy back onto the vowel.

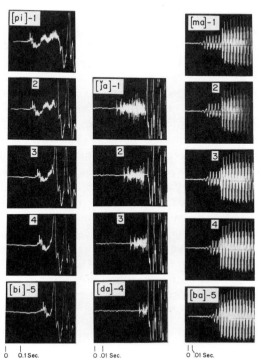

Figure 9. Test series generated by removing increasingly longer segments of energy just prior to the onset of the vowel. Note that syllables in each series have identical onsets.

TABLE 2   Sample Adaptation Sentences

Type of sentence	Sentence
Containing a predominance of voiceless stops	The Card Place sold pretty writing paper, pencils in sets of ten, penny candy, and all sorts of teasers to tempt those with plenty of cash to spend.
Containing a predominance of affricates	The Joneses, Jane and Chuck, joined Chelsea and John Champi after lunch. Jane chose cherries jubilee, Chuck chose German chocolate cake, and Chelsea and John just chose jello.
Containing a predominance of nasals	Norman was mentally nearly a moron. Nevertheless he had a natural knack for maintaining his new motorcycle. The mechanic from North Newton noted that his knowledge of the machine's motor much exceeded that of most "normal" men.

Examples of the adapting sentences used in each experiment are shown in Table 2. It can be seen that a "voiceless" adapting sentence contains words beginning with /p/, /t/, and /k/ and no words beginning with the voiced stops /b/, /d/ or /g/. "Affricate" sentences contained words beginning with /č/ and /ĵ/ and no words beginning with voiced stops. "Nasal" sentences contained words beginning with /m/ and /n/ and no words beginning with voiced stops.

In each experiment, subjects first identified (by number) syllables from one of the test series (e.g., 1 = clear /ti/, 5 = clear /di/) and then identified these same syllables after listening to sets of 2 adapting sentences. For example, subjects in the "voiceless" experiments first identified each of the five syllables in the /ti/–/di/ series 10 times each and then listened to 10 different pairs of "voiceless" adapting sentences. After listening to each pair of sentences, subjects identified five randomly presented syllables from the /ti/–/di/ series. Thus, each test syllable in the /ti/–/di/ series was identified 10 times before presentation of the sentences and 10 times after presentation of the sentences.

The results of these experiments are shown in Figure 10. The predicted adaptation effect was observed in each experiment. Presentation of voiceless sentences, for example, resulted in a general decrease in the mean integer response (i.e., syllables were rated as more /d/-like) to syllables in the /ti/–/di/ series.[4] These results suggest that adaptation to speech is not limited to repeated presentation of isolated syllables, but may be observed with fairly natural, ongoing speech.

The experiments reviewed in this section provide strong preliminary support for the notion that speech perception is at least partially mediated by analyzers that respond to phonetically relevant parameters of the acoustic signal. Selective adaptation has been shown to be an extremely robust effect that has been observed for a variety of synthetic and natural speech syllables as well as for connected speech.

---

[4] Although it appears from Figure 10 that adaptation in these experiments was nonselective, this is due to the fact that even the endpoint stimuli were acoustically quite close to the phoneme boundary.

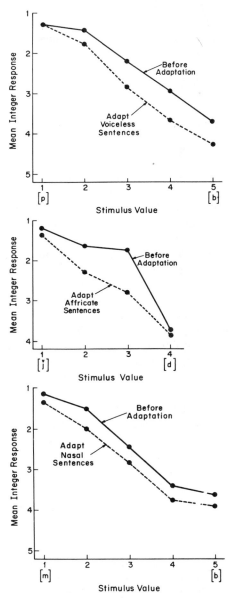

Figure 10. Mean integer response to syllables in the test series presented in Figure 9 before and after presentation of adaptating sentences.

The boundary shift observed following adaptation has been shown to be a true sensory effect and not the result of response bias. At the time of this writing, the best bet seems to be that adaptation of speech provides empirical support for the existence of feature detectors for speech.

DEVELOPMENTAL IMPLICATIONS

Phonetic Feature Detectors in Infants?

Experiments with adult listeners have repeatedly verified that humans perceive certain phonetic distinctions *categorically*. For example, English speakers presented with syllables from a /b/−/p/ continuum cannot discriminate between stimuli with VOT values of 0 and 20 msec, which are both perceived as /b/, or among stimuli with VOT values of 40 and 60 msec, which are both perceived as /p/. However, they are readily able to discriminate among stimuli with VOT values of 20 versus 40 msec since the former are perceived as /b/ and the latter as /p/. Thus, listeners are only able to discriminate among synthetically produced stop consonants when they are able to assign the stimuli to different phonetic categories. Categorical perception has been demonstrated for stop consonants along the voiced−voiceless dimension (/b/ versus /p/, /d/ versus /t/, and /g/ versus /k/), and the place of articulation dimension (/b/ versus /d/ versus /g/).

In a most provocative series of experiments, Eimas and his collaborators (Cutting & Eimas, 1975; Eimas, 1974; Eimas, *et al.,* 1971) have shown that infants respond to synthetic stop consonants in precisely the same fashion as adults. Using the nonnutritive, high-amplitude sucking paradigm described by Entus (Chapter 6, this volume), Eimas *et al.* (1971) found that infants perceive VOT differences in stop consonants only when the stimuli belong to different phonetic categories according to adult identification functions. In subsequent experiments, Eimas (1974) and Cutting and Eimas (1975) found that infants respond categorically to synthetic stop consonants differing in place of articulation.

One of the main implications of the finding that infants perceive certain speech sounds in a categorical manner is that perception of these sounds is mediated by finely tuned auditory feature detectors. Cutting and Eimas (1975) suggested this possibility:

> To explain the infant's ability to discriminate variations in the cues for voicing and place of articulation by reference to phonetic feature values, we need first to assume the presence of appropriate phonetic feature analyzers. These analyzers, by inference from our infant studies, must be operative shortly after birth, perhaps having been set in operation merely by experiencing speech. Given the passive nature of a feature detector analysis, the presentation of a signal with sufficient linguistic information to activate the speech processing mechanisms will excite each of the phonetic feature analyzers for which there is an adequate stimulus. The repeated presentation of the same stimulus, which occurs in the infant studies, will result in the adaptation of the activated detectors (see also Eimas and Corbit, 1973). Adaptation of the detectors, which presumably

results in the diminution of their output signals, may well be related to the decrement in the reinforcing properties of novel stimuli and the subsequent decrement in the infant's response rate. The presentation of a second speech stimulus, which, although acoustically different, excites the same set of detectors, will not be experienced as a novel stimulus by the infant. Consequently, there will be no increased effort to obtain this stimulus. Introduction of a second stimulus that activates one or more different detectors, on the other hand, yields a different set of phonetic feature values and will be experienced as novel. Our notion is that the infant increases his response rate in order to obtain this new perception. [From Cutting, J., & Eimas, P.D., Phonetic feature analyzers and the processing of speech in infants. In J.F. Kavanagh & J.E. Cutting (eds.), *The role of speech and language,* 1975, Cambridge, Mass., M.I.T. Press, p. 59].

Feature Detectors in Infants: Nature or Nurture?

Does categorical perception in 1-month-old infants demonstrate an innate mechanism? Cutting and Eimas (1975) suggest that it does: "With respect to the younger infants, in particular, there is no reason to believe that they have learned much, if anything, about their to-be-native language between birth and four weeks [p. 52]."

I think it is important to keep another hypothesis in mind: that feature detectors can be "tuned" within a very short time after birth by mere exposure to language. This possibility is suggested by a recent series of experiments performed by Condon (1974) and Condon and Sander (1974). These investigators have shown that the movement patterns of infants as young as 1-day-old are entrained to the speech rhythms of their language. Using a frame-by-frame analysis of infants' movements during exposure to speech, Condon found that infants' movements are precisely synchronized to the articulated structure of adult speech. The segmentation of the infants' motion was found to correspond to the segmentation of the adult's speech at both phoneme and syllable boundaries. The same pattern of results was not observed in a control condition in which the infants' movements were compared to a randomly selected sample of speech. Condon (1974) speculates:

If the infant, from the beginning, moves in precise, shared rhythm with the organization of the speech structure of his culture, then he participates developmentally through complex, sociobiological entrainment processes in millions of repetitions of linguistic forms long before he later uses them in speaking and communicating. By the time he begins to speak, he may have already laid down within himself the form and structure of the language system of his culture. [From Condon, W.S., Neonate movement is synchronized with adult speech: Interactional participation and language acquisition, *Science, 183,* p. 101.]

It is thus possible that, by 1 month of age, the infant's perceptual system has become finely tuned to the acoustic parameters of his language environment.

Streeter (1975) has provided evidence that at least one phonetic distinction may be *acquired* by 2 months of age. Streeter tested 2-month-old African infants exposed to Kikuyu, a language of Kenya, for their ability to discriminate bilabial stops with VOT values of −30 versus 0, 10 versus 40, and 50 versus 80 msec.

Streeter found that—similar to the American infants tested by Eimas—Kikuyu infants were able to discriminate between stops having VOT values of 10 versus 40 msec (/b/ versus /p/ in English) but were unable to discriminate stops with VOT values of 50 versus 80 msec (both /p/ in English). Since stops with VOT values over 0 msec do not occur in the Kikuyu language, it appears that perception of the 10 versus 40 msec VOT difference by Kikuyu infants was mediated by an innate perceptual mechanism. Apparently children are able to distinguish between stops having short versus long VOT values without exposure to a linguistic system where this distinction is relevant.

On the other hand, Kikuyu infants, unlike American infants, are able to discriminate prevoiced stops from stops with 0 msec VOT, and, in the Kikuyu language, the presence or absence of sufficient prevoicing signals the voiced—voiceless distinction for stop consonants. American infants, who are not exposed to prevoiced stops, are unable to make this discrimination (Eimas, et al., 1971). It thus appears that exposure to a language in which stops are prevoiced is necessary for discrimination of prevoicing by 2-month-old infants.

Whatever the relative contribution of nature versus nurture, it is clear that infants are quite sophisticated listeners. Infants are able to perceive differences among synthetically produced stop consonants differing in place and manner of articulation (Eimas et al., 1971; Eimas, 1974; Morse, 1972), as well as differences among naturally spoken stops (Trehub & Rabinovich, 1972), fricatives (Eilers & Minifie, 1975), and vowels (Trehub, 1972).

IMPLICATIONS OF INVARIANCE FOR NEUROLOGICAL THEORIES OF SPEECH PERCEPTION

The research reviewed in the previous sections may be summarized as follows: (a) There are at least two sources of information about phonemes—*invariant features*, such as the nasal resonance that accompanies /m/ and /n/, and *context-conditioned* features, such as the vowel transitions that signal the distinction between /m/ and /n/. Both invariant and context-conditioned cues should be thought of as acoustic features. (b) Experiments using the selective adaptation paradigm provide independent support for the existence of phonetic feature detectors for both invariant features (Cole et al., 1975) and context-conditioned features (e.g., Cooper & Blumstein, 1974; Cooper et al., 1976). (c) Infants distinguish among certain speech sounds *as if* their perception were mediated by finely tuned feature detectors.

I would like to conclude with a brief discussion of the question: What kind of neurological theory of language development is best suited to handle the data reviewed here?

There are currently two major theories of speech perception: "motor theories" and "feature detector" theories. The motor theory of speech perception discussed earlier was originally proposed to explain how listeners could perceive segmental phonemes without reference to invariant features. Feature detector models of speech perception have since been proposed as an alternative to the motor theory of speech perception (e.g., Abbs & Sussman, 1971; Cole & Scott, 1972; Cooper & Nager, 1975; Cutting & Eimas, 1975; Eimas, 1974; Eimas & Corbit, 1973). Feature detector models assume that phoneme identification is based on the activation of analyzers sensitive to specific configurations of acoustic energy.

Feature detector models have certain advantages over the motor theory of speech perception. First, while there is no independent evidence for the neuro-motor invariants proposed by the motor theory, there is now independent evidence for phonetic feature detectors. Second, feature detector models, unlike the motor theory, allow for the direct perception of phonetic segments based on either invariant or context-conditioned features present in the speech wave. Third, feature detector models are able to explain the infant speech perception data, while these same data raise certain problems for the motor theory, as described in an earlier section.

Finally, it should be noted that the major stumbling block to feature detector theories has been the presumed lack of invariant features for phonemes. In fact, the motor theory of speech perception was originally proposed in order to account for this presumed lack of invariance. In this chapter I have attempted to demonstrate that this is not really a problem, for two reasons. First, most phonemes are accompanied by invariant acoustic features. Second, even such context-conditioned cues as vowel transitions may be regarded as specifiable acoustic features. Recent evidence suggests finely tuned feature detectors responsive to both types of cues may mediate perception of speech for both infants and adults.

ACKNOWLEDGEMENT

I thank William Cooper and Peter Eimas for their comments on an earlier draft of this chapter.

REFERENCES

Abbs, J.H., & Sussman, H.M. (1971) Neurophysiological feature detectors and speech perception: A discussion of theoretical implications. *Journal of Speech and Hearing Research, 14,* 23–26.

Blumstein, S.E., & Stevens, K.N. (1976) Perceptual invariance and onset spectra for stop consonants in different environments. Journal of the Acoustical Society of America., *60,*(1) 90.

Carlson, R., Granstrom, B., & Pauli, S. (1972) Perceptive evaluation of segmental cues. The 1972 Conference on Speech Communication and Processing, Boston, April 24–26.

Cole, R.A., Cooper, W.A., Allard, F., & Singer, J. (1975) Selective adaptation of English consonants using real speech. *Perception & Psychophysics, 18,* 227–244.

Cole, R.A., & Scott, B. (1972) Phoneme feature detectors. Paper presented at the meeting of the Eastern Psychological Association meeting, Boston, April.

Cole, R.A., & Scott, B. (1973) Perception of temporal order in speech: The role of vowel transitions. *Canadian Journal of Psychology*, *27*(4), 441–449.

Cole, R.A., & Scott, B. (1974a) The phantom in the phoneme: Invariant cues for stop consonants. *Perception & Psychophysics*, *15*, 101–107.

Cole, R.A., & Scott, B. (1974b) Toward a theory of speech perception. *Psychological Review*, *81*, 348–374.

Condon, W.S. (1974) Neonate movement is synchronized with adult speech: Interactional participation and language acquisition. *Science*, *183*, 99–101.

Condon, W.S., & Sander, L.W. (1974) Synchrony demonstrated between movements of the neonate and adult speech. *Child Development*, *45*, 456–462.

Cooper, W.E. (1974) Adaptation of phonetic feature analyzers for place of articualtion. *Journal of the Acoustical Society of America*, *56*, 617–627.

Cooper, W.E., & Blumstein, S. (1974) A "labial" feature analyzer in speech perception. *Perception & Psychophysics*, *16*, 591–600.

Cooper, W.E., Ebert, R.R., & Cole, R.A. (1976) Perceptual analysis of stop consonants and glides. *Journal of Experimental Psychology: Human Perception and Performance, 2*, 92–104.

Cooper, W.E., & Nager, R.M. (1975) Perceptuo-motor adaptation to speech: An analysis of bisyllabic utterances and a neural model. *Journal of the Acoustical Society of America*, 1975, *2*, 105–114.

Cutting, J., & Eimas, P.D. (1975) Phonetic feature analyzers and the processing of speech in infants. In J.F. Kavanagh & J.E. Cutting (eds.) *The role of speech and language* Cambridge, Mass.: M.I.T. Press.

Dorman, M.F., Raphael, L.J., & Studdert-Kennedy, M. (1975) Cues for stop consonants in natural speech: The role of bursts and formant transitions. *Journal of the Acoustical Society of America*, *58*(1), 58.

Eilers, R.E., & Minifie, F.D. (1975) Fricative discrimination in early infancy. *Journal of Speech and Hearing Research*, *18*, 158–167.

Eimas, P.D. (1974) Auditory and linguistic processing of cues for place of articulation by infants. *Perception & Psychophysics*, *16*(3), 513.

Eimas, P.D., & Corbit, J.D. (1973) Selective adaptation of linguistic feature detectors. *Cognitive Psychology*, *4*, 99–109.

Eimas, P.D., Sequeland, E., Jusczyk, P., & Vigorito, J. (1971) Speech perception in infants. *Science, 171*, 303–306.

Fant, G. (1967) Auditory patterns of speech. In W. Wathen-Dunn (Ed.), *Models for the perception of speech and visual form.* Cambridge, Massachusetts: M.I.T. Press.

Fischer-Jørgensen, E. (1972) Tape cutting experiments with Danish stop consonants in initial position. (Annual Report VIII) Copenhagen: Univ. of Copenhagen, Institute of Phonetics.

Gerstman, P. (1957) Perceptual dimensions for the friction portion of certain speech sounds. Unpublished doctoral dissertation, New York Univ.

Grimm, W.A. (1966) Perception of segments of English spoken consonant-vowel syllables. *Journal of the Acoustical Society of America, 40*, 1454–1461.

Halle, M., Hughes, G.W., & Radley, J.P.A. (1957) *Journal of the Acoustical Society of America*, *29*, 107–116.

Harris, K.S. (1958) Cues for the discrimination of American English fricatives in spoken syllables. *Language and Speech, 1*, 1–7.

Just, M., Suslick, S., Michaels, S., & Shockey, L. (in preparation) Acoustic cues for the perception of stop consonants.

Liberman, A.M. (1957) Some results of research on speech perception. *Journal of the Acoustical Society of America, 29*, 117–123.

Liberman, A.M. (1970) The grammars of speech and language. *Cognitive Psychology, 1*, 301–323.

Liberman, A.M., Cooper, F.S., Shankweiler, D.P., & Studdert-Kennedy, M. (1967) Perception of the speech code. *Psychological Review, 74,* 431–461.

Malécot, A. (1956) Acoustic cues for nasal consonants. *Language, 32,* 274–284.

Moffitt, A. (1971) Consonant cue perception by twenty to twenty-four-week-old infants. *Child Development, 42,* 717–731.

Morse, P. (1972) The discrimination of speech and nonspeech stimuli in early infancy. *Journal of Experimental Child Psychology, 14,* 477–492.

Rudnicky, A.I. & Cole, R.A. (1977) Adaptation produced by connected speech. *Journal of Experimental Psychology: Human Perception and Performance, 3*(1), 51–61.

Scott, B. (1971) The verbal transformation effect as a function of embedded sounds. Unpublished masters thesis, Univ. of Waterloo, Ontario, Canada.

Sharf, D.J., & Hemeyer, T. (1972) Identification of place of consonant articulation from vowel formant transitions. *Journal of the Acoustical Society of America, 51,* 652.

Stevens, K.N. (1972) Segments, features, and analysis by synthesis. In J.F. Kavanagh and I.G. Mattingly (Eds.), *Language by ear and by eye.* Cambridge, Massachusetts: M.I.T. Press.

Stevens, K.N. (1973) Potential role of property detectors in the perception of consonants. M.I.T. Research Laboratory of Electronics, QPR No. 110, July 15.

Stevens, K.N., & Blumstein, S. (1976) Context-independent properties for place of articulation in stop consonants. *Journal of the Acoustical Society of America, 59*(1), 40.

Stevens, K.N., & Halle, M. (1967) Remarks on analysis by synthesis and distinctive features. In W. Wathen-Dunn (Ed.), *Models for the perception of speech and visual form.* Cambridge, Massachusetts: M.I.T. Press.

Streeter, W. (1975) Language perception of two-month-old infants shows effects of both innate mechanisms and experience. Bell laboratories research report.

Trehub, S. (1973) Infants' sensitivity to vowel and tonal contrasts. *Developmental Psychology, 9,* 91–96.

Trehub, S., & Rabinovich, M. (1972) Auditory-linguistic sensitivity in early infancy. *Developmental Psychology, 6,* 74–77.

Winitz, H., Scheib, M.E., & Reeds, J.H. (1972) Identification of stops and vowels for the burst portion of [p, t, k] isolated from conversational speech. *Journal of the Acoustical Society of America, 51,* 1309–1317.

19

The Identification of Four Vowels by Children 2½ to 3 Years Chronological Age as an Indicator of Perceptual Processing

JOHN H. V. GILBERT

One of the continuing questions that bedevil those workers interested in verbal language acquisition, particularly phonology, is whether the child's perception of the speech signal is the same as, or different from, an adult's perception of the same signal. Does the child "first distinguish in what it hears only the coarser contrasts between the sounds which reach its ear"—a view stated by Leopold (1953, p. 3) and slightly refined by Kornfeld (1971, 1974) to "children hypothesize abstract segment representations that may be different from mature forms [Kornfeld, 1974, p. 210]"? Or does the child, in fact, start with the fine contrasts because he is, in effect, able to perceive them, gradually working these contrasts into some larger unit of the speech code—a view that might be commensurate with the infant studies of Eimas (1974), Morse (1974), Trehub (1973), and others? Or is the question of *speech* perception in children so fraught with theoretical and experimental problems that it is virtually insoluble?

In this chapter, I present data that concern one very small part of this larger issue of adultlike or unadultlike speech perception, that is, children's identifications and productions of a set of four vowels, produced by an adult speaker and by themselves. These data relate to a general hypothesis, which is that, at least by 2½ years of age, the perception of speech by the child (represented by their own and adult vowel tokens) is no different from that of an adult. Using data from this experiment and those of other investigators, I shall speculate that although productive phonological deviancy (in a nonpathological sense) may persist in children past the age of 2½ years, the child's *perceptive* capacities for speech segments are in fact fully matured by this time. It is, in effect, only the articulatory mechanism that goes on "hunting" to achieve the correct outputs of perception, it is not the process of perception itself that changes.

The seemingly simple vowel sounds can be described using three parameters: First, articulatory: by tongue hump position and degree of constriction; second, acoustic: by frequency and sound pressure level; and third, linguistic: by distinctive features that underline articulatory and acoustic information. In this way, vowel sounds have a multidimensional character, which the child perceives and maps (normalizes) very early in the acquisition process, perhaps because the dimensions of the perceptual space of the vowel system seem to be essentially the same as the physical dimensions: tongue advancement equals tongue hump and tongue height equals degree of constriction (Lindau, Harshman, & Ladefoged, 1971; Pols, van der Kamp, & Plomp, 1969).

EXPERIMENTAL METHOD

Subjects

Subjects for the experiment were 11 preschool children between 2½ and 3 years of chronological age, who were recruited from a university community. All were white, middle-class, and free of any known pathology. They attended from four to six sessions over a period of 1 month, the times of attendance being randomized across mornings and afternoons to minimize time-of-day effects. No direct reward was given for cooperative participation, although refreshment was provided at the end of each session. There were six boys and five girls in the group.

Stimulus Tapes

A trained male phonetician produced three tokens each of the vowels /i, a, æ, u/ in an h-d context. One token of each CVC was selected as most acceptable by two trained listeners, and was transferred to tape loops. A master tape of 80 items was constructed (20 tokens of each of the CVCs) which was used to elicit verbal responses from the child subjects. These verbalizations were later used as a test for children's perceptions of their own utterances.

Response Mode

One of the major constraints on perceptual tests with children is the children's obvious inability to respond in an adult mode, that is, by writing responses or scoring response sheets. A second major problem is in deciding whether a verbal versus a pointing response will greatly influence the outcome of the experiment. In the present experiment, a verbal mode of response was chosen over some form of pointing—for example, to a nonsense drawing. The latter method necessarily involves "teaching" the child which "stimulus" goes with each nonsense picture, since the child would need this information in order to be able to respond appropriately. (The "Catch-22" problems involved in testing perception in children are discussed elsewhere. See Gilbert, 1976.)

STIMULUS PRESENTATION

Children Listening to Adult Speakers

All original adult speaker stimuli were presented on high quality tape, from a Revox 877, over Sennheiser HD 414 headphones in a laboratory room with very low ambient noise level (NC22). A "warm-up" period preceded each session and subjects were not tested until they had become quite comfortable with the test environment. Since parental or caretaker cooperation was vital, the entire experiment was always explained in full to the caretaker prior to testing and caretakers were allowed to remain with the children throughout the test sessions.

Since attention getting, and retaining, can present a major experimental problem, stimuli were usually presented in sets of 10 items with a break between sets. Sometimes it was possible to present a greater number of items at one time. Children were seated at a kindergarten table approximately 12" from a B & K 1-inch microphone suspended above the table and associated with a Revox 877 tape recorder. A Dynaco loudspeaker was situated approximately 5 feet in front of the child. At each session, all the children were told what they would hear over the loudspeaker and how they were to respond; every effort was made to ensure that the instructions were simply phrased and part of a general conversation. Stimuli were presented at a comfortable listening level. Responses were recorded on high-quality magnetic tape on a Revox 877 tape recorder at 7 1/2 ips.

Each verbal response was checked by an observer, who noted especially those responses that were obviously at variance with the stimulus items. Notes taken on each child's performance proved helpful in the second part of the experiment, as will be apparent from what follows.

Theoretically, each child *could* have given 20 responses to each of the four vowel items; this would have given the possibility of 220 responses (summed across subjects) in each vowel category. Unfortunately 220 was to remain the theoretical number! For, following testing, item analysis and auditory observation on acceptability criteria of the response tapes by two experienced phoneticians gave only 100 tokens of each vowel in the h-d context. Many verbal response items proved unacceptable and were therefore dropped from tapes, chiefly on account of unintelligibility.[1] Although the 400 items to be used in the child: Child test (100 tokens of each vowel) were selected at random from across the 11 subjects, a surprisingly even distribution of tokens was obtained among those speakers.

---

[1] Acceptable identifications were obtained on a "closed-set" response sheet, i.e., two judges had to assign tokens to one of five categories /i/, /a/, /æ/, /u/ or "unacceptable" (i.e., unintelligible). A Pearson r correlation coefficient of 0.94 was obtained between judges.

Children Listening to Child Speakers

Of the 400 items (representing 100 tokens of each vowel in the h-d context), 20 of each vowel were now randomly selected and randomized into a tape of "child speakers." This consisted of 80 items and was presented to the same group of children in the same manner as the adult tape. By this time in testing the children had experienced considerable practise in the mechanics of the task and were surprisingly good at attending and responding. For the most part it took four sessions to collect all the identification—production responses. During this part of the experiment, the investigators benefited from prior experience, but still not to an extent large enough to prevent a major loss of data.

On listening to the children's responses to child speakers, it was possible for two experimenters clearly to identify the following number of responses to each vowel category /i/: 103; /a/: 197; /æ/: 90; /u/: 108. Since 90 was the minimun number of responses to one of the four vowel stimuli (/æ/), I decided to select 90 items at random from each of the other vowel categories, in order to arrive at an equal number of observations for each vowel for data analysis.

RESULTS

Since children's responses to the adult utterances were contaminated (by unintelligibility) as indicated above, *two* sets of results were computed: Set 1 consisted of changes in children's fundamental frequencies $(F_0)^2$ format two frequencies (F_2) and duration of tokens when *repeating* tokens spoken by: (a) adult speakers and (b) child speakers. Set 2 consisted of a confusion matrix of children's responses to child speakers.

Set 1

The means, standard deviations, and ranges for F_0, F_2, and duration of tokens for children responding to adults are given in Table 1. This means, standard deviations, and ranges for F_0, F_2, and duration of tokens for children responding to children are given in Table 2.

Set 2

A confusion matrix of children responding to children's utterances is given in Table 3. Although a *t*-test for the difference between the F_0 for /æ/ of children responding to children and children responding to adults was significant, I have no immediate explanation for it. A possible notion is that, for this vowel only, children were making greater attempts at a productive match with the utterances of children. A subjective observation for the significant *t* for duration of /a/ is that a number of

---

[2] We were most interested in determining whether F_0 changes in the direction of a perceived voice, a point often made in the literature on "input" or motherese. F_0 is also relatively easily measured on spectrograms, thus providing quick and useful information.

TABLE 1 F_0, F_2, and Duration of Vowels Produced in h-d Context by Children Responding to Adult Speakers

	F_0 (Hz)	F_2 (Hz)	Duration (sec)
/hid/			
Mean	287.0	3345.0	.367
SD	42.2	428.7	.155
Range	199.0	2740.0	.681
/had/			
Mean	266.0	1574.0	.413
SD	23.3	205.1	.097
Range	97.0	810.0	.421
/hæd/			
Mean	281.0	2422.0	.416
SD	38.6	230.2	.137
Range	170.0	860.0	.559
/hud/			
Mean	285.0	1509.0	.352
SD	34.7	242.6	.130
Range	185.0	1110.0	.316

TABLE 2 F_0, F_2, and Duration of Vowels Produced in h-d Context by Children Responding to Child Speakers

	F_0 (Hz)	F_2 (Hz)	Duration (sec)
/hid/			
Mean	287.0	3063.0	.319
Standard Dev.	30.5	813.5	.084
Range	145.0	2660.0	.344
/had/			
Mean	262.0	1478.0	.357
Stan. Dev.	27.2	200.1	.084
Range	99.0	800.0	.320
/hæd/			
Mean	260.0	2241.0	.377
Stan. Dev.	26.3	514.9	.108
Range	128.0	1790.0	.426
/hud/			
Mean	288.0	1430.0	.363
Stan. Dev.	42.6	241.5	.074
Range	207.0	1070.0	.237

the subjects tagged this vowel with the remark "That's what the doctor says." A study of vowel duration in this environment by children at this age might elucidate this point, although the "fis–fish" problem, discussed later in the chapter, is a difficult one to disambiguate.

TABLE 3   Confusion Matrix of Children Responding to Vowel Tokens
Produced by Children[a]

		Vowel				
		/i/	/a/	/æ/	/u/	
Stimulus	/i/	90				90
	/a/	1	76	11	2	90
	/æ/		1	88	1	90
	/u/	1		3	86	90
			Response			

[a]Σ = 90; subjects = 11

TABLE 4   *t*-Tests for Differences between Means of Acoustical and
Durational Data of Children Responding to Child Speakers versus
Children Responding to Adult Speakers (*df* = 10)

	F_0	F_2	Duration
/hid/	$t = 0$	$t = 1.749$	$t = 1.753$
	(n.s.)	(n.s.)	(n.s.)
/had/	$t = .66$	$t = 2.033$	$t = 2.678$
	(n.s.)	(n.s.)	($p < .05$)
/hæd/	$t = 2.703$	$t = .01$	$t = 1.389$
	($p < .05$)	(n.s.)	(n.s.)
/hud/	$t = .323$	$t = 1.4$	$t = .472$
	(n.s.)	(n.s.)	(n.s.)

DISCUSSION

Within the severe limitations of this small experiment, two very general points
may be made with respect to the identification and production of vowels presented
in h-d context to children between 2½ and 3 years of chronological age. First, that
the age of speaker does not appear to affect F_0, F_2, or duration when children of
this chronological age are responding to stimuli from child and adult speakers;
second, that the child appears to have no difficulty in identifying four broadly
spaced vowel tokens produced by children (and by inference from acoustical
analyses, by adults), as demonstrated in the confusion matrix.

Now, although the results of the present experiment can only be considered as
minimal evidence if used alone to support notions concerning perception of speech

processes in children, I should like to use them in conjunction with other data to speculate about what might be going on in perception and why this process might have to be considered separately from production.

A paper by Locke and Kutz (1975) using a /w/ and /r/ voiced perception task with children between 5:3 and 5:10 demonstrated very clearly how well children at that age can make virtually error-free perceptual responses on a simple pointing task, despite the fact that they produce /w/ for /r/ in running speech, and despite the fact that these same children experienced significantly more /w—r/ confusions in recall than children who characteristically produced a correct /w/ and /r/. Data supporting the notion that children perceive speech in terms of the adult system, while production is affected by motor difficulties, is presented by Gallagher and Shriner (1975) in a study of inconsistent production of /s/ and /z/. The inconsistent production of /s/ and /z/ was found to be related to motor sequencing constraints *independent* of word boundaries. In an interesting experiment conducted with children between 2:3 and 4:7, the ability of young children to understand their own and other children's deviant phonological forms was tested by Dodd (1975). Dodd found that children were better at understanding an unfamiliar adult's speech than they were at understanding their own or other children's speech. Their understanding was found to be related to the degree to which the deviant speech resembled the adult phonological form. Dodd concluded that children do not store their own deviant phonological form for recognition in the same way that they store the adult forms.

It is apparent that the phonetic inventory of the child is elaborated very early, phonological discriminative processes having been shown by Graham and House (1971) to be acquired by 3 years.

Although sketchy, the evidence at the present time would seem to demonstrate a *perceptual* system which appears very early in childhood and is very akin to that of the adult. The infant discrimination studies at least demonstrate that the *auditory* system (which is the cornerstone of speech perception) is operative in a discrimination mode virtually at birth. It would be difficult to negate arguments that proposed a rapidly developing perceptual system, at least for speech signals. The issue of the linguisticality of such signals is a far larger, far more complex problem.

Allowing sufficiently for these observations, the linguisticality of the speech signal would appear to be buried in that confusing no-man's-land between crying—cooing on the one hand and babbling on the other. Claims for "linguistic" processing at an earlier age are, as yet, debatable.

For the ongoing fluctuations in the *output* (noisy) signals of the neonate—infant must, in the child, have to be adjusted (or normalized) to its language environment by its own sense system. It is evident that the successful emergence of the child's speech—language is dependent on this normalizing process across maturational change—that the input—output process is both caretaker initiated and child initiated. Caretaker and child each operate a physiologically similar mechanism to originate sound and a complex interactive device to transform each other's code.

Whether this device works (in the perceptual sense) from top-down or bottom-up deserves attention.

Let me use one example to illustrate the complexities in such a view. It is a commonplace observation that breathing must have something to do with output from the vocal mechanism. Every study on the first year of life makes appropriate mention of intonation. It should therefore be apparent that the breathing cycle must ultimately impose its particular constraints on the signal, those constraints being in the time domain. Yet only as recently as 1975, in a rather interesting study by Prescott, has a reasonably accurate method of interpreting breath group measures been proposed. If any sense is to be injected into the continuity—discontinuity argument, the data will have to come from examining the acoustic signal in parallel with other physiological—psychological processes. For the developing patterns of durational change and variability in fundamental frequency (which are themselves associated with timing changes) would appear to be the *first* indicators of the child's attempt at mapping the signals, which most observers then record as intonation. Timing (Allen, 1973; Hawkins, 1973) in the one domain, breathing, enters information into the perceptual—physiological system, with which we have to contend in describing (or theorizing about) the onset of linguisticality.

On the other hand numerous studies (Di Simoni, 1974, 1975; Hawkins, 1973; Kewley-Port & Preston, 1974; Kornfeld & Goehl, 1975; Tingley & Allen, 1975) would appear to support a productive phonological development process sometimes at variance with that of the adult speaker. We might speculate that such variance is a consequence of a developing physiological system with all its attendant timing problems and constraints. There are abundant basic physiological data (i.e., height, weight, frame size, etc.) to support this view, although there are no direct physiological data of the EMG and high-speed cine tape that might corroborate its effect on the production of speech.

I would propose that what we are witnessing in acquisition of language is that the process of speech sound *discrimination* occurs very early in development, within the first few months as indicated by the studies of Eimas (1974), Trehub (1973), and Fodor, Garrett, and Brill (1975); furthermore, that this process fast becomes one of speech sound *perception,* allowing the infant to start vocally tagging its environment within the first 4 or 5 months of life, and that that perception remains relatively unchanged from then onward, largely because the ear and auditory system have defined the limits of the speech signals that the infant is able to process by frequency, intensity, and durational transformation. This proposal, for which there is now accumulating evidence, is not a novel idea, having been spoken for by, among others, Dennis Fry (1966).

Based on a much broader analysis of data than I have presented here, I hope I may be forgiven some slight speculation about the neurological—physiological—linguistic interaction.

Obviously, the sense organs of the system set limits on the *kind* of information that can be registered. Their ways of orienting, adjusting, and exploring are partly constrained by anatomy but partly free. The basic neural circuitry for making such adjustments is built into the nervous system by the time of birth but continues to develop in man for a long time afterward.

All the developmental data we have to the present time indicate that the child cannot be expected to perceive certain "facts" about the world until he is ready to perceive them. He is not simply an adult who does not have any experience but, as Piaget has clearly shown, develops by passing through various stages. The ability to select and abstract information about the world grows as he grows.

The environment at the same time provides an inexhaustible reservoir of information. The ears, for example, are not analogous to microphones, which would imply a fixed relationship to the brain. "Listening" (and all that it implies) continues to improve with experience, so that higher order variables can still be discovered, even in old age. It therefore comes as no surprise that the speech in the infant's environment is a product of carefully adjusted, interactive processes.

In J. J. Gibson's (1966) terminology, perceptual learning associated with the act of speaking might be conceived of as a process of differentiation—of learning what to attend to, both overtly and covertly, within the limitations of each of the sense systems. A system "hunts" to achieve clarity, and the process occurs at more than one level. First, the pickup of information reinforces the exploratory adjustments of the organs that make pickup possible. And second, the registering of information reinforces whatever neural activity in the brain brings about the registering.

Speech sound production, on the other hand, is dependent on a physiological system (for speech) that undergoes continuous change at least until puberty is passed, by which time the coarticulatory patterns underlying speech output are well established. Thus phonological errors which occur after that time are a result of lexical retrieval, as outlined by Fromkin (1973), rather than of misdirection at a lower, physiological level. Whatever misadventures occur to the perception of speech by children over 2 years are most probably part of the totality of language coding, rather than the result of something as discrete as speech sound misperception.

ACKNOWLEDGMENTS

This research and preparation of this chapter was supported by grant number MT-4217 from the Medical Research Council of Canada.

REFERENCES

Allen, G.D. (1973) Segmental timing in speech production. *Journal of Phonetics, 1*, 219–237.
Di Simoni, F.G. (1974) Evidence for a theory of speech production based on observations of the speech of children. *Journal of the Acoustical Society of America, 56*, 6, 1919–1921.
Di Simoni, F.G. (1975) Perceptual and perceptual-motor characteristics of phonemic development. *Child Development, 46*, 243–246.

Dodd, B. (1975) Children's understanding of their own phonological forms. *Quarterly Journal of Experimental Psychology, 27,* 165–172.

Eimas, P.D. (1974) Linguistic processing of speech by young infants. In R.L. Schiefelbusch & L.L. Lloyd (Eds.), *Language perspectives-acquisition, retardation and intervention.* Baltimore: University Park Press. Pp. 55–73.

Fodor, J.A., Garrett, M.F., & Brill, S.L. (1975) Pi ka pu: The perception of speech sounds by pre-linguistic infants. *Perception and Psychophysics, 18,* 2, 74–78.

Fromkin, V.A. (1973) Slips of the tongue. *Scientific American* (Dec.), 110–117.

Fry, D.B. (1966) The development of the phonological system in the normal and the deaf child. In F. Smith & G. Miller (Eds.), *The genesis of language,* Cambridge, Massachusetts: MIT Press.

Gallagher, M., & Shriner, T.H. (1975) Articulatory inconsistencies in the speech of normal children. *Journal of Speech and Hearing Research, 18*(1), 168–175.

Gibson, J.J. (1966) *The senses considered as perceptual systems.* Boston: Houghton Mifflen.

Gilbert, J.H.V. (1976) Some observations on the unresolvable "fis-fish" conundrum.

Graham, L.W. & House, A.S. (1971) Phonological oppositions in children: A perceptual study. *Journal of the Acoustical Society of America, 49,* 2, (Part 2), 559–566.

Hawkins, S. (1973) Temporal coordination of consonants in the speech of children: Preliminary data. *Journal of Phonetics, 1,* 181–217.

Kewley-Port, D., & Preston, M. (1974) Early apical stop production: A voice onset time analysis. *Journal of Phonetics, 2,* 195–210.

Kornfield, J.R. (1971) What initial clusters tell us about a child's speech code. MIT Research Lab. of Electronics, *Quarterly Progress Report, 101,* (15 April), 218–221.

Kornfield, J.R., & Goehl, H. (1974) A new twist to an old observation: Kids know more than they say. *Chicago Linguistic Society, 10,* 210–219.

Leopold, W.F. (1953) Patterning in children's language learning,. *Language Learning, 5,* 1–14.

Lindau, M., Harshman, R., & Ladefoged, P. (1971) Factor analysis of formant frequencies. *Journal of the Acoustical Society of America, 50,* 1 (1), 117.

Locke, L., & Kutz, K.J. (1975) Memory for speech and speech for memory. *Journal of Speech & Hearing Research, 18* (1), 176–191.

Morse, P.A. (1974) Infant speech perception: A preliminary model and review of the literature. In R.L. Schiefelbusch and L.L. Lloyd (Eds.), *Language perspectives-acquisition, retardation and intervention,* Baltimore: Univ. Park Press. Pp. 19–53.

Pols, L.C.W., van der Kamp, L.J., & Plomp, R. (1969) Perceptual and physical space of vowel sounds. *Journal of the Acoustical Society of America, 46,* 2, (2), 458–467.

Prescott, R. (1975) Infant cry sounds: Developmental features. *Journal of the Acoustical Society of America, 57,* 5, 1186–1191.

Tingley, Beth M., & Allen, G.D. (1975) Development of speech timing control in children. *Child Development, 46,* 186–194.

Trehub, S.E. (1973) Infants' sensitivity to vowel and tonal contrasts. *Developmental Psychology, 9,* 91–96.

20

The Development of Speech Timing

WILLIAM E. COOPER

Since the publication of Jakobson's *Kindersprache* (1941), studies of children's speech have focused primarily on two structural problems: (a) the chronological order in which different speech sounds are first mastered in meaningful contexts and (b) the development of hemispheric specialization for speech in the brain. The research on these two problems provides background for formulating a theory of speech development and for the diagnosis of certain abnormalities. Yet, it should be recognized that such research provides only the barest hints about how one might provide an account of speech development that is *predictively adequate,* in the sense of Chomsky (1965, 1975) or, in addition, how one might apply therapy to cases of speech abnormality. In order to approach these latter goals, greater emphasis must be placed on study of the processes that underlie development—the maturational and learning processes that are responsible for enabling the child to master aspects of speech previously absent from his repertoire. In this chapter, questions about such underlying attributes will be discussed, first in light of general characteristics of speech development and then with respect to the development of timing rules for speech, an area in which a fair amount of progress has been made.

GENERAL ASPECTS OF SPEECH DEVELOPMENT

In this introductory section I briefly sketch the course of speech development and point out some possible maturational and learning processes. For more extensive reviews of speech development, the reader is referred to McNeill (1970), Menyuk (1971), and Ferguson and Slobin (1973).

In the earliest days of infancy, sound production is restricted to crying. The acoustic study of infant crying has proved to be a useful diagnostic tool for detecting a variety of abnormalities, including brain tumors, anoxia, and Down's syndrome (Vuorenkoski, Lind, Wasz-Hockert, & Partanen, 1971). The characteristics of crying also appear to provide an index of general neurological maturity. Tenold, Crowell, Jones, Daniel, McPherson, and Popper (1974) have shown that the crying of premature infants contains greater variability in the acoustic spectrum than the crying of term neonates. Aside from its use as a diagnostic, the study of infant crying might be of some predictive value for determining the subsequent course of an infant's speech development. This intriguing possibility has, however, never been seriously studied.

When an infant does begin to produce recognizable speech sounds, at the age of about 6 months, the sounds do not have a specific referential meaning, and this stage of development is accordingly referred to as *babbling* (Jespersen, 1925). During this stage, the child's speech includes a large array of possible speech sounds (Irwin, 1947a, b, c, 1948). With some exceptions (e.g., Bever, 1961; Gruber, 1966; Cruttenden, 1970; Oller & Smith, 1976; Oller, Wieman, Doyle, & Ross, 1976), the babbling stage has not been studied systematically, and it remains largely unknown to what extent babbling provides the child with speech opportunities that are essential for later language development. The child might begin at this stage, for example, to build an internalized map of his vocal tract, important for the correct production of vowels (Lindblom & Sundberg, 1971). In addition, the child might learn to coordinate tongue and jaw movements with one another and with laryngeal movements as an aid to consonant production (a possibility that is discussed later in this chapter). It is reasonable to suppose that babbling does serve such purposes, but the empirical work required to test these possibilities has not been conducted, and, in some cases, it cannot be conducted, given the ethical limitations rightly imposed against controlling an infant's environment.

When the child begins to speak referentially, speech is marked by a severe restriction on the range of sounds produced (Jakobson, 1941; Ferguson & Farwell, 1975). According to Jakobson, the acquisition of phonetic distinctions at this stage proceeds in an orderly fashion by successive differentiation, whereby the first contrasts mastered among vowels and consonants are maximally distinct. Later, the child masters sound contrasts that are less distinct. To take an example, the first vowel contrasts typically mastered by children are /i/ and /a/. These two vowels represent extremes of oral constriction and tongue height within the vowel space dimensions of the human vocal tract. For /i/, the oral region of the vocal tract is in a relatively constricted position (a greater constriction would result in the production of a consonant), with the tongue's highest point nearing the roof of the mouth (Stevens, 1972). For /a/, on the other hand, the amount of constriction in the oral cavity is minimal, with the jaw and tongue lowered. Only after the contrast between these extreme vowels is mastered do children typically learn to differentiate these vowels from a vowel like /ɛ/, for which the amount of oral constriction and tongue height lie about midway between /i/ and /a/.

Jakobson's principle of successive differentiation may be considered a special case of a general principle of learning. Both children and animals learn a difficult contrast more easily if they first learn a contrast involving more highly discriminable stimuli along the same dimension. For instance, a pigeon can be taught to respond differentially to small differences in visible wavelength by first being trained to differentiate larger wavelength differences (Reynolds, 1968; Riley, 1968). It is likely that the child makes use of this same principle of learning in acquiring mastery of at least some speech contrasts. It should be noted that, while the principle invoked here is placed within the realm of *learning,* the neural machinery responsible for its widespread and perhaps universal appearance in early development is probably innately determined in man and lower animals (see Chomsky, 1975, Chapter 1, for discussion of innateness and language acquisition).

As pointed out by Kiparsky and Menn (1976), Jakobson's theory was proposed to account for the development of phonetic *contrasts,* not the development of attaining a particular phonetic target. However, the early mastery of extreme vowels like /i/ and /a/ could be accounted for in terms of their target configuration by relying on Stevens' (1972) quantal theory of speech production, accompanied by some additional assumptions about the child's use of template matching. The quantal theory was originally based on acoustic properties of the output from a two-tube approximation to the adult vocal tract. Stevens observed that the vocal tract configuration required for a vowel like /i/ or /a/ yielded regions of acoustic stability for which small differences in the tract configuration yielded only slight differences in the acoustic output. Lesser stability accompanied a vowel like /ɛ/. If Stevens's observations apply as a first approximation to the smaller vocal tract of the child, then the child should be able to produce vowels like /i/ and /a/ with greater reliability in early production than a vowel like /ɛ/, since slight errors in reaching the ideal target positions for /i/ and /a/ would result in a less severe acoustic change.

The applicability of the quantal theory to speech development rests on the assumption that the child's early intentional speech is restricted to those sounds that are most easily reproduced. In fact, the immediate reproduction of syllables appears to be a major characteristic of early speech (Gunnilstam, 1974; Moskowitz, 1971), as in /dada/, /mama/, and it is reasonable to suppose that such reproductions serve a useful purpose. At this stage, the child may reproduce syllables in order to check the degree to which the acoustic properties of the syllables match some internalized representation, or *template,* which is itself genetically predetermined. Template matching by auditory feedback has been proposed in the case of birdsong acquisition (Konishi, 1965; Marler, 1970, 1974), and the assumptions required for template matching seem to be satisfied with regard to human speech. The template-matching notion requires that auditory templates of speech sounds exist in children prior to the onset of speech production. This assumption is satisfied in large part by the recent discovery that preverbal infants are capable of discriminating speech sounds in a manner similar to that of adults (Eimas, Siqueland, Jusczyk, & Vigorito, 1971; Eimas, 1974; Trehub, 1973; for a review, see Cole, Chapter 18, this volume). In addition, the template-matching scheme relies on the assumption that auditory feedback is essential to speech development, an assumption that receives general support from the inability of congenitally deaf children to achieve normal speech.

Based on these considerations, Stevens' quantal theory may provide a reasonable account of the child's early mastery of vowels like /i/ and /a/. In effect, the child might restrict early vowel productions, to /i/ and /a/ just because these sounds can be reliably reproduced, with these vowels providing the best initial test cases for the child's template-matching scheme.

We turn now to consider the mastery of consonants. The first consonants typically acquired in intentional speech include stop consonants (e.g., /b/ and /p/) and nasals (e.g., /m/ and /n/) (Menyuk, 1968). Both classes are characterized in speech production by a complete obstruction of airflow at some location in the supralaryngeal tract. Mastery of stridents (e.g., /f/ and /s/) and of liquids (e.g., /r/ and /l/) appears conspicuously later.

An account of the early mastery of stops and nasals may be provided by either of the principles reviewed earlier for vowel acquisition. For example, Jakobson's principle of successive differentiation predicts the early appearance of stops and nasals as opposed to stridents and liquids because the former consonants are maximally distinct from vowels in terms of vocal constriction and consequent acoustic quality. Similarly, the quantal theory cum template-matching scheme proposed for vowels predicts the early appearance of stops and nasals based on the view that the articulatory precision required to reach these consonant targets is less strict (and hence less subject to large error in the acoustic output) than is the precision required for stridents and liquids.

Aside from these general accounts, other proposals have been advanced to explain the order of acquisition of certain classes of consonants. To mention one, Salus and Salus (1974) proposed to account for the late acquisition of stridents like /f/ and /s/ by appeal to a constraint on the child's perception. They argued that young children are perceptually unable to distinguish among stridents because, due to incomplete myelination, they are unable to hear the high frequency components of the acoustic signal that differentiate these sounds (e.g., Hughes & Halle, 1956). In effect, Salus and Salus proposed that young children are perceptually limited by high frequency sensorineural hearing loss like that typically found in cases of nerve degeneration in adults. However, recent work has indicated that young infants are capable of perceiving distinctions among the stridents /s/ versus /š/ (/š/ as in "fish"), which differ primarily in their energy distribution at high frequencies (Eilers & Minifie, 1975), indicating that the Salus and Salus proposal cannot be applied to the late acquisition of stridents as a class. It appears rather that, as in the case of distinctions among stop consonants and vowels, the neural machinery required for the perception of stridents is available to the child at birth or at some early stage of development well before the onset of speech production. According to the template-matching scheme proposed earlier, the early perceptual capabilities of the child would not be established *coincidentally* by the time that speech production begins; rather, the early appearance of perceptual capabilities would be necessary to the later operation of template matching as a means for continual refinement of the child's own speech.

To summarize the discussion of the general course of vocal development, it can be said that very little is known about the earliest stages of vocal development, including crying and babbling, but some proposals can be advanced to account for general aspects of the course of referential speech. In particular, Jakobson's principle of successive differentiation or Stevens' quantal theory coupled with the template-matching scheme provide reasonable first-order accounts of the chronological order in which certain vowels and consonants are mastered. Not surprisingly, however, such phonetically based principles of speech development may interact with, or even be overruled by, concurrent development of syntactic and semantic attributes. In cases where the chronological order of speech sound mastery departs from that predicted on the basis of phonetic regularities (e.g., Ferguson & Farwell, 1975; Curtiss, Fromkin, Krashen, Rigler, & Rigler, 1974), it is quite possible that interactive effects with semantics or syntax or both are responsible. The disentangling of isolable and interactive effects remains a formidable task, but at present it still seems appropriate to regard the course of phonetic development in terms of a neurological subsystem of language that operates quasi-independently of subsystems that involve syntactic and semantic domains.

THE DEVELOPMENT OF TEMPORAL COORDINATION IN CONSONANT PRODUCTION

In order to focus more closely on processes that underlie the acquisition of speech sounds, we turn to consider the development of a particular phonetic contrast involving stop consonants. In English, the distinction between stop consonants like /b/ and /p/, /d/ and /t/, and /g/ and /k/ can be signaled in syllable-initial position by a temporal relation known as voice onset time (VOT), defined as the interval between the consonant's closure release (in the case of /b/ or /p/, for example, the release of lip closure) and the onset of vibration of the vocal folds of the larynx (Lisker & Abramson, 1964). The VOT value of a /d/ in adult English may range from about −180 msec to +25 msec, with negative VOT values signifying that vocal fold vibration precedes the consonant release. A high percentage of the adult VOT values for /d/ occur in the range from 0 to +20 msec VOT. For /t/, on the other hand, the VOT values occupy a range extending from about +40 to +120 msec VOT. The distribution of VOT values for /t/ can be approximated by a normal curve for adult speakers (Lisker & Abramson, 1964; Cooper & Lauritsen, 1974).

In effect, then, the VOT value for a stop like /d/ is considerably shorter than the value for /t/, produced at the same place of articulation (the closure interval for both consonants is produced by touching the alveolar ridge, lying behind the upper teeth, with the tongue). The earlier onset of vocal fold vibration for /d/ than /t/

corresponds to the traditional phonetic distinction between such consonants as voiced versus voiceless or unaspirated versus aspirated.

The development of the contrast between /d/ and /t/ in syllable-initial position has been studied longitudinally for three English-speaking children from age 6 months to 2.5 years by Kewley-Port and Preston (1974). Their findings appear to have a bearing on possible neural models of speech development and will thus be reviewed here in some detail. At the age of 6 months, children produced values of VOT along a broad range covering both the /d/ and /t/ regions of adult speech. At this early stage, the child apparently exercised no control over the timing of consonant release and the onset of vocal fold vibration.

At a later stage, the children began to produce VOT values consistently in the short-lag range from 0 to +20 msec VOT, corresponding to the typical VOT region of an adult's [d]. During this stage, the children rarely produced either long-tag [t] or prevoiced [d] VOTs. Finally the latter types of VOT values emerged in the children's speech, in accordance with the speech of adults.

The main problem is to account for the earlier emergence of short-lag VOT values in children's speech, as opposed to both long-lag and prevoiced VOTs. Kewley-Port and Preston were able to provide a first-order account in terms of the degree of complexity of neural control required for producing the three types of VOT values.

To present this account, it is first necessary to review some aspects of vocal fold vibration. Three major conditions must be met in order for the vocal folds to vibrate: The folds must be relatively near one another (adducted), they must be relative slack, and a sufficient drop in pressure across the larynx must be maintained (Halle & Stevens, 1971). The neural control required to meet these conditions differs for the three types of VOT. For short-lag VOTs, a speaker must simply adduct the vocal folds at some time prior to the actual release of consonant closure and keep the folds relatively slack. As the consonant closure is released, a sufficient drop in pressure across the larynx occurs as an automatic consequence of the equalization of mouth pressure (Ohala, 1970), enabling vocal fold vibration to begin shortly after the release. The point to emphasize here is that a relatively broad temporal interval exists during which the speaker can issue a motor command to adduct the vocal folds in order to produce a short-lag VOT value, acoustically well defined in terms of small variability. This relative ease with which the short-lag VOT value can be produced with consistency may be advantageous to the child in early template-matching tests.

In contrast, the other two types of VOT—prevoiced and long-lag—require neural commands in addition to those required for short-lag VOTs. For prevoicing, special musculature must be used to maintain a sufficient pressure drop across the larynx during the interval when the vocal folds are vibrating while the consonant closure is simultaneously maintained (Rothenberg, 1968). For long-lag VOTs, the timing of vocal fold adduction must be initiated at a relatively precise moment in relation to the consonant release. At the time of the release itself for a long-lag VOT, the vocal folds must be in an *ab*ducted or spread position to permit the passage of turbulent airflow, corresponding to the production of aspiration (an "h"-like noise which can be observed in exaggerated form by releasing the closure of /t/ more slowly than normal). The command to adduct the vocal folds must be initiated so that the folds will be approximated typically within 80 msec after the release.

It is reasonable to explain the difference in chronological mastery for the three different VOT regions in terms of a difference in the complexity of neural commands. Simply put, the early emergence of short-lag VOTs as opposed to both prevoiced and long-lag VOTs is attributed to the relative simplicity of the commands that accompany the short lag. But perhaps of greater interest is the question of how children make the transition from producing short-lag VOTs almost exclusively to producing the three regions of VOT values found in adult speech. Whereas the difference in chronological mastery per se seems attributable to the neural machinery that controls the onset and maintenance of vocal fold vibration—machinery that is part of the child's innate genetic endowment—an account of how the child makes the transition from producing primarily short-lag VOTs rely on principles of maturation or learning. We will discuss one possible learning account for the acquisition of long-lag VOTs.

Klatt (1973a) suggested that children learn to produce long-lag VOTs by using peripheral feedback from the oral pressure drop that automatically accompanies the release of a stop consonant. According to this view, the detection of a pressure drop would trigger a command to adduct the vocal folds reflexively, yielding a VOT lag greater than 40 msec. Although the actual time required for this feedback loop is not known, we might suppose that the use of such feedback by children might yield relatively longer long-lag VOTs in comparison with adult speech, under the assumption that in later speech development children acquire centralized, open loop, control of the commands for producing the long lag. Some support for this possibility has been provided by Menyuk and Klatt (1975), who found that long-lag VOTs are somewhat longer on the average for children than adults in the same speech contexts.

But the pressure feedback hypothesis also appears to apply to at least some extent in adult speech. Perkell (1976) has conducted experiments for a single speaker in which the normal pressure drop accompanying consonant release was artificially regulated during consonant production without the speaker's awareness. Regulating the pressure drop exerted some control over the voicing onset for a voiceless (i.e., long-lag VOT) consonant. Perkell's preliminary findings suggest that pressure feedback may serve as a cue for initiating commands to facilitate voicing onset in adults, strengthening the likelihood that such feedback also plays a role in the acquisition of long-lag VOTs. We are still left with the question of why the feedback loop appears in speech development when it does, but an answer to this question may depend on a genetically determined course of maturation whose schedule we cannot yet guess.

We have discussed the order of appearance of short-lag and long-lag VOTs in terms of one difference—in complexity of the neural commands that control speech production. But recent research has opened up the possibility that a difference in neural complexity of a different sort might account for the earlier appearance of short-lag VOTs as well. According to this hypothesis, the late acquisition of long-lag VOTs is accounted for by the late development of a fully integrated system subserving both speech production and perception. The evidence for a centralized perceptuo-motor processor, operative in the case of long-lag but not short-lag VOTs, is provided by experiments in perceptuo-motor adaptation (Cooper, 1974; Cooper & Lauritsen, 1974; Cooper & Nager, 1975), in which repetitive listening to a consonant + vowel syllable with a long-lag VOT produced a small but systematic shortening of long-lag VOT values in speech production. This effect could not be accounted for in terms of mimicry of the VOT value of the adapting stimulus (Cooper, 1974). Whereas a perceptuo-motor adaptation effect was observed for long-lag VOTs, no such effect was observed for short-lag VOTs, for which the VOT value is determined by simple coupling (Ohala, 1970). It is possible that the relatively late acquisition of long-lag VOTs is attributable to the extra maturation typically required to develop perceptuo-motor processing.

The neural circuitry believed to be involved in the perceptuo-motor system for long-lag VOTs has been sketched by Cooper and Nager (1975). This circuitry appears in Figure 1. The model is comprised of excitatory and inhibitory neural

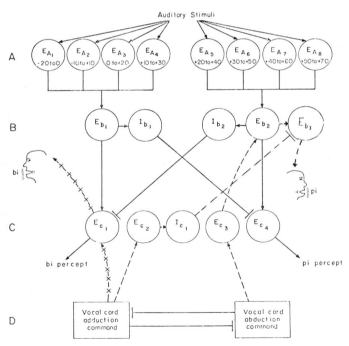

Figure 1. Neural model of the perceptuo-motor system for voiced–voiceless distinctions in initial stops (from Cooper & Nager, 1975).

elements with exclusively lateral connections. Each neural element can be regarded as either an individual cell or as a cell aggregate.

For present purposes, we will consider only the circuit route taken during speech production. At level D, commands originate for the production of short-lag and long-lag VOTs. These commands include the *ab*duction of the arytenoid cartilages for long-lag VOTs and the *ad*duction of these cartilages for both short-lag and long-lag VOTs. The commands may also include tensing of the vocal folds for long-lag VOTs. Each of these commands may in turn involve a sophisticated set of instructions to intrinsic laryngeal muscles and, in some cases, to extrinsic laryngeal muscles as well, but the model can be illustrated simply in terms of commands for abduction and adduction of the arytenoids.

According to Cooper and Nager (1975), the opeartion of the model is viewed as follows:

> The neural command to adduct the arytenoids accompanies the production of both voiced and voiceless prestressed plosives, since without such adduction the vocal folds are sufficiently spread to prevent the onset of voicing. For the articulation of voiced plosives, the adduction command is the only command necessary for lateral arytenoid movement. In the case of most short-lag VOTs, it is simply necessary that the timing of this command be controlled so that the vocal folds are in adducted position by the time of oral release. For the articulation of voiceless plosives, the situation is more complicated.
>
> Prior to the initiation of the adduction command, an *ab*duction command must be transmitted to the laryngeal control system when producing voiceless plosives. We speculate that this abduction command is transmitted through the neural system via Eb_2, a proposed site of perceptual adaptation. The strength of this abduction command is weakened to some extent as a function of repetitive listening to a voiceless plosive, resulting in a smaller amount of total abduction of the arytenoids. Assuming that the rate of glottal adduction is constant, the end result of this decrease in total abduction is a shorter delay in the onset of vocal fibration relative to the release of oral closure. With this circuitry, we can thus account for the shortening effects of VOT that accompany perceptuo-motor adaptation with voiceless plosives as adapting stimuli and test utterances.
>
> Since the abduction command is involved in the production of voiceless plosives but not voiced plosives, the model accounts for why perceptuo-motor adaptation is observed for voiceless but not voiced utterances. In addition, since the structures fatigued by repetitive listening to a voiced plosive are not part of the circuitry postulated for abduction, the model also accounts for why perceptual adaptation with a voiced plosive does not alter the VOTs of voiceless plosive utterances. The only perceptuo-motor effect permitted under the present model is a net shortening of VOTs for voiceless plosives, the only perceptuomotor effect observed thus far experimentally [pp. 263–64].

Although we have indicated how differences in the neural commands for short-lag and long-lag VOTs may account for their order of appearance in language acquisition, much remains to be known about VOT development. For example, the VOT relation is subject to a number of contextual effects, including influences of consonant place of articulation, vowel environment, and speaking rate (Lisker &

Abramson, 1967; Klatt, 1973a; Coker, Umeda, & Browman, 1973), and little information has been obtained about possible developmental trends for these effects (cf. Eguchi & Hirsh, 1969). Another problematic area involves developmental changes in VOT as a function of second-language learning, an area recently studied by Williams (1974).

SOME CONTEXTUAL RULES OF SYLLABLE TIMING

The influence of context on speech timing can be observed more readily by considering the distinction between voiced and voiceless consonants in syllable-final position. Here, the voicing of the final consonant exerts a large influence on the duration of a preceding vowel. House and Fairbanks (1953) noted that a vowel duration was longer when it appeared in the environment of a voiced consonant in adult speech. This effect could be accounted for by two very different physiological operations, depending on whether one regards the influence on vowel duration as a matter of vowel shortening before voiceless consonants or as vowel lengthening before voiced consonants. Lengthening might be attributed to an effect of voicing assimilation (Heffner, 1969), allowing the speaker to render the presence of a voiced consonant more perceptible. On the other hand, shortening might be attributed to a physiological need to halt vocal fold vibration abruptly in anticipation of a voiceless consonant. A priori, there is no way to decide between these two alternatives.

A developmental study by Di Simoni (1974a) appears to have strong bearing on the issue of directionality of this voicing context rule. Di Simoni studied the development of vowel duration with voiced and voiceless consonants in children aged 3, 6, and 9 years. The duration of vowels /i/ and /a/ increased systematically with age in the environment of the voiced consonants /b/ and /z/, but the duration of the same vowels in the environment of voiceless consonants /p/ and /s/ did not vary with age. The asymmetry in development noted by Di Simoni suggests that the timing rule should be regarded as a rule for lengthening before a voiced consonant rather than as a shortening rule before a voiceless consonant (Di Simoni, 1974b).

We have found here a case in which developmental data can be used to help improve our understanding of adult speech. Recently, Raphael (1975) has provided physiological support for regarding the voicing effect on vowel duration as a lengthening rule before voiced consonants in adults. Raphael noted in electromyographic experiments that the peak level of EMG activity was sustained for vowels when they preceded voiced versus voiceless consonants, even though the peak activity in the two environments was reached at approximately the same time.

The likelihood that the voicing context rule is a lengthening rather than shortening rule may call for a reinterpretation of durational studies in which a shortening gesture was assumed. For example, Klatt (1973b) studied the possible interaction between the voicing rule and a rule involving the shortening of a stressed vowel before an unstressed syllable. He found that the two rules did not produce a linear subtractive shortening effect in combination, and this departure from linearity was accounted for by a principle of incompressibility. However, it may be that the nonlinearity was attributable to the possibility that the two rules were not in fact both shortening rules.

If the voicing rule is in fact a lengthening rule, as suggested by the developmental data of Di Simoni (1974a) and the physiological data for adults of Raphael (1975), we would suspect that children should show a tendency to produce voiceless consonants more easily than voiced consonants in syllable-final position. And, in fact, available data, though fragmentary, support this claim (Braine, 1974; Stampe, 1969; Velten, 1943). At an early stage of development, Velten found, for example, that syllable-final consonants were voiceless in the speech of his daughter, such that words like *bet* and *bed* were pronounced indistinguishably as /bɛt/. At a later stage of development, the two words were distinguished only by vowel length /bɛt/ versus /bɛːt/), and not until a later stage did the child attain the adult pronunciation (/bɛt/ versus /bɛːd/) by producing a syllable-final voiced consonant.

In addition to the influence of consonant voicing on vowel duration, Di Simoni has studied possible developmental trends for two other effects of syllable context. In one study (1974c), he attempted to determine whether differences in vowel context would alter the duration of consonants. Schwartz (1969) had found for adults that the duration of /s/ was slightly longer when it preceded /i/ than /a/. This finding was interpreted in terms of a rule of anticipatory coarticulation (cf. MacNeilage & DeClerk, 1969), whereby speakers shortened the consonant before /a/ in order to begin the larger tongue motion required to reach the steady-state vowel /a/ versus /i/. However, Di Simoni found no differences in consonant duration of this sort for children aged 3, 6, and 9 years. Perhaps the coarticulatory effect was not observed for these children because their smaller orofacial cavity reduced the difference in extent of tongue motion required to reach the two vowel targets.

Another contextual effect studied by Di Simoni involved the possibility of temporal compensation for a consonant and vowel duration within the same syllable. Kozhevnikov and Chistovich (1965) observed in the speech of Russian adults that the durations of consonants and vowels within the same syllable were negatively correlated across repetitions of the syllable, such that longer-than-average vowels were accompanied by shorter-than-average consonants, and vice versa. The variance of the duration of the entire syllable was therefore less than the sum of the variances of the consonant and vowel segments within the syllable. This finding favored the syllable as a basic unit of speech-timing control (but see Ohala, 1970). Di Simoni (1974d) examined the possibility of a temporal compensation effect in English-speaking children aged 3, 6, and 9 years. He found no such effect for any of the three age groups tested. However, it is difficult to interpret this null result in terms of speech development, since Di Simoni's study included no data for English-speaking adults, leaving open the possibility that the null effect was attributable to a difference in the particular language or measurement technique. The issue is further clouded by the possibility that the original result for Russian speech may have been attributed to negatively correlated measurement errors for adjacent segments (Ohala, 1970).

RULES FOR SENTENCE TIMING

We have thus far considered timing rules pertaining to two domains—the phonetic segment and the syllable. A number of timing effects in adult speech operate at the sentence level as well, and we turn now to consider the development of such effects. One influence concerns the relation between utterance length and the length of individual segments. For adult speech, the relation is such that the longer the utterance, the shorter the individual segments (Jones, 1948; Lindblom, 1968; Malmberg, 1944; Schwartz, 1972). Di Simoni (1974e) studied the effect in children and found that this relation was present in the speech of children as early as 3 years of age, the youngest age group tested. The finding indicates that young children can preplan the timing of segments within utterances to some extent, presumably in order to facilitate the coordination of breathing with speech (Lieberman, 1967; Lindblom & Rapp, 1973). The shortening of segments in long utterances allows the speaker to minimize breath pauses, of possible advantage to the speaker's long-term utterance planning, and of possible advantage to the listener, who may associate breath pauses with the location of major grammatical boundaries (Maeda, 1976).

Another line of research on durations in sentence contexts has been conducted by Tingley and Allen (1975), who studied the ability of children to repeat the same utterance with a reliable rhythm. They asked children aged 5, 7, 9, and 11 years to repeat the sentence "Twinkle, twinkle, little star, how I wonder what you are," and found that children's variability decreased as a function of age, approaching the minimal variability found for adults by age 11. The finding of a gradual long-term increase in timing precision is in accord with the general maturation of motor skills. Tingley and Allen in fact found that the variability of a child's timing for the sentence was correlated with his ability to tap his finger in a steady rhythm, suggesting that a common maturational process might be responsible for the development of precision in both speech and nonspeech rhythmic tasks.

Tingley and Allen also analyzed their data to determine the possible role of peripheral feedback in timing control. Applying Allen's (1973) quantitative model of speech-timing factors, they found no significant sequential dependencies in the rate of the children's sentences. This result suggested that the children did not adjust their timing on a trial-by-trial basis by feedback from the previous utterance. Thus, while peripheral feedback may well play a role in timing control at the segmental level (see the first two sections of this chapter), there is no available evidence to suggest that it plays a role in timing effects ranging over the domain of an entire utterance.

There exists one major area of research on sentence timing that has yet to be studied developmentally. It has been shown for adult speech that the durations of segments in sentences vary considerably as a function of syntactic and semantic context (Coker *et al.,* 1973; Cooper, 1976; Klatt, 1975; Lindblom & Rapp, 1973; Martin, 1970). For example, segment lengthening is observed for words in clause-final position and for content words. It is conceivable that children would show developmental trends toward greater reliance on such syntactic and semantic influences of timing as these latter aspects of language are expanded and refined in development. If so, the developmental study of syntactic and semantic effects on speech timing should provide a fruitful way of studying systematic interplay among the major subsystems of language acquisition.

CONCLUDING REMARKS

Research on speech development has provided some clues about the kinds of maturational and learning processes that underlie such development, although it has not provided as many clues as we might have wished. In some cases, as with Jakobson's principle of successive differentiation, a process that appears to mediate speech development can be viewed as a special case of a general learning principle. In other cases, as with the neural system of voice-onset timing control, an aspect of speech development can be accounted for in terms of a specialized neural apparatus, presumably innately present. Some developmental studies appear to have a bearing on a theory of adult speech, as indicated by the relevance of Di Simoni's (1974a) results for voicing context in assessing the directionality of a durational rule. Such findings suggest that further work[1] on the development of speech timing will be of some value not only to practitioners of research on child language but also to those who typically confine their interests to studying the language of adults.

ACKNOWLEDGMENT

This work was supported by an NIH Postdoctoral Fellowship. I thank Professor Kenneth N. Stevens for helpful comments.

[1] Since the writing of this chapter, three relevant articles have appeared in the *Journal of Speech and Hearing Research:*

Kent, R.D. (1976) Anatomical and neuromuscular maturation of the speech mechanism: Evidence from acoutic studies, *19,* 421–447.
Zlatin, M.A., & Koenigsknecht, R.A. (1975) Development of the voicing contrast: Perception of stop consonants, *18,* 541–553.
Zlatin, M.A., & Koenigsknecht, R.A. (1976) Development of the voicing contrast: A comparison of voice onset time in stop perception and production, *19,* 93–111.

REFERENCES

Allen, G.D. (1973) Segmental timing control in speech production. *Journal of Phonetics, 1,* 219–237.

Bever, T.G. (1961) Pre-linguistic behavior. Unpublished honor's thesis, Department of Linguistics, Harvard Univ.

Braine, M.D.S. (1974) On what might constitute learnable phonology. *Language, 50,* 270–299.

Chomsky, N. (1965) *Aspects of the theory of syntax.* Cambridge, Massachusetts: M.I.T. Press.

Chomsky, N. (1975) *Reflections on language.* New York: Random House.

Coker, C.H., Umeda, N., & Browman, C.P. (1973) Automatic synthesis from ordinary English text. *IEEE Audio and Electroacoustics, AU-21,* 293–297.

Cooper, W.E. (1974) Perceptuomotor adaptation to a speech feature. *Perception and Psychophysics, 16,* 229–234.

Cooper, W.E. (1976) Syntactic control of timing in speech production. Unpublished doctoral thesis, Department of Psychology, M.I.T.

Cooper, W.E., & Lauritsen, M.R. (1974) Feature processing in the perception and production of speech. *Nature, 252,* 121–123.

Cooper, W.E., & Nager, R.M. (1975) Perceptuo-motor adaptation to speech: An analysis of bisyllabic utterances and a neural model. *Journal of the Acoustical Society of America, 58,* 256–265.

Cruttenden, A. (1970) A phonetic study of babbling. *British Journal of Disorders of Communication, 5,* 110–118.

Curtiss, S., Fromkin, V., Krashen, S., Rigler, D., & Rigler, M. (1974) The linguistic development of Genie. *Language, 50,* 528–554.

Di Simoni, F.G. (1974a) Influence of consonant environment on duration of vowels in the speech of three-, six-, and nine-year old children. *Journal of the Acoustical Society of America, 55,* 362–363.

Di Simoni, F.G. (1974b) Evidence for a theory of speech production based on observations of the speech of children. *Journal of the Acoustical Society of America, 56,* 1919–1921

Di Simoni, F.G. (1974c) Effect of vowel environment on the duration of vowels in the speech of three-, six-, and nine-year old children. *Journal of the Acoustical Society of America, 55,* 362–363.

Di Simoni, F.G. (1974d) Some preliminary observations on temporal compensation in the speech of children. *Journal of the Acoustical Society of America, 55,* 360–361.

Di Simoni, F.G. (1974e) Influence of utterance length upon bilabial closure duration for /p/ in three-, six-, and nine-year old children. *Journal of the Acoustical Society of America, 55,* 1533–1534.

Eguchi, S., & Hirsh, I.J. (1969) Development of speech sounds in children. *Acta Otolaryngolica,* Supplement No. 257.

Eilers, R.E., & Minifie, F.D. (1975) Fricative discrimination in early infancy. *Journal of Speech and Hearing Research, 18,* 158–167.

Eimas, P.D. (1974) Auditory and linguistic processing of cues for place of articulation by infants. *Perception & Psychophysics, 16,* 513–521.

Eimas, P.D., Siqueland, E.R., Jusczyk, P., & Vigorito, J. (1971) Speech perception in infants. *Science, 171,* 303–306.

Ferguson, C.A., & Farwell, C.B. (1975) Words and sounds in early language acquisition. *Language, 51,* 419–439.

Ferguson, C.A., & Slobin, D.I. (Eds.) (1973) *Studies of child language development.* New York: Holt.

Gruber, J.S. (1966) Playing with distinctive features in the babbling of infants. *Quarterly Progress Report of the M.I.T. Research Laboratory of Electronics, 81,* 181–186.

Gunnilstam, O. (1974) The theory of local linearity. *Journal of Phonetics, 2,* 91–108.

Halle, M., & Stevens, K.N. (1971) A note on laryngeal features. *Quarterly Progress Report of the M.I.T. Research Laboratory of Electronics, 101,* 198–213.

Heffner, R-M.S. (1969) *General phonetics.* Madison, Wisconsin: Univ. of Wisconsin.

House, A.S., & Fairbanks, G. (1953) The influence of cosonant environment upon the secondary acoustical characteristics of vowels. *Journal of the Acoustical Society of America, 25,* 105–113.

Hughes, G., & Halle, M. (1956) Spectral properties of fricative consonants. *Journal of the Acoustical Society of America, 28,* 303.

Irwin, O.C. (1947a) Infant speech: Variability and the problem of diagnosis. *Journal of Speech and Hearing Disorders, 12,* 287–289.

Irwin, O.C. (1974b) Infant speech: consonant sounds according to place of articulation. *Journal of Speech and Hearing Disorders, 12,* 397–401.

Irwin, O.C. (1974c) Infant speech: consonantal sounds according to manner of articulation. *Journal of Speech and Hearing Disorders, 12,* 402–404.

Irwin, O.C. (1948) Infant speech: Development of vowel sounds. *Journal of Speech and Hearing Disorders, 13,* 31–34.

Jakobson, R. (1941) *Kindersprache, Aphasie, und allgemeine Lautgesetze.* Uppsala: Almqvist & Wiksell. [English trans. *Child Language, Aphasia, and Phonological Universals.* The Hague: Mouton, 1968].

Jespersen, O. (1925) *Language.* New York: Holt.

Jones, D. (1948) Chronemes and tonemes. *Acta Linguistica.*

Kewley-Port, D., & Preston, M.S. (1974) Early apical stop production: A voice onset time analysis. *Journal of Phonetics, 2,* 195–210.

Kiparsky, P., & Menn, L. (1976) On the acquisition of phonology. Unpublished ms., M.I.T.

Klatt, D.H. (1973a) Voice onset time, frication, and aspiration in word-initial consonant clusters. *Quarterly Progress Report of the M.I.T. Research Laboratory of Electronics, 109,* 124–136.

Klatt, D.H. (1973b) Interaction between two factors that influence vowel duration. *Journal of the Acoustical Society of America, 54,* 1102–1104.

Klatt, D.H. (1975) Vowel lengthening is syntactically determined in a connected discourse. *Journal of Phonetics, 3,* 129–140.

Konishi, M. (1965) The role of auditory feedback in the control of vocalization in the white-crowned sparrow. *Zeitscrift fur Tierpsychologie, 22,* 899–902.

Kozhevnikov, V.A., & Chistovich, L.A. (1965) *Speech: Articulation and perception.* Joint Publications Research Service, 30. U.S. Department of Commerce.

Lieberman, P. (1967) *Intonation, Perception, and Language,* Cambridge; MIT Press.

Lindblom, B. (1968) Temporal organization of syllable production. Speech Transmission Laboratory, Royal Institute of Technology, *Quarterly Progress and Status Report,* Stockholm, Sweden (October).

Lindblom, B., & Rapp, K. (1973) Some temporal regularities of spoken Swedish. *Papers from the Institute of Linguistics,* University of Stockholm, Publication 21.

Lindblom, B., & Sundberg, J. (1971) Neuropsychological representation of speech sounds. Paper presented at the XV World Congress of Logopedics and Phoniatrics, Buenos Aires, Argentina, August.

Lisker, L., & Abramson, A.S. (1964) A cross-language study of voicing in initial stops: acoustical measurements. *Word, 20,* 384–422.

Lisker, L., & Abramson, A.S. (1967) Some effects of context on voice onset time in English stops. *Language and Speech, 10,* 1–28.

MacNeilage, P.F., & DeClerk, J.L. (1969) On the motor control of coarticulation on CVC monosyllables. *Journal of the Acoustical Society of America, 45,* 1217–1233.

Malmberg, B. (1944) Die Quantitat als phonetisch-Phonologischer Bergriff. *Lunds Universitests Arsskrift, 41,* 104.

Marler, P. (1970) Bird song and speech development: Could there be parallels? *American Scientist, 58,* 669–673.

Marler, P. (1974) On the origin of speech from animal sounds. In J.F. Kavanagh & J.E. Cutting (Eds.), *The role of speech in language.* Cambridge, Massachusetts: MIT Press.

Maeda, S. (1976) *A characterization of intonation in American English.* Unpublished doctoral dissertation, M.I.T.

Martin, J.G. (1970) On judging pauses in spontaneous speech. *Journal of Verbal Learning and Verbal Behavior, 9,* 75–78.

McNeill, D. (1970) *The acquisition of language.* New York: Harper.

Menyuk, P. (1968) The role of distinctive features in children's acquisition of phonology. *Journal of Speech and Hearing Research, 11, 138*–146.

Menyuk, P. (1971) *The acquisition and development of language.* Englewood Cliffs, New Jersey: Prentice-Hall.

Menyuk, P., & Klatt, M. (1975) Voice onset time in consonant cluster production by children and adults. *Journal of Child Language, 2,* 223–231.

Moskowitz, A. (1971) Acquisition of phonology. Unpublished doctoral dissertation, Univ. of California, Berkeley.

Ohala, J.J. (1970) Aspects of the control and production of speech. *Working Papers in Phonetics,* No. 15, Los Angeles: U.C.L.A. Phonetics Laboratory.

Oller, D.K., & Smith, B. (1976) Syllable timing as a function of position-in-utterance in infant babbling. *Journal of the Acoustical Society of America, 60,* S26 (Abstract).

Oller, D.K., Wieman, L.A., Doyle, W.J., & Ross, C. (1976) Infant babbling and speech. *Journal of Child Language, 3,* 1–11.

Perkell, J.S. (1976) Responses to an unexpected suddenly induced change in the state of the vocal tract. *Quarterly Progress Report of the M.I.T. Research Laboratory of Electronics,* in press.

Raphael, L.J. (1975) The physiological control of durational differences between vowels preceding voiced and voiceless consonants in English. *Journal of Phonetics, 3,* 25–33.

Reynolds, G.S. (1968) *A primer of operant conditioning,* Glenview, Illinois: Scott, Foresman.

Riley, D.A. (1968) *Discrimination learning.* Boston: Allyn and Bacon.

Rothenberg, M. (1968) The breath-stream dynamics of simple-released, plosive production. *Bibliotheca Phonetica, 6.*

Salus, P.H., & Salus, M.W. (1974) Developmental neurophysiology and phonological acquisition order. *Language, 50,* 151–160.

Schwartz, M. (1969) Influence of vowel environment on the duration of /s/ and /ʃ/. *Journal of the Acoustical Society of America, 46,* 480.

Schwartz, M. (1972) Influence of utterance length upon bilabial closure duration for /p/. *Journal of the Acoustical Society of America, 51,* 666.

Stampe, D. (1969) The acquisition of phonetic representation. *Papers from the Ninth Regional Meeting.* Chicago: Chicago Linguistic Society. Pp. 433–444.

Stevens, K.N. (1972) The quantal nature of speech: Evidence from articulatory-acoustic data. In E.E. David, Jr. and P.B. Denes (Eds.), *Human communication: A unified view.* New York: McGraw-Hill.

Tenold, J.L., Crowell, D.H., Jones, R.H., Daniel, T.H., McPherson, D.F., & Popper, A.N. (1974) Cepstral and stationarity analyses of full-term and premature infants' cries. *Journal of the Acoustical Society of America, 56,* 975–980.

Tingley, B.M., & Allen, G.D. (1975) Development of speech timing control in children. *Child Development, 46,* 186–194.

Trehub, S. (1973) Infants' sensitivity to vowel and tonal contrasts. *Developmental Psychology, 9,* 91–96.

Velten, H.V. (1943) The growth of phonemic and lexical patterns in infant language. *Language, 19,* 281–292.

Vuorenkoski, V., Lind, J., Wasz-Hockert, O., & Partanen, T.J. (1971) Cry score. A method for evaluating the degree of abnormality in the pain cry response of the newborn and young infant. Speech Transmission Laboratory, Royal Institute of Technology, *Quarterly Progress and Status Report,* Stockholm, Sweden (January-March). Pp. 68–75.

Williams, L. (1974) Speech perception and production as a function of exposure to a second language. Unpublished Doctoral Dissertation, Harvard Univ.

Subject Index

375